IN MEMORY OF

ANDREAS CHRISTIAN GERLACH,

LATE DIRECTOR OF THE ROYAL VETERINARY INSTITUTE,

BERLIN, PRUSSIA,

TO WHOSE EXAMPLE, LOVE, AND SYMPATHY

THE AUTHOR OWES WHAT LITTLE ABILITY HE POSSESSES,

THIS BOOK IS AFFECTIONATELY

Dedicated.

ISBN 978-0-428-95770-4
PIBN 10124411

THE RELATION

OF

ANIMAL DISEASES TO THE PUBLIC HEALTH,

AND THEIR PREVENTION.

BY

FRANK S. BILLINGS, D. V. S.,

GRADUATE OF THE ROYAL VETERINARY INSTITUTE OF BERLIN; MEMBER OF THE ROYAL VETERINARY ASSOCIATION OF THE PROVINCE OF BRANDENBURG; HONORARY MEMBER OF THE VETERINARY SOCIETY OF MONTREAL, CANADA, ETC.

NEW YORK:

D. APPLETON AND COMPANY,

1, 3, AND 5 BOND STREET.

1884.

PREFACE.

THIS book is written for the benefit of the people of the United States. Its purpose is to introduce to every thinking man and woman of the country a new subject, the higher purposes of Veterinary Medicine. It is a work which treats of the *Prevention* of Diseases, not their *Treatment.* While at times the language of the author may appear unnecessarily severe to the casual reader, he should not forget that the author is an enthusiast; that he has given his life and energies to the subject of the establishment of Veterinary Science in this country; and that the evils so severely combated are not "straw men," the creations of a vivid imagination, but actual evils that, unless prevented, will work most serious injury to the country in the not distant future. All that the author asks is calm reflection and an honest verdict upon his work.

CONTENTS.

PART I.

PART II.

PART III.

PART I.

THE DISEASES OF DOMESTIC ANIMALS.

THE subject of the relation of animal diseases to the public health, while not by any means unknown to hygienists, is still one which has not until the last few years attracted the scientific study which its importance demands. This is mainly due to the practical tendency which has prevailed in all veterinary schools, and which has been pushed, to the undue neglect of scientific investigation. Thankfully, the day of the school empiric is fast drawing to a close, and the rising sun of scientific research is beginning to dispel the fogs of tradition and the apathy of self-content which has rested upon veterinary medicine.

The day has come when veterinary medicine is beginning to make its power felt, and to take its true place as a scientific institution among the nations of the world.

We have all been taught that the first commandment is "to have no other gods besides me." But without desiring to enter into the discussion of religious questions, the hygienist may say that, while this may be very important to the spiritual man, the earthy man has also certain positive responsibilities to himself, which find their expression in the command, "Man, know thyself." This commandment seems to be a stranger to the minds of most men, for how little do we know of the physiological laws which control that complicated machine, the animal organism, or of the means by which we can in a large measure prevent diseases, not only among ourselves, but among our animals! The majority of our people assume that the nucleus of all knowledge is to be found somewhere in that record of Jewish history, the Christian Bible.

With reference to the prevention of human diseases from causes to be sought in the animal world, either directly or indirectly, we find, however, but little of practical value in that book. The instructions of Moses to the Jews have far more to do with certain superstitious ideas of the cleanliness or uncleanliness of certain species of animals as unfitting them for food than with any true knowledge of their non-hygienic character. Enthusiastic but blind worshipers have even gone so far as to assert that Moses must have known that trichinæ existed in pork, hence his forbidding its use as food. But they do not stop to think that these parasites require a microscope for their detection, an instrument which was not known to man until thousands of years after the books of Moses were written. That the flesh of diseased animals was unfit for human food did not entirely escape the attention of the Israelitic legislator; but his restrictive utterances were limited to his own people. He tells the chosen of the Lord that: "*Ye shall not eat of anything that dieth of itself; thou shalt give it unto the stranger that is in thy gates, that he may eat it; or thou mayest sell it unto an alien; for thou art an holy people unto the Lord thy God.*"—*See* Deut. xiv, 21.

Numerous passages, which command that all blood must be removed from the body before using it, lead us to infer that all such articles were to be well cooked before being eaten, and that raw or underdone meats were an abomination to the Jews, as they should be to all people.

Plutarch asks: "Why is it that the priests of Jupiter are forbidden to touch raw flesh?" And answers: "Raw flesh is no more a living creation, and is unfit to eat. Cooking gives it another form."

Not only is human life endangered by the consumption of products from previously diseased animals, or from the consumption of improperly cooked flesh, but quite a number of animal diseases are capable, by intentional or accidental means, of transmission to man. Virchow has said that "man is far more susceptible to infection from animal diseases than the latter from similar diseases of man."

TRICHINIASIS OF MAN AND ANIMALS.

THERE is, perhaps, no one disease of our domestic animals which enjoys a more sensational reputation, or which has been more thoroughly investigated, than the disease of swine caused by the parasite *trichina spiralis*. There is none more worthy of the attention of the public or the hygienist. Although the literature * treating upon

* The American student will find the best compilation that exists on this subject in the "Report on Trichinæ and Trichinosis," Glazier. 1881. Published by the United States Marine-Hospital Service.

this disease is of comparatively modern date, still we have no justifiable reason for doubting the presence of these parasites in swine at a very early date, and also that the consecutive disease in man must have existed for years, if not centuries, before it came to scientific recognition; I am inclined to think, almost coeval with the consumption of pork as food. In this opinion I find myself opposed by many distinguished observers; but the fact that trichinæ were not discovered earlier than 1831 does not at all militate against my conclusions. They simply were not suspected. Every fact in connection with the history of the parasite—its minuteness, the uncertainty of its pathognomonic phenomena in man, and still more so in the hog, which render difficult the correct diagnosis of trichiniasis—supports my hypothesis.

Hiller * says: "The history of this disease can be appropriately divided into three periods, the first beginning with the discovery, or observation, of the capsule—the parasite not being recognized—in 1821–'28, including the description of the same by Dr. Hilton, of Guy's Hospital, London, England, in 1835.

"The second period extends from 1835, when Paget discovered the encapsulated parasite and Owen described it, giving to it its name, 'trichina spiralis,' to the first authentic observation of the disease in a human being, and the direct establishment of its connection with a parasitic disease of swine which took place in 1860.

"This begins the third period in the history of trichina spiralis—the period of active scientific investigation—which is by no means at an end, and which awaits its conclusion in the discovery of the original source whence swine derive the parasite."

In the mean time, Professor Leidy, of Philadelphia, was the first to discover the parasite in the flesh of the hog in 1867. It is a singular fact that this discovery should have been made by means of an American hog.

The principal workers in this important field of helminthic research have been Owen, Cobbold, Bristow, and others, in Britain; and Leuckart, Virchow, Zenker, Küchenmeister, and the veterinarians Gerlach and Fürstenberg, in Germany.

Cobbold † describes the parasite as follows: "Trichina spiralis is an extremely minute nematode helminth, the male in its fully developed and sexually matured condition measuring only one eighteenth of an inch, while the perfectly developed female reaches a length of about one eighth; body rounded and filiform, usually slightly bent on itself, rather thicker behind than in front, espe-

* Ziemssen's "Encyclopædia of Medicine," vol. iii.

† "Entozoa," p. 335.

cially in the males; head narrow, finely pointed, unarmed, with a simple, central, minute oval aperture; posterior extremity of the male furnished with a bilobed caudal appendage, the cloacal or anal aperture being situated between these divergent appendages; penis consisting of a single spicule, cleft above, so as to assume a V-shaped outline; female stouter than the male, bluntly rounded posteriorly, with genital outlet placed forward at about the end of the first fifth of the long diameter of the body. Eggs measuring $\frac{1}{1270}$ of an inch from pole to pole; mode of reproduction viviparous."

"The shell-less ova develop into minute embryos immediately on fructification, and completely fill the uterus of the female, and are born in immense numbers." * "The embryos measure, previous to birth, about ten micrometres in length, and five to six in transverse diameter. The study of the structure of the embryo is almost impossible so long as it is retained within the body of the maternal parasite. Here it resembles a delicate thread, having a somewhat uniform granular appearance, which becomes less distinct as development progresses. In the older embryos—extra-maternal—we may perceive a very delicate cuticle and an axial line running through the body; the extremities are more or less blunt, and not easily to be distinguished as to which is the posterior or anterior end of the parasite. In the intestines the embryos measure about 0·1 mm. in length, sometimes more, and have a transverse diameter of about 6 μ." (Pagenstecker.)

"Within the abdominal cavity they may be found to measure from 0·12 to 0·16 mm. in length, with a transverse diameter of 8 μ. They have scarcely ever been seen less than 0·12 mm. in length when in the muscles. Comparison with mature trichinæ indicates that the slenderer of the two extremities is the head."

"The posterior extremity possesses more rigidity than the anterior, and also seems to have a backward and forward motion. The rigid condition of the terminal end of the parasitic embryo corresponds with the situation, or limits, of the axial line, which is looked upon as the rudimentary alimentary canal. The anterior portion of the embryo is not granulous, but clear, being only modified by a delicate chitin thread which is continuous with the cuticle, and constitutes the first indication of the chitinous lining of the oval cavity. As development progresses, this axial line divides into two parts; the anterior portion corresponds to the so-called cell-body of the mature parasite, and the posterior to the stomach, intestines, etc. The sexual organs can not, as yet, be distinguished. The embryos

* Leuckart, "Die menschlichen Parasiten," vol. ii, p. 512.

may be met with not only in the abdominal cavity of the autosite, but also in the thoracic and pericardial sac, and in such numbers that these places may be looked upon as normal resting-places for the embryos on their migrations over the infected organism. In general we find them far more numerously represented in the abdominal cavity, which corresponds exactly with our knowledge of their activity, for it is here that they must first come after passing the intestinal parietes on their migrations. From here they pass on to the other cavities by means of the natural openings, or ostia, through which the œsophagus and large vessels pass through the diaphragm. These vessels are loosely surrounded by connective tissue, which offers favorable conditions for the passage of the parasites. From these cavities the embryos follow the course of the larger vessels and nerves over the body, the loose connective tissue offering the favorable conditions. The duration of the migratory period can not be determined with any great degree of accuracy; but it is undoubtedly very short, as embryos have been found in the thoracic cavity, the pericardial sac, and adjoining muscles, as early as in the abdomen. The majority of observers seem to agree in considering the ninth or tenth day of invasion as terminating the migratory period—that is, when but a single invasion has taken place."

"The embryos display no distinguishable changes either in size or structure during the period of migration. The first appreciable changes occur after they have reached the muscles, and have become lodged in their fibers."

"When they have penetrated the fiber—that is, become intra-sarcolemmatous—the protoplasma of the muscle-cell undergoes certain pathological changes, which exactly correspond to the fatty degeneration observed in parenchymatous myositis. A proliferation of the nuclei is quite common, if not an invariable phenomenon. Like all tissues which have undergone fatty degeneration of their plasma, such fibers are darker, less refracting, than those which have not been subjected to parasitic invasion. Such fibers lose their contractility. When cut transversely, the swollen parenchyma extends beyond the sarcolemmatous sheath, and if the trichina be near the section, it often extends free, or becomes free, with the protruded plasma. It is doubtful whether the trichinæ live upon the elements of the plasma while lodged in the fiber, as they are in an apparently chrysalis condition. This fatty degeneration of the parenchyma seems to offer no impediment to a second invasion of the fiber."

"While previous to migration the embryo shows a somewhat slender form, it soon becomes thicker, or more rotund, its transverse diameter being nearly double that which it had before migration. Its anterior portion becomes more slender and resembles that of the mature parasite. The posterior end becomes more blunt. Progressive changes also take place in the axial line, the different organs becoming distinct; especially is this the case in the cell-body. The primitive sexual gland is to be seen as an elongated sac; the pointed anterior end extends beyond the stomach in the females, and turns abruptly backward in the males. The oval cavity has a proportionate length, and over its middle distinctly shows the first traces of a nervous system, which in the form of an oval enlargement, cervical ganglion, is to be distinguished from the cylindrical mass."

"With the progressive development of the internal organs comes a corresponding increase of the external dimensions of the parasite. It increases more in length than thickness, and its previous rotund form becomes more slender. At the same time the body becomes curved, and after a while assumes an irregular, spiral position—trichina spiralis. They begin to assume this position the earliest in the larger fibers; but it occurs in all, even when the lumen scarcely exceeds the transverse diameter of the parasite. In the vicinity of the parasite the sarcolemmatous sheath invariably becomes distended, owing to the lateral pressure exerted by the parasite. The spindle shape of the tube is due to the elasticity of the sarcolemma; but, as it becomes thicker and clouded, proliferation must take place as well. The intra-sarcolemmatous, or capsular, development of the parasite terminates in about three weeks from the time of its invasion of the fiber."

"The enlargements of the sarcolemma—capsules—vary much in form and size. Sometimes they are far more cylindrical and elongated than at others, and again one end may be elongated and the other bluntly rounded."

"The capsules are surrounded by a *rete* of capillaries, which can be injected. A growth in length and thickness, due to the irritation caused by the parasite, gives them a very ramified character."

In this condition the parasites are known as "muscle trichinæ"; but when in the intestines of an autosite, as "intestinal trichinæ." In the first form they make their abode entirely in the striated, or motory, muscles—the flesh. They have not been met with in an encapsulated condition, either in the non-striated muscles or in purely adipose tissue.

While this seems to be the opinion of almost all observers, during my observations in 1879, and again in 1881, I frequently found encapsuled trichinæ in the midst of purely adipose tissue, *between muscle-fibers of very fat hogs; never*, however, in the adipose tissue which lies upon musculature. Since then, other observers have reported the same thing. In a letter, read at the ninth annual meeting of the American Public Health Association, held at Savannah, Georgia, in 1881, emanating from the Department of Agriculture, dated October 29, 1881, the author, with the customary ignorance and consequent impudence of an American politician, says, in answer to the question, "Are trichinæ found in the fat?" "I have until now thought not. Professor Taylor, of this department, tells me that in the 'Journal of the Microscopical Association' *he has recently seen that they have been found in fat. I should rather see than believe without so doing.*"

I think this is easily explained. The great amount of fatty infiltration had caused absorption of the plasma, and atrophy of the fibers by compression, which was, however, resisted by the greater density of the sarcolemma in the vicinity of the parasite, and also by the latter itself. No other explanation seems to me possible, for the capsules were comparatively perfect.

The encapsuled parasites may be met with in the striated muscles of all parts of the body, such as the digital muscles, those of the abdominal walls, of the extremities, the eye, the ear, the larynx and pharynx, the tongue, œsophagus, and the diaphragm; but the heart seems to be a favored locality, for they have only been found in its flesh in very isolated cases.

In making examinations of the œsophageal muscles of a rabbit that had been fed with infected pork, I was much struck with the abruptness with which I met trichinæ, in passing in review a microscopical section of the œsophageo-cardiac portion of the stomach, when one passed from the fibers proper to the stomach to those of the œsophagus; in fact, trichinæ could be seen in the striated fibers of the latter, where they intruded between the non-striated of the former; but in no case were there any to be seen in the smooth, or inorganic fibers.

These parasites are not, however, equally distributed over the musculature of the autosite, but, on the contrary, appear to have their favorite places of abode. They have a predilection for the muscles of the anterior part of the body; of these, those of the tongue, larynx and pharynx, and masticatory muscles are especially favored. The muscles of the rump are more profusely invaded than those of the extremities. Very few have been discovered in the tail of any animal. In the extremities, the parasites are found to be more abundant where the muscle-fibers begin to lose themselves in their tendinous extension than in the body of the muscle. Numerous estimates have been published by different observers as to the percental invasion of the different muscle-groups, several of which may be given here.

Microscopic specimens,* of an average length of two centimetres and a width of one centimetre, were taken from the flesh of several hogs which had been found trichinous.

Eighty specimens taken from hog No. 1 gave the following:

a.	Pillars of diaphragm	12 trichinæ.
b.	Muscles "	4 "
c.	" larynx	1 "
d.	" ribs	None.
e.	" tongue	"
f.	" neck	"
g.	" eye and overarm	"

Sixty specimens from hog No. 2:

a.	Pillars of diaphragm	10 trichinæ.
b.	Muscles "	6 "
c.	" larynx	2 "
d.	" ribs	None.
e.	" tongue	"
f.	" eye	"
g.	" overarm and neck	"

Forty from hog No. 3:

a.	Pillars of diaphragm	40 trichinæ.
b.	Muscles "	25 "
c.	" larynx	4 "
d.	" ribs	6
e.	" tongue	8
f.	" neck, eye, and overarm	2

Forty from hog No. 4:

a.	Pillars of diaphragm	40 trichinæ.
b.	Muscles "	30 "
c.	" larynx	10 "
d.	" ribs	10 "
e.	" tongue	6 "
f.	" overarm	2 "

* "Mittheilungen aus. d. thierärzlichen Praxis im Preussischen Staate," 1877–'78, p. 99.

According to Gerlach: *

One grain of flesh taken from the			
Psoas muscle	contained	161	trichinæ.
Diaphragm muscle	"	129	"
Laryngeal "	"	126	"
Tongue "	"	105	"
Orbital "	"	64	"
Abdominal "	"	54	"
Masseter "	"	45	"
Lips, near snout	"	43	"
Serratus magnus	"	39	"
Pectoralis major	"	33	"
Œsophagus, anterior to the diaphragm	"	31	"
" posterior "	"	1	"
Pelvi-femoral muscle	"	26	"
Tibial "	"	26	"
Longissimus-dorsi muscle	"	20	"
Scapulo-humeral "	"	18	"
Radio-ulnar "	"	17	"
Metatarsal "	"	9	"
Intercostal "	"	8	"
Small muscle of ear	"	2	"
" tail	"	1	"

Krämer † gives the following as the results of examining one gramme of flesh from different parts:

From the biceps	contained	420	trichinæ.
" masseter	"	213	"
" genio-glossus	"	188	"
" gastrocnemius	"	186	"
" sterno-mastoid	"	171	"
" pectoral	"	148	"
" diaphragm	"	129	"
" crico-thyroid	"	124	"
" intercostal	"	113	"
" rectus abdominis	"	106	"
" psoas	"	105	"
" tongue	"	58	"
" laryngeal	"	21	"

Not having any opportunity to make detailed examinations of the muscles of any whole or single hog, I could not make any personal observations of the percental dispersion of the trichinæ over the different muscle-groups or parts of the organism.

Coming upon a piece of a pillar of the diaphragm which was wonderfully infected, I made the following numerical observation

* "Die Trichinen." † "Deutsche Klinik," July and August, 1872.

(in fact, I never saw among all my examinations a piece of pork so completely filled with these pests; capsules with four trichinæ in them were by no means seldom): ·05 (5 centigrammes) contained at least 50 trichinæ. One gramme would therefore contain 1,000, and 4 grammes, or a drachm, 4,000, and a pound of such pork would contain at least 400,000, and, if we assume the muscles of a hog to weigh 100 pounds, its organism—were equal dispersion possible—would contain 40,000,000.

The immense multitude of these parasites which may be found infecting a single organism is still more wonderful than their wide dispersion over the autosite.

Leuckart estimates that, in some of the cases which have come under his observation, a single gramme of flesh lodged from twelve to fifteen hundred; and assuming the muscles of a man to weigh forty pounds, the number of these parasites infecting a human organism at such a ratio would sum up some thirty millions.

In Zenker's case—to be especially noticed later—Fiedler calculated that the woman must have lodged some *ninety-four millions;* and Cobbold assumes that *one hundred millions* of the encapsulated parasites may sometimes infect one organism at the same time.

Leuckart again says that no one would look upon the foregoing as exaggerated estimates who, like himself, had found some sixty trichinæ in ten milligrammes of muscle.

In a report of the Chicago Academy of Sciences, it was estimated that one cubic inch of pork, examined under its auspices, contained some *ten thousand*, and that a person consuming the ordinary amount of such flesh, taken at a single meal, would introduce into his organism more than *one million* trichinæ.

Rauch found numerous trichinæ infecting the muscles of a hog. Of three hundred microscopic specimens, they failed in but three. In some he found thirty in one focus; in others, but five or six examples. As in seventy specimens weighing one gramme three hundred and fifty trichinæ were found, one pound would contain one hundred and seventy-five thousand; and one hundred pounds, seventeen million five hundred thousand. In many cases, however, the parasites are much less frequently met with; and one has to search through many microscopic specimens before meeting with any, and then only with isolated examples.

When sufficient time has elapsed from the invasion of the muscles and formation of the capsules, the same may be recognized microscopically as small, white specks. Such muscles appear as if sprinkled with grains of white salt or sand. The calcification of the capsule begins about the fifth month subsequent to the invasion of the muscles.

It has been said by some observers that the trichinæ capsules in the hog do not calcify; others affirm the contrary. The polariscope, however, will reveal the presence of calcareous salts in the capsule if sufficient time has elapsed since invasion. The reason they may not be easily recognized microscopically must be sought in the influence on the salts of the fatty oils in the porcine organism, which renders the crystals less visible.

The Intestinal Trichinæ.

So long as the trichinæ remain encapsulated in the fibers of the muscle, their condition remains unchanged. They make no progress in their development, irrespective of the number of years that they may have been imprisoned. They have been seen in an active—i. e., capable of progressive—development, under favorable conditions, thirteen, twenty, and even twenty-four years from the time invasion took place.

a. In 1861 a woman was admitted into the hospital at Altona, Germany, suffering from a mammary cancer, which had been developing some twelve years. On its removal and subjection of its tissues to microscopic examination, the presence of trichinæ in the muscle-fibers was manifested. On inquiry, it was ascertained that in 1856 the woman had resided at Davenport, Iowa, where she was taken suddenly very ill, gastric and rheumatic phenomena being the most prominent of any, together with œdema of various parts and paralytic phenomena. Her brother, with whom she resided, was attacked in a similar but less severe form at the same time. The woman died at the Altona Hospital in 1864, and an examination of her muscles revealed the presence of great numbers of encapsulated trichinæ. A cat fed with pieces of these muscles died in the course of sixteen days, its muscles being repletely infected with these parasites.

b. Virchow reports a case where, after the *lapse of thirteen years and a half*, the parasites moved in their capsules on prolonged exposure to the heat of the sun.

c. Klopsch reports a case of trichiniasis, with complete recovery, which took place in 1842. The parasites were discovered in the muscles of the individual twenty-four years afterward. This discovery was also made on the excision of a mammary cancer. At the same time that this woman was ill, two persons in the same house became sick under similar conditions. Both died. (Virchow's "Archiv," Bd. 35, p. 609.)

d. Professor Dammau,* formerly of the Eldena Agricultural Academy, reports a very interesting case, illustrating the longevity and tenacity of life of embryonal trichinæ in the muscles of a hog.

This hog was fed with trichinous meat in November, 1864, and in February, 1865, presented to the experiment station at Eldena. Since that time the animal had been kept isolated, unless removed from its pen for examination. On February 3, 1875, and February 12, 1876, Dammau removed a small piece of flesh from the shoulder. At both times trichinæ were found. A considerable piece of flesh was removed and fed to two rabbits, and eighteen days subsequently their muscles were found to be plentifully invaded with trichinæ.

This case demonstrates, beyond all question, the presence of living trichinæ, which were capable of maturing, fructifying, and developing young when fed to other animals, after a period of eleven years and a quarter from the time that the invasion of the hog took place.

Although the encapsulated trichinæ suffer no changes while confined in the muscles of an autositic organism, yet the introduction of portions of such muscles into the intestinal tract of man, or other suitable animal, causes rapid changes in their condition. The processes of digestion soon set the imprisoned parasites free from their capsules, three to four hours being sufficient for the purpose. The freed parasites rapidly complete their development to mature trichinæ, thirty to forty hours being enough. In cases of fresh invasion, when the capsules have not become very hardened, twenty-four hours have been found sufficient to demonstrate the presence of sexually matured trichinæ in the intestines of animals fed with such flesh by way of experiment. Still, we may often find trichinæ inclosed in their capsules on the third day after feeding infected flesh to an animal.

There is scarcely another helminth by which this matured stage in its development is reached in so short a period.

Under these circumstances it is self-evident that the changes necessary to maturity by these parasites must be of a very insignificant character.

As a rule, sexual connection takes place within two days from the time the trichinæ become free.

The parasite increases in length and thickness, and in the female the uterus fills with fructified ova, which soon develop into embryos still inclosed in the maternal worm.

* "Zeitschrift für prac. Thierheilkunde," 1876, vol. iii, p. 92.

The female intestinal or matured parasite lives from five to six weeks, and produces at least fifteen hundred embryos. (Leuckart.)

The newly born embryos are at first buried in the mucus which lines the intestinal canal; a microscopic examination of such mucus, at this time, will reveal them as free and movable parasites. The embryos soon begin their migration and dispersion over the organism, the first act being the penetration of the intestinal parietes. It seems to be still a matter of discussion as to the means or ways by which further migration takes place. Some authorities, in fact, all the most eminent, favor the view that the parasites proceed by the way of the mesenterium and connective-tissue tracts over the organism, and penetrate the sarcolemma, or sheath of the muscle-fibers.

Another view, the possibility of which is conceded by the above-named authors to a minor degree, is that the embryos gain access to the circulation, and are transported over the organism by the moving fluid, boring the smaller vessels at convenience, and thus gaining access to the muscles. (Thudicum.)

Were this the principal path of dispersion, we ought to be able to discover numerous examples of the parasite in the circulating blood of living animals that have been subjected to feeding experiments. This has not been the case, however.

Thus it is evident that the host, or consumer of trichin-infected flesh, provides the means for its own invasion.

While this is, in general, the manner in which invasion takes place, it by no means excludes the possibility of the infection of an animal taking place by intestinal trichinæ (embryos), which have passed from an already infected organism with its fæces. In this way an infected swine may infect others, or, in fact, give occasion to a secondary invasion of itself, by rooting in the manure of its pen. In the same way swine may become infected from infected human beings where, as is too often the case, the out-houses for the family are placed over the pig-pen, or lead into it, or where the contents of the same are thrown into the piggery for the swine to work over.

Thus we see the cycle of invasion may frequently continue from swine to man, and from man to swine.

Trichinæ may be assumed to be regular cosmopolitans. Whether Noah took a pair of them with him into the ark will probably continue to be an open question. They have been discovered in Germany, England, Scotland, Denmark, Sweden, Russia, France, Italy, North and South America, Africa, India, Australia, Spain, Egypt, and Syria.

In fact, it may truly be said that they have been found infecting pork in whatever land, and wherever they have been sought for.

As to their presence in other animals than man and the hog, they have only been unquestionably found in warm-blooded animals, such as cats, dogs, rabbits, rats, mice, the marmot, the wild hog of Europe, and even the hippopotamus.

Gerlach has produced invasion in calves and horses, while Leisering was unable to in the latter animal.

Several reports have been published with reference to the discovery of trichinæ in the flesh of fish and other cold-blooded animals, but they all fail of experimental proof, and are non-conformable with our knowledge of the physiological activities of the parasite, which becomes torpid in a temperature a few degrees below that of the ordinary living mammal.

For some unknown reason they do not seem to be able to invade the muscles of fowls, though some authors claim to have found them in the intestines. A case is reported of invasion of some soldiers from eating a goose ("Philadelphia Medical Times," April 13, 1878), the accuracy of which is very questionable, as pigs are fully as easily stolen as geese; and no evidence exists that they were seen in the flesh of the goose.

With regard to hens, I made quite a series of experiments.

1. I fed them with highly infected pork, in the natural way. Results negative. No trichinæ, either in the intestines or muscles.

2. Assuming that the triturating powers of the gizzard might be sufficient to destroy the parasites before they could gain access to the intestines, I caused a quantity of infected pork to be chopped for several hours, until it became a veritable mush; microscopic examination of this mass revealed the presence of numerous free trichinæ. This mass was stirred up with warm water, so that it could be drawn into a coarse syringe; the intestines of the fowls were then washed out as cleanly as possible with warm enemas, and time given for the water to flow off again. Several syringefuls of the mass were then injected, and the outflow stopped artificially. After forty-eight hours this obstruction was removed. Results absolutely negative, so far as producing muscle-invasion was concerned, at an examination made four weeks from the time of the experiment. No trichinæ in intestines.

3. The abdominal cavity of six other fowls was opened, and two tablespoonfuls of the watery mass, but thicker than the preceding, poured in. The aperture was then sewed up. The hens drooped

a few days, but recovered, and ate well. Examination at the same time with the others gave negative results, although a queer-looking condition of the abdominal cavity existed. Why these hens did not die of septicæmia I do not know.

I had hoped to carry on numerous feeding and therapeutic experiments during my examinations of pork in 1881, but lack of means on my own part, as well as on the part of the Board of Health of Massachusetts, prevented their accomplishment.

Trichiniasis in Swine.

As we have previously mentioned, the disease was discovered in swine by Leidy, in 1847.

It is to German observers that we must look almost entirely for any authoritative statements with reference to the percental infection of swine with these pests, for in no other country is there at present anything approaching a systematic examination of pork, and even in Germany there is much room for improvement.

To make the statistics valuable, it is necessary that the law should require that, at least so far as domestic consumption goes, all hogs should be examined before being cut up, and that only one part—viz., the pillars of the diaphragm, or psoas muscles—should be used for examination. There is no evidence that this is the case in Germany, hence I much doubt whether it would not be possible to largely increase their present ratio of infection. The following statistics have been gathered at random, with no attempt at completeness, but simply as illustrations, from the books in my own library, such as Virchow's "Archiv," the "Vierteljahrsschrift für gerichtliche Medicin," the "Deutsche Zeitschrift für Thiermedicin," "The Veterinary Reports of Saxony and Hanover," the "Magazin für Thierheilkunde" (Gurlt u. Hertwig), the "Archiv für Thierheilkunde," and the "Mittheilungen aus d. Praxis d. Preussischen Staate."

For Rostock, Germany, Petri gives the following:

1869.............	Number	hogs	examined,	5,457;	trichinous,	1
1871.............	"	"	"	6,520	"	2
1872.............	"	"	"	6,555	"	0
1873.............	"	"	"	6,441	"	3
1874.............	"	"	"	6,731	"	2
1875.............	"	"	"	7,222	"	5
1876.............	"	"	"	7,165	"	0
1877.............	"	"	"	7,562	"	2
Total............................				53,653		15

Trichinous, 1·3543.

For Braunschweig, Uhde reports: Whole number examined between 1866 and 1880, 111,806; trichinous, 29.

1866–'67	there was found	1	hog of every	6,700	examined,	trichinous.
1867–'68	"	"	1	"	5,700	"	"
1868–'69	"	"	1	"	14,500	"	"
1869–'70	"	"	1	"	15,300	"	
1871–'72	"	"	1	"	13,387	"	
1872–'73	"	"	1	"	4,874	"	
1873–'74	"	"	1	"	5,129	"	
1874–'75	"	"	1	"	7,004	"	
1875–'76	"	"	1	"	13,183	"	
1876–'77	"	"	1	"	7,127	"	
1877–'78	"	"	1	"	5,879	"	
1878–'79	"	"	1	"	10,397	"	
1879–'80	"	"	1	"	3,857	"	

PRUSSIAN STATE STATISTICS.

	No. examined.	Trichinous.	Measles.	No. of state examiners.
1876............	1,728,595	800	4,705	11,915
1877............	2,057,272	701	5,434	12,865
1878............	2,524,105	1,222	6,165	16,251
1879............	3,164,656	1,938	9,669	17,413
1880............	3,342,303	2,284	11,379	18,332
Total.......	12,816,831	6,945		

Trichinous, 1 to 1,845.

Eulenburg's report for 1880 deserves some special consideration. The ratio of trichinæ in swine in Prussia has, we see, constantly advanced with each year since 1876. In 1879 it was 1 to 1,632; and in 1880, 1 to 1,460; which must be attributed to greater exactness in the observations. The great number, constantly increasing, of appointed examiners is also worthy of notice: from 11,915 in 1876, they have been increased to 18,332 in 1880. In Berlin they found 1 to 1,247 swine trichinous, while in Posen the ratio was 1 to 138, which more nearly corresponds to the conditions in this country. There does not seem to be at present any endeavor on the part of the Government to make investigations into the cause of these things. Three hundred and twenty-nine cases of trichiniasis among human beings, and four deaths, are reported. In all cases it was traced to the consumption of either uncooked or improperly examined pork. In Berlin there were but sixteen cases during the year, a much smaller number than in previous years, which is attributed to the greater stringency with which the examinations are carried out. One of these cases is interesting from the fact that the person who died, consumed, raw, a piece of pork known to be trichinous, in order to show that the idea that trichinæ caused disease in man was a fallacy. Of examinations of American pork, the report says 3,030 trichinous pieces, sides, were found. Such an examination has no statistical value, as it does not show whether the sides were all from different hogs or not; further, were they *all* American? The average of trichiniasis in American PIECES, not hogs, was found to be 4 to 100. It was found that the abdominal muscles were only serviceable for examination, or such as were attached to the shoulders. More than twenty sides a day should not be examined by one person (?).

In Schleswig, of 782 "Amerikanischen Rouladen," 8 were found trichinous; of 1,952 sides, 64; 3,903 hams, 66; and 13 shoulders, 3.

In Stettin, of 72,230 sides, 1,124 were found trichinous.

The number of swine affected with measles was 1,710 more than in the former year.

From Hamburg, Germany, we have a few statistics which may have an instructive comparative value:

In 1878, of 35,510 American hams examined, 397 trichinous.
" " 14,003 " sides " 85 "
" " 17,113 European hams " 3 "
" " 222 " sides and 10,838 hogs examined, none trichinous.
In 1879, of 79,864 American hams examined, 1,087 trichinous.
" " 22,749 " sides and shoulders examined, 196 trichinous.
" " 28,710 European hams examined, 2 trichinous.
" " 16,204 " hogs " 1 "
In 1880, of 55,008 American hams examined, 566 trichinous.
" " 23,589 " sides " 270 "
" " 49,943 European hams, sides, and hogs examined, none trichinous.

At Blankenburg, from 1864–'65, 7,000 to 8,000 hogs examined, and but 1 infected.

At Hanover, from 1865–'66, 18,656 hogs examined, and 12 trichinous.

In Sachsen-Weimar, from March, 1868–'69, 19,611 examined, and 1 found trichinous.

In 1875–'76, at Frankfort, 8,000 hogs examined, 4 trichinous.
" " Gulen, 1,600 to 1,800 hogs examined, 1 trichinous.

At Copenhagen, 1867, 8,174 examined, 15 trichinous.

At Charkow, Russia, 1876, 3,550 examined, 5 trichinous.

These statistics could be multiplied *ad libitum*, but they are sufficient to show the results of Continental examinations. It is to be regretted, however, that we have no reliable statistics from either England, Scotland, Ireland, or France, or other Continental countries, since they have commenced to lay so much stress upon the infected condition of American pork.

Trichinæ in American Pork.

We have already noticed the examinations of American pork made at Hamburg during several years, and will follow with a few more quotations of the same nature:

At Rostock, 12 of 622 American sides were found trichinous.

At Gothenburg, 8 of 210 American sides were found trichinous.

At Ebbing, 2 per cent of the pieces examined were found trichinous.

In Schleswig-Holstein, of 5,673 pieces examined, 47 were found trichinous.

In 1877, 343 cases of infected American pork were reported, and 183 cases of the disease in human beings.

In the early part of the year 1881, badly infected American pork was reported as having been found at Lyons, France.

Professor Mueller, of the Berlin Veterinary Institute, wrote me, under date of December, 1880, that of eighty-eight live American hogs (constituting a part of a shipment) that had been slaughtered at Dresden, *fourteen* were found trichinous.

Dr. Loring* says, "I do not know that Germany or France has even examined for this disease *in live hogs*."

The foregoing was reported by me in American papers at the time, and subsequently in the report of the Imperial Board of Health of Germany, and several German medical reviews; and *could* have been as well known to our agricultural department as the presence of pleuro-pneumonia in the District of Columbia, a fact that ocular demonstration of diseased lungs could scarcely force upon our agricultural commissioner.

At Turin, Italy, February, 1879, four per cent of a lot of Cinciunati hams were found trichinous, which led to the Government putting restrictive examinations on all further importations.

A continual recurrence of such facts has caused a more or less strong feeling on the Continent against our pork, a feeling which nationalism and the public prints have fostered to the fullest extent.

The result has been that in many countries restrictive measures regulating the importation of American pork have been introduced, which to a certain measure have acted as an embargo against further importations. In some countries these measures have even been extended to American lard, and a great alarm created about some kind of hydraulic pressing out of the same instead of trying it out; in fact, everything possible is being done to keep out the competition of American products.

* Letter to Health Congress, Savannah, 1881.

With regard to our pork, I think the assertions of the Germans and their restrictive measures are just.

Naturally enough the old adage, "Touch a man's pocket and you touch his heart," found an illustration on this side of the Atlantic.

The pork-producers of every variety became very much alarmed, and called upon the Government to assist them.

Our consuls all over Europe were requested to make inquiries as to the true nature of these reports, and to report to their own Government. It is not within the nature of my work to consider these reports in detail; but, suffice it to say that they displayed fully as much patriotism for the purity of American pork as the Continentals did for their own. Some went so far as to call the whole thing a humbug. A real desire to know the truth pervaded neither our representatives at home nor abroad.

As with pleuro-pneumonia of our cattle, so with trichiniasis of the hog, our Government adopted a prevaricating and false course. It sought to "bluff down" the results of foreign examinations, and either did not seek to discover, or ignored the results of, home examinations.

In the face of a report of the State Board of Health of Massachusetts—numerous copies of which were sent to Washington—which contained a paper on the subject of trichiniasis, and statistics of the examination of the largest number of hogs which had until then been made in the country, the State Department published a singular document, which requires attention. It utterly ignored the statistics of the above report.

Clauses 8, 9, and 10 are as follows:

8. That the percentage of American hogs infected with trichinæ is, *in all probability*, *by reason of the superiority of the breed* (which?) *and feeding*, *much less than that among the hogs of any other country*.

9. That freedom from trichiniasis of the *two great pork-consuming centers of the West*, Chicago and Cincinnati, furnishes the strongest possible evidence of the purity of American pork. In Chicago, of forty thousand deaths, with causes, reported for a series of years, only two were from trichiniasis. During the same time none were reported in Cincinnati.

10. The reported cases of trichiniasis among human beings have resulted from eating uncooked pork, etc.

With regard to trichinæ in American hogs, the above-quoted sections from a state document have no foundation whatever. They have nothing to stand upon.

In clause 8 it does not stand upon facts, but upon a mere assertion—that "probably," etc.

Again, the person who instructed the Government knew absolutely nothing about trichinæ. Neither the breed of the hogs nor corn-feeding, or any manner of feeding as commonly practiced, aside from swill-feeding, need have anything to do, *pro* or *con*, with trichinæ in the hog. The hogs at the two great packing centers have never been thoroughly examined for trichinæ, and at the time this document was published neither the Interior nor any other department had organized any proper examination of American pork.

The percentage of deaths among human beings has nothing to do with the percentage of infection among swine.

Luckily for the American people, it has not. Even though cooking will kill trichinæ, and thus render infected pork harmless, it does not prove that American hogs have "much less trichinæ than those of any other country." A German has as much right to indulge a taste for uncooked smoked ham or spiced hashed pork as an American or Englishman has for rare or raw, warm or cold roast beef. The German may be invaded by trichinæ for his cannibalism, and the American by a tape-worm (*tænia medio-canalata*).

Examinations of American Pork.

At Chicago, April, 1881, a Dr. Paton is said (newspaper report) to have examined twenty specimens each, from *four hundred hogs*, and found NONE trichinous.

The Chicago Academy of Sciences ("Boston Medical and Surgical Journal," vol. lxxiv, p. 136) reports the examination of *thirteen hundred and ninety-four* hogs, and finding *twenty-eight trichinous.*

Health Commissioner De Wolff reported (1879) finding eight out of a hundred trichinous.

In 1879 I commenced my examinations of pork for the State Board of Health of Massachusetts, and again during three months of the summer of 1881. These examinations were not made upon any selected lots of swine, but the specimens were taken at random from the hogs as they hung up.

No attempt was made to discover whence the hogs originally came, though, with the exception of about fifty, they were all bought at Chicago, and hence *were emphatically Western hogs.* In making these examinations, the pillars of the diaphragm were invariably used, one pillar representing one hog. But three microscopic specimens were taken from each pillar—a rule which I invariably adhered to.

1879.

LOT.	Number examined.	Non-infected.	Trichinous.
1	47	44	3
2	48	46	2
3	72	62	10
4	60	56	4
5	226	210	16
6	192	179	13
7	100	96	4
8	81	80	1
9	95	94	1
10	93	89	4
11	98	90	8
12	300	275	25
13	201	188	13
14	192	187	5
15	200	184	16
16	257	252	5
17	238	225	13
18	163	154	9
19	26	25	1
20	12	11	1
	2,701	2,547	154

Trichinous, 1 to 17·54.

From the same source as the preceding:

1881.

LOT.	Number examined.	Non-infected.	Trichinous.
1	127	120	7
2	130	127	3
3	153	150	3
4	120	115	5
5	124	123	1
6	100	99	1
7	119	113	6
8	127	123	4
9	160	152	8
10	125	118	7
11	127	122	5
12	122	118	4
13	124	118	6
14	100	100	0
15	122	115	7
16	120	114	6
	2,000	1,929	71

Trichinous, 1 to 28.

From another source:

LOT.	Number examined.	Non-infected.	Trichinous.
1	129	120	9
2	130	123	7
3	140	130	10
4	105	102	3
5	73	71	2
6	130	125	5
7	119	115	4
8	127	120	7
9	132	130	2
10	182	175	7
11	93	93	..
12	128	125	3
13	112	110	2
14	124	120	4
15	81	80	1
16	84	80	4
17	120	117	3
18	59	57	2
	2,068	2,199	75

Trichinous, 1 to 27.

From a third source:

LOT.	Number examined.	Non-infected.	Trichinous.
1	105	105	..
2	45	45	..
3	65	64	1
4	80	78	2
5	61	60	1
6	63	60	3
7	96	92	4
8	100	99	1
9	100	99	1
10	98	96	2
11	90	86	4
12	101	98	3
13	121	121	..
14	103	100	3
15	76	75	1
16	102	100	2
17	130	124	6
18	130	125	5
19	131	128	3
20	122	120	2
21	85	84	1
	2,004	1,959	45

Trichinous, 1 to 44.

RÉSUMÉ.

	Number of hogs examined.	Non-infected.	Trichinous.
1879	2,701	154	1 to 17
1881. Same source	2,000	71	1 to 28
" Second source	2,068	75	1 to 27
" Third source	2,004	45	1 to 44
Total	8,773	345	1 to 25

The above figures do not certainly serve to support the words of our state document, that there are "less trichinæ in American pork than in that of any other country." They do speak in no uncertain terms that our Government has a duty which it owes to a large national interest, and that is, to spare no expense until the original source whence our swine become invaded be discovered.

As has been already said, all but about fifty of these eighty-seven hundred hogs were bought at Chicago, hence were Western hogs, though killed and examined at Boston. They were purchased at the same yards whence the Chicago packing-houses get that pork which our State Department declares to be so "free from trichinæ."

Further, the percentage of infection of the hogs from the different sources is interesting, but not very instructive. In 1879 we had a ratio of infection of 1 to 17 hogs, and from the same place 1 to 28 in 1881; while by the hogs from a third source we had an infection of 1 to 44. Yet they were all Western hogs.

This variation in the ratio of infection between those examined in 1879 and 1881 called forth the following remarks from Dr. Loring, the present Commissioner of Agriculture:

"A veterinarian of New England informed me on the 14th of April last that he had examined portions from 2,701 Western hogs, obtained in Boston, 154 of which he found infected, i. e., one case to each $17\frac{54}{100}$ hogs examined. He tells me that he will make a statement to this meeting that he has examined portions of 8,773 Western animals, and has found one case to every 25 animals. *You will see that there is a great difference between his first (April) examination and this one, and his result is so greatly different from the English examination of our hogs, above mentioned, and so much above any known proportion among animals of every other country, that I can not but entertain doubts of the value of his examination.*" *

* See letter to Health Congress, Savannah, 1881.

The English examination spoken of reads as follows:

"*The inspectors of the Veterinary Department examined two hundred and seventy-nine separate portions of swine's flesh, which were sent from Liverpool, and detected living trichinæ in three specimens*" (1 to 93).

As to the discrepancy spoken of between the results of my examinations, made about a year apart: it is not greater than that between any two lots taken at random in the same examination, nor so great as between very many lots examined on two consecutive days; for instance, in my series of 1881, lot 14 (source the same as in 1879) consisted of 100 pieces, of which NONE were infected, while of lot 13, 124 pieces, *six were trichinous.*

In two different epidemics of small-pox, the number of deaths is never the same, or even the number of cases. Are we, then, to say a later invasion is not small-pox, because the number of cases or deaths is less or more than in a previous? I never for a moment expected similar results, and should have been as pleased to find none as any one in the country.

With reference to the English examination, 1 to 93, *it is greater by far than the ratio of infection found in the hogs of any other country, and greater than I found in some lots examined by me; for instance, lots* 1, 2, 3, 4, *of my third series,* 1881, *contained, respectively,* 105, 45, 65, *and* 80 *specimens, representing* 295 *hogs, of which three were trichinous,* 1 to 98. Further, we do not know the parts that the English examined; had they been pillars of the diaphragm, the proportion might have been greater.

As to the *correctness* of my results, I will simply say that Dr. Folsom, of the Massachusetts Board of Health, went over a large part of those examined in 1879, and that competent physicians and a gentleman whom I educated to work with me, continually revised my other specimens as I examined them.

Again, if the Commissioner of Agriculture doubts my results, let him send a competent man, or men, here, and examine with me the same specimens, be it one or ten thousand, and I venture to say we shall find a percentage of infection *larger than that reported in any other country, and large enough to satisfy any one.*

Further, the Germans might well doubt the figures of their own examinations, as, from the Prussian statistics, we see the ratio of infection is steadily augmenting.

I wish now to refer to the report of Dr. Jansen T. Payne,* from which I quote the following:

* Report of the American Public Health Association, 1881.

"The method of conducting the researches was as follows: 'The examples procured one afternoon were examined the following day by the aid of a good microscope, capable of magnifying objects *two hundred diameters. A low power was found to give greater satisfaction than a higher one could have done, and observers in this field would do well to bear this in mind. When it is taken into account that each of the specimens had to be separated into minute shreds before they were placed upon the stage of the microscope, and consider the number of fibers examined in such cases*'" (he examined in all 21,600 specimens from 5,400 hogs), "'*it will readily be perceived that it is impossible to make anything like an accurate guess as to the whole number of pieces of muscle-fiber examined.*'"

Result: Number examined, 5,400; trichinous, 22.

"*By this series of examinations, it has been ascertained that Southern-bred hogs are free from trichinæ.*"

If there is anything I dislike to do, it is to criticise the work of another observer; but one would like to know if *two hundred diameters* is considered a *low* power. For myself, when looking for trichinæ, should I use such a power, I should not expect to find many trichinæ, but boa-constrictors; in fact, many would escape me. The male trichina measures one eighteenth, the female one eighth of an inch, in length—magnified two hundred diameters, what would one have?

Again, dividing specimens into shreds may be highly technical, but eminently unpractical; for with crush-specimens one can easily recognize the parasite, and it is done quickly; while in this way, and with such a high power as two hundred diameters, one would be sure to miss many.

I doubt the statement that "*Southern hogs are free from trichinæ*" as much as I do that "*corn-feeding*" *has anything to do* with trichiniasis.

But Boston is not the place for anything but statistical examinations. We must go nearer to the fountain-head. At Chicago it would be possible to examine large lots of hogs that have come directly from the breeder or fattener to the packer. Here *lots* could be examined and traced to the breeder. If highly infected, it would be easy to go to such places and make all manner of examinations of the remaining hogs, of the earth, worms, grubs, etc. Some unknown living thing lodges trichinæ before they enter the porcine organism. The scientific questions are: What is it? where is it? and what are its modes of life?

These things discovered—and they *must* be—we can put an end to porcine trichiniasis, and every other kind.

AMERICAN HOGS MUCH MORE INFECTED THAN CONTINENTAL.

A comparison of the statistics here given shows beyond all question that American hogs are more liable to trichiniasis than those of Germany; for we have seen that in those examined at Rostock we had but 1 to every 3,543; at Braunschweig, 1 to 8,963; in Prussia, 1 to 2,032, as trichinous; while of the American examinations, from authentic sources, we have 28 out of 1,394, or 1 to 50; 8 out of 100, and 345 out of 8,773, or 1 to 25, as infected. These were Western hogs, yet no one well acquainted with the circumstances would, I think, assert that the hygienic conditions under which our Western swine are raised are not superior to those of the famed "home-fed porkers" of the small New England farmer, raised, as they only too often are, in dark, loathsome, poorly ventilated pens, only too frequently under stables, with the house-vaults and sink-drains emptying into them.

I should here mention that it has seemed impossible to make any valuable examinations of Massachusetts-raised hogs, there being no authorities to co-operate with me in procuring specimens. It will finally become necessary for each State to organize an exact statistical examination of the hogs raised within its limits, as to the proportion infected with trichinæ.

As to German hogs, whoever has been upon a tour of observation through the agricultural districts of Germany, must have been most forcibly struck with the absurd non-hygienic conditions under which, not only hogs, but all the domestic animals are, in general, raised, in comparison with those of our own country, especially of the great stock-raising West.

In making examinations of hogs, with reference to tracing them back to the raiser, an important question will be whether the greatest proportion of trichiniasis is found among the hogs fed at the large distilleries, or under the apparently more favorable open-air feeding of the farmer; or, again, as many farmers pasture their hogs in woods, etc., before the corn is ready for fattening, is it among such that we find more trichiniasis than among those kept constantly in pens? It would also be of interest, and perhaps of practical value, to know if the wild swine of our Southern forests are much invaded, as well as the peccaries of Mexico and South America. The following freely made translations of published remarks of an eminent German, will show the opinions which are gaining ground in Germany with regard to our pork, and also how well posted even specialists are with reference to the true conditions in this country.

Bollinger * (pathologist of the Veterinary School at Munich), writing on the "Trichinæ in American Pork," in a review of an article by Roeper on the same subject, says: "The author of the paper 'Die Trichinen der americanischen Schinken' has made numerous examinations in order to contradict the opinion held in America" (by whom?) "that the trichinæ of American pork are an entirely different species from those found in the swine of Germany, and are harmless. Also to contradict the opinion that the peculiar process which 'American sugar-cured hams' are passed through, is sufficient to render the parasites harmless."

He found both these assertions without foundation. The curing process does not in all cases kill the trichinæ in the deeper seated parts of the ham.

The following absolutely erroneous explanation is given for the greater proportion of trichiniasis in our hogs in comparison with those of Germany:

"The swine that are BROUGHT to the LARGE *American slaughter-houses are allowed to feed upon the refuse from slaughtered swine, and in this way have* TIME *and* OPPORTUNITY *to infect themselves. Such infected swine are themselves slaughtered, and again give cause to infection of those that remain, which may have arrived later. Accordingly, this evil must go on constantly extending, and all persons must earnestly be warned against the consumption of raw American pork.*"

This German author certainly betrays ignorance of the true conditions at any large American packing-house. The refuse from the *slaughtered swine* is never fed to other swine that may be at such places, at any large packing-house in this country. It is sold for fertilizing purposes, or prepared for that purpose, and that only.

According to the best German authorities, it takes from five to seven days for the newly introduced trichinæ to bring forth young. No large American packing-house keeps a lot of swine on hand for from five to seven days, for they are killed as soon after arrival as possible. It would be impossible for them to kill from one to three thousand a day and do otherwise. While these assertions are absolutely false with reference to the large packing-houses, they are as strictly true, not only of many smaller establishments, where hogs

* "Deutsche Zeitschrift f. Thiermedicin," vol. i, p. 220.

are killed for home consumption, but also where they are fattened and killed by the farmer, or raised for the use of his family.

This report says further: "*This refuse from slaughtered swine at such large establishments is sold to the neighboring farmers as food to fatten their swine, and thus helps to swell the percentage of trichiniasis in American hogs.*"

This is false also!

The report ends as follows: "It is therefore right to warn the people against the consumption of American pork"—and recommends the most stringent microscopic examination of the same.

The Disease in Swine.*

Numerous feeding experiments with trichinous flesh were made at the Berlin school, the results being given in an able paper by Professor Mueller. It was proved that the consumption of such flesh by swine, with the sequential development of the embryos in their intestines, and their migration and lodgment in the muscles, may indeed cause disease, but that the phenomena of the same have neither that constancy nor distinctness of character which will admit of its recognition during the life of the animal.

All the swine thus fed became ill within a few days after consuming the meat.

The following were the most constant phenomena presented:

Diarrhœa, but not constant, being frequently interrupted by the passage of more solid fæces; sometimes it did not come to pass at all.

Phenomena, indicating abdominal pains, were frequently observed; such as uneasiness, burying themselves in the straw, etc.

Such phenomena, either singly or collectively, may be observed in swine, entirely aside from any anticipatory trichin-infection. They simply indicate the action of some irritant within the intestinal canal, and in this case, it being trichinæ, if the swine die, or are killed, we should have the same phenomena as in an intestinal catarrh of like grade, plus the trichinæ, which could not, however, be recognized macroscopically.

With the gradual cessation of the migration by the trichinæ, the abdominal symptoms become less marked, and finally disappear, to be followed by those indicating some disturbance of the motor functions. If the latter do not lead to death, they in their turn gradually cease with the encapsulation of the parasites.

Although the presence of trichinæ within the intestines causes

* Taken from the "Magazin f. d. gesammte Thierheilkunde," vol. xxxi, p. 6.

diarrhœa, yet, in these animals, it was impossible to find any embryos in their fæces.

This by no means excludes the possibility of finding them in other cases; yet their passage away with the fæces must in a measure be retarded from their being buried in a profuse layer of mucus, which is the product of the irritation caused by them.

In none of these swine was it possible to discover anything resembling the subcutaneous œdema which comes to pass in man under the same circumstances, and which serves essentially to the confirmation of the diagnosis.

Leisering, of Dresden, has also made numerous experiments with swine, of the same nature.*

He says: "One can not speak of a trichin-disease in swine, which is characterized by distinct and pathognomonic phenomena. In this regard the trichinæ deport themselves similarly to the cysticerci, measles."

Gerlach † says:

a. "About two fifths of the hogs fed were either not affected or but slightly indisposed; the remaining three fifths were visibly sick.

b. "The light cases presented nothing of diagnostic value, while in the severe ones the symptoms were of such a character that, *with* the aid of the scalpel and microscope, a diagnosis could be made."

(This is no more than saying that, with diarrhœa and abdominal pains, followed by disturbances in the motor functions, the scalpel and microscope would reveal the true cause, if trichinæ.)

c. "After an attack of trichiniasis, the hog again becomes well, and can be raised and fattened, as if nothing had happened.

d. "In cases which apparently pass over symptomless, as the animal betrays but slight constitutional disturbances, the infection is still sufficient to make the flesh a dangerous article of food.

e. "Hogs are most susceptible to trichin-invasion in early age. Old hogs are not easily infected; i. e., the muscles are not very much invaded by the parasites.

f. "Death results in over one half of the extremely severe cases.

g. "Death is caused by means of intestinal irritation, as well as the severe muscular disturbances. Forty-one per cent die by the former, and fifty-nine by the latter."

That trichinæ can only gain entrance to an organism by means of the mouth and alimentary canal is beyond all question.

* "Bericht u. d. veterinair Wesen im Sachsen," 1862, p. 118.

† "Die Trichinen."

Notwithstanding the apparent negation of the quoted Berlin experiments, we have the very highest authorities affirming, on the strength of positive observations, *that intestinal and embryonal trichinæ do leave the invaded organism with the fæces.*

Leuckart says: "As the usually matured trichinæ accumulate in great numbers in the intestines, and as the irritation caused by them leads to the development of a more or less intense diarrhœa, it is evident that the young must be taken up and pass off with the fæces; and not only free embryos, but also pregnant females, are subjected to this removal, which has been sufficiently attested by my own observations and those of Vogel, Kuhn, Gerlach, and others. This form of migration, under favorable circumstances, also contributes to the further distribution of trichinæ. Haubner and Gerlach give cases where they intentionally caused the invasion of young—non-infected—swine by causing them to live in the same pens with known infected ones. Such embryos and pregnant females become mixed with the manure and bedding of the hog-pens or on the grass of pastures, and may be taken up by other swine, or even by the original autosites, thereby leading to renewed invasion."

In the above we have a course of invasion in which the swine are the only factors.

Is there no other factor (or factors) in the question? We have previously remarked that wild swine have been found trichinous; also that rats, dogs, foxes, and other wild animals serve as autosites to them.

Of all animals in which these parasites have been found, none have that interest, aside from swine, to the hygienist and pathologist which is enjoyed by the rat, on account of a *hypothetical* etiological connection between the trichinæ which infest them and those in swine.

Leisering appears to have been the originator of this hypothesis.

The following statistics will suffice to show that the rat is even more favored with trichiniasis than swine:

Of 704 rats from different parts of Germany, 59 were found trichinous—8·3 per cent.

Of 208 rats from German knackers, 46 were found trichinous—22·1 per cent.

Of 224 rats from German slaughter-houses, 12 were found trichinous—6 per cent.

Of 272 rats from other places, 1 was found trichinous—0·3 per cent.

Of 326 rats from other places, 39 were found trichinous—11 per cent.

Of 51 rats caught at a knacker establishment at Spectacle Island, Boston Harbor, I found 39 trichinous.

The proprietors of this place kindly gave me opportunity to examine twenty-eight hogs, which had been kept and fattened by them at the island in question. *None were found trichinous. These hogs received no city swill of any kind. What flesh they received had been subjected to the heat necessary to extract the fats; otherwise, they received nothing but corn-meal.*

Forty rats caught at one of the large packing-houses near Boston were all found trichinous.

Of sixty rats caught for me at different stables in the city of Boston, where no hogs were or had been kept, but six contained trichinæ.

I can not see any just grounds for accepting the rat-infection theory; i. e., that swine become invaded in the majority of cases from eating trichin-invaded rats. In fact, I am strongly inclined to think that quite the contrary is the case; though I willingly admit that an occasional hog may become invaded in this manner. My own observations would seem to prove that whenever rats have opportunity to get at the trimmings or refuse of slaughtered hogs, there the rats will be found to be most profusely trichinous; while in other localities it will not be so.

Admitting that an occasional rat may lead to trichin invasion among hogs, we have still the open question, *Is there no common source from which not only swine and rats, but wild animals, may derive this parasite?* As, according to my own observation upon American pork, and my very limited examinations of American rats, they are both more largely invaded by trichinæ than similar animals in Germany, it seems as if here in America were THE place to study and decide these important questions.

It will not do for us to falsify or ignore true facts. The manner hitherto adopted of asserting, by way of pure negation, that "*American pork has no* trichinæ," as the pork interest has done, will not do. We must stand on facts gained by accurate and trustworthy observers. We must accept them. We must search for the cause. Any other course is absurd, and equally ruinous to self-respect.

Prevention of Trichinæ in Swine.

1. Boards of health should take means, looking to the better education of the people in relation to hog-raising, as well as all the principles of animal hygiene.

2. Boards of health should instigate exact statistical *researches* into the percentage of trichiniasis among swine raised in their respective States, as well as the hygienic conditions under which hogs *are* raised, in relation to this and other diseases.

3. Continued examinations of rats should be made in all parts of the country, and their slaughter encouraged in every legal way. In this regard we can look upon the rat-pit as serving a public purpose; and the rat-invasion theory, with reference to hogs, will receive a final settlement.

4. All sick swine should be peremptorily isolated from healthy ones, under the supervision of a competent veterinary inspector.

5. All swine suffering from diarrhœa should be isolated, and singly. The greatest care should be taken in cleansing the pens of such swine from all fecal masses and refuse.

a. The fæces from such swine should be subjected to microscopic examination.

b. On cessation of the diarrhœa, whether motor disturbances appear or not, the muscles, tongue, etc., should be harpooned, and the specimens thus gained subjected to microscopic examination.

6. Hogs in which trichinæ had been found should be branded and fattened singly, or together; but they should never be allowed to be sold for human food. Their lard could be tried out and sold.

7. All hog-pens should be kept scrupulously clean, and the turning of compost-heaps, or the drains from water-closets or houses, into hog-pens should be forbidden by law.

8. Feeding the offal from slaughtered swine to others, cooked or uncooked, or having slaughter-houses over places where swine are kept, should be forbidden by law.

9. Each State should have a board of animal hygiene, and a corps of competently educated veterinary police.

The Microscopic Examination of Pork.

Numerous elaborate essays have been written upon this subject; but the entire process is so easy and simple, that such extended labor can well be looked upon as useless.

Among the first, and at the same time most profusely invaded muscles, are the so-called "pillars of the diaphragm." They are always to be found as two small stumps of muscles—flesh—immediately below the kidneys in the dressed hog when hung up to "cool out," or in front of them when the hog is laid down. If there are any trichinæ in the organism, examples will surely be found here. These pieces belong to the trimmings, and their removal in no way interferes with the value or appearance of the dressed hog.

Although a power of fifteen to twenty diameters is sufficient to demonstrate the presence of trichinæ to a proficient examiner, still it is much easier and safer to use one of from fifty to seventy-five.

Fair microscopes, but by no means as convenient as the Hartnach model of Continental makers, are to be had from Americans at from fifteen to twenty dollars. A large table to the microscope is a convenience.

A few glass slides, or object-glasses, and some strong covering-glasses, a pair of small curved scissors, and two teasing-needles, are all that is necessary to complete the outfit.

The first step is to take a piece of muscle and cut into its substance, in order to have it as moist as possible, and with the curved scissors cut several thin slices lengthwise to the fibers, and with a needle place them on the object-glass a little distance apart; the

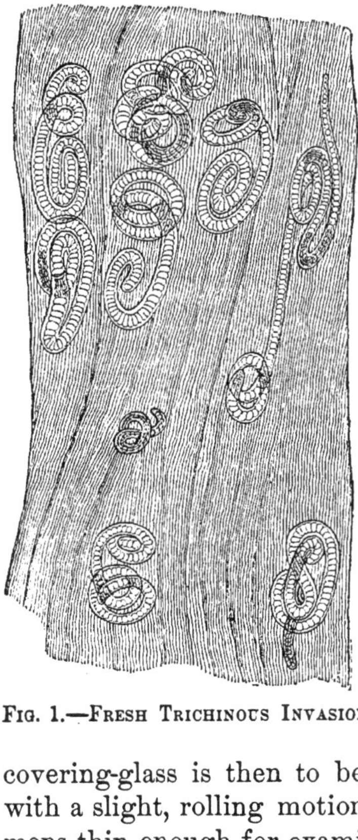

FIG. 1.—FRESH TRICHINOUS INVASION.

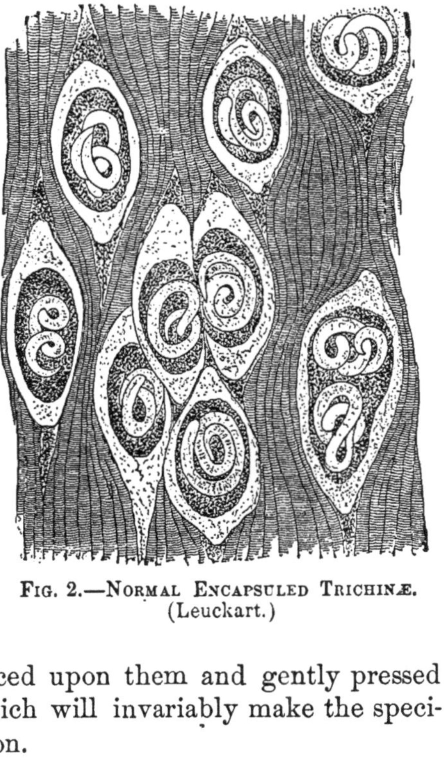

FIG. 2.—NORMAL ENCAPSULED TRICHINÆ. (Leuckart.)

covering-glass is then to be placed upon them and gently pressed with a slight, rolling motion, which will invariably make the specimens thin enough for examination.

It is not necessary to cleanse the glasses for each specimen to be examined.

To determine if the trichinæ still live, place the object-glass over heat—a spirit-lamp—for a second, enough to warm the slide, and then place it under the microscope, and they will be seen to move in their capsules.

Salted pork is best examined by cutting it into thin pieces and soaking for a time, although the specimens can be at once placed in water for a few moments.

Objects which may be mistaken for Trichinæ, or not recognized as such.

It not unfrequently happens that the capsules become abnormally thickened, and the parasites dead within them. They do not then present the same appearances that are generally observed under normal conditions.

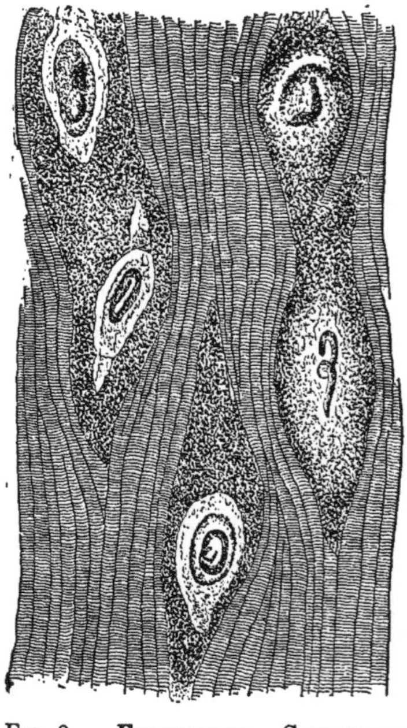

Fig. 3. — Encapsuled Concretions with Dead Embryos in them.

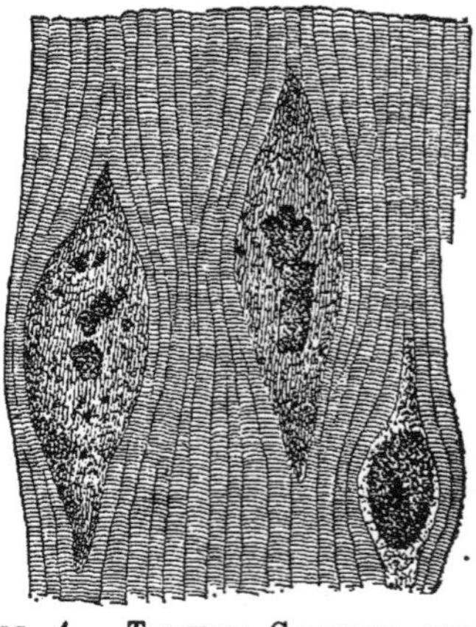

Fig. 4. — Trichina-Capsules with Calcified and Disintegrated Contents.

In other cases the calcification is of such a character as to almost entirely change the appearance of both capsule and contents.

Treatment of such capsules with hydrochloric acid will render the diagnosis easier.

In some cases cysticerci, measles, perish and become calcified. These objects are somewhat larger than trichina-capsules, and often contain a caseous mass.

The sacs of Rainey, or, as they are also termed, "psorospermiæ," are elongated granulous bodies, like the trichinæ, situated *within* the sarcolemma of the fiber. Their true nature or pathological importance is not yet well determined.

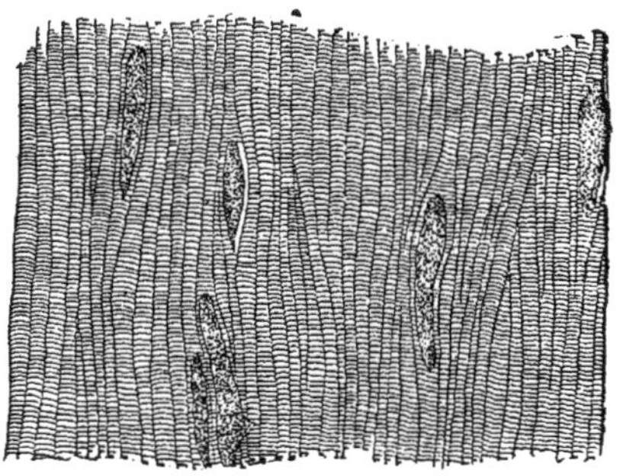

FIG. 5.—PSOROSPERMS IN A HOG'S MUSCLE. (Leuckart)

Some valuable diagnostic points are, that in the latter—trichinæ—the striation of the fiber is entirely destroyed within the capsule, while by psorosperms it is retained, limiting the objects laterally, and continuing directly from their extremities.

Bruch, Virchow, and Leuckart have described peculiar roundish or oval objects of a whitish color, having varying dimensions, which sometimes appear in the flesh of hams, and which have been demonstrated to consist of agglomerates of needle-like crystals. They fill the fiber to a variable degree without otherwise disturbing its contents, and disappear upon the addition of muriatic acid, the normal striation again becoming visible.

TRICHINIASIS IN MAN.

It is not my purpose to write an essay on the pathology of trichiniasis, either in man or animals, but to give the necessary natural historical facts of its life, and to illustrate its prevalence, with short notices of the phenomena of the disease in the above species. Treatment being so unsuccessful, it would be folly to notice it, and it also belongs more to works on medicine than in an essay on hygiene, or a contribution to preventive medicine.

It has been previously mentioned that the honor of confirming the causal nexus between trichinæ in pork and in man belongs to Dr. Zenker of Dresden, Germany. This was in the case of a servant-girl, admitted to the city hospital at Dresden, *as a typhus patient.* She died, her muscles being found completely infected with trichinæ. At the same time that she became ill, other persons of the same family, and the butcher that slaughtered a hog for them, were ill also, but in a modified form. An examination of the pork at the house revealed the presence of numerous trichinæ.

Thudicum * sums up the principal phenomena of trichiniasis in man as follows: "Sudden swelling of the face, particularly of the eyelids, after the patient has for some days felt prostrate and lost his appetite—the swelling causes only a sense of tension, but no pain—fever, quick pulse, copious perspiration, which not rarely has a repugnant odor; painfulness and immobility of the arms and legs; the muscles are swelled and contracted, and give great pain on being moved, or pressed severely; in the worst cases the entire body is perfectly immovable and highly sensitive; there is diarrhœa, with a red, somewhat coated tongue, inclined to dryness; when the swelling of the face has subsided, œdema of the feet, legs, and thighs comes on. Shortly afterward anasarca and swelling over the trunk makes its appearance."

From the time of Zenker's case, numerous others have come to pass in different countries, and epidemics have caused a shudder of horror among reflecting people.

Epidemics have been reported at Corbach, 1860; Plauen, 1861–'62; Calbe, 1862; Hallstadt, 1862–'63; Hanover, 1864; Dresden, 1864; and other places in Germany. The most remarkable outbreak is that of Hedersleben, a place of some two thousand inhabitants, of whom 337 became sick at one time, and 101 died.

Cobbold communicated to Heller that the first authentic case of the disease, during life in man, occurred in England in 1871.

We have mentioned several cases illustrating the intra-vital discovery of the parasites in human beings on the excision of tumors, and numerous others are reported in medical literature.

Forty persons became infected with trichinæ at one time at Bremen from, it is said, eating American pork.

At Lissa,† five members of one family became infected from eating of a ham which, it was said, had been pickled, smoked, and boiled for two hours.

A poor woman ‡ became trichinous from eating the flesh of a dog, to which her necessities had driven her.

At Linden,# a suburb of Hanover, four hundred persons were diseased at one time, and twenty-one died from eating trichinous pork.

Dr. Keifer, ‖ of Detroit, reports a fatal case of this disease, the patient dying at the end of the fourth week.

* "Seventh Report of the Privy Council," London, 1865.

† "Boston Medical and Surgical Journal," vol. xc, p. 491; vol. xci, pp. 471 and 627; vol. l, p. 208.

‡ Ibid.

Ibid.

‖ Ibid.

Dr. Herr, of Dubuque, Iowa, reports fifteen cases and five deaths from eating raw smoked ham made into sausages.

Several cases are reported for Philadelphia in the "American Journal of Sciences."

In January, 1881, a case occurred at Blackwell's Island, New York. Two cases were reported at Chicago during the same month, and two at Milwaukee.

Dr. Germer, health-officer at Erie, Pennsylvania, reports by letter of January 27, 1881, that the preceding Christmas he discovered seven cases in a place eight miles distant, which were traced to the eating of home fed and cured pork.

The most interesting American case is one that occurred at Brooklyn, Long Island, September, 1879. Seven of a family were affected, and two persons died from the disease. This case came to trial at Brooklyn, the family suing a packing-house from which they had bought a portion of a ham two days previous to the eruption of the disease. As they had been continually in the habit of eating raw ham and sausages, and as they had purchased the ham only two days previous to the first appearance of illness, it was self-evident that the plaintiffs did not have any case, especially as no microscopic examination of the ham had taken place. Further, it does not seem as if retailers of pork can be held responsible for its containing trichinæ in a country where neither the law nor the community recognize any such disease of the hog. Even our boards of health simply recognize the existence of trichinæ in pork as a scientific fact. All the hogs, specimens from which I examined, were cut up and sold, even though the Massachusetts Board of Health knew that I was continually finding them trichinous. Until the public becomes alive to its own interests, we may be sure that no steps toward prevention will be taken by the State.

A German judge has ruled differently. A provision-dealer at Berlin was declared "guilty" for selling trichinous pork, which had not been subjected to microscopic examination, but which had caused disease among a number of persons, some of whom died. The judge ruled that such a decision was justifiable, even though the microscopic examination of pork was not then made imperative by law. The objection that the seller had no knowledge of its injurious character was ruled out.

Dr. Sutton,* of Aurora, Indiana, reports nine cases of trichiniasis with three deaths from the consumption of uncooked sausage. The meat of the same was found to be trichinous. A cubic inch of the

* "Lancet," vol. ii, 1875.

flesh, taken from the bone of one of the persons that died, was assumed to contain one hundred thousand trichinæ.

Dr. Sutton says that "microscopic examination of *thousands of swine slaughtered* in Indiana reveals three to sixteen per cent of them as trichinous." This is an unfounded statement, there being no authentic statistics of the examination of thousands of swine in Indiana even now, nor at the time the above was written.

The "Rochester Democrat," May 1, 1879, reports several cases of trichiniasis in that vicinity.

Cases have also been reported in the "Annals of the Michigan Board of Health," at Otsego, Detroit, Port Huron, and other places, several of which terminated fatally.

In Saxony,* from 1860 to 1875, 39 different eruptions of the disease had taken place. The whole number of cases reported was 1,267, with 19 deaths; of the 19 that died, 3 out of 8 acquired the disease from eating raw meat; 2 out of 630 diseased from cold sausage; 8 of 340 from fried sausage, and 2 of 48 from eating raw ham.

Of the 6,959,964 swine which were slaughtered in Saxony in these sixteen years, *only 39*, 1 to 180,000, gave occasion to trichiniasis in human beings.

TABLE GIVING THE OBSERVED CASES OF TRICHINIASIS IN BAVARIA.

No.	Place.	Year.	Number of cases.	Author.	Where described.	Nature of trichinous meat.
1	Wurzburg.	1853	2†	Virchow.	"Virchow's Archiv," vol. lxxxi, 1853.	Fresh meat and raw ham. (Nos. 1–5)
2	"	1861	1†	Kölliker.	"Wurz. med. Zeit.," vol. ii, 12, 1861.	
3	Erlangen.	1870	8‡	Maurer.	"Deutsch. Arch. f klin. Med," vol. viii, 368, 1871.	
4	"	(?)	1†	Zenker.	Ibid., p. 388.	
5	Zweibrücken.	1870–'71	1†	Friedreich.	Ibid., vol. ix, p. 459, 1872.	
6	Speyer.	1873	5	David.	Communicated to Dr. Göring.	Swine from Baden.
7	Hof.	1878	6	Roth.	"Ref. Aerztekammer v. Oberfronken."	Home-made pork.
8	Bamburg.	Feb., 1878	30, 1 died.	"	" "	
9	Nürnberg.	May, 1878	10			
10		May, June.	3	Merkel. (Nos. 9–10)	" "	Salted pork.
11	Treuchtlingen.	"	4	"	" "	Sausage-meat.
12	Marktlenten.	July.	19	Roth.	" "	Partly-fried sausage.
13	Burgsinn.	Feb., 1879	7, 3 died.	"	"Mittheile polit. Zeitung."	

* Reinard, "Archiv d. Heilkunde," p. 241, 1877. † Accidentally found at the autopsy.
‡ "Deutsche Zeitschrift für Thiermedicin," Bollinger, Bd. 5, Hefte 3 u. 4, p. 204.

Glazier, in his report, has collected a list of 3,044 cases of disease among human beings, and 231 deaths, in Europe. For this country, 77 cases and 24 deaths.

He has also endeavored to get at the prevailing opinion of doctors as to its extension among the people in this country, as revealed in autopsies, but, while many report having seen cases, the reports are in general of so vague a nature as to be next to valueless.

An Epidemic of Trichiniasis on the Jordan.*

By Dr. John Wortahet.

The outbreak of the disease was traced to a wild hog which had been shot in the swamps adjoining the village of El Khiam, on the 25th of November, 1880. It was a very large boar, and I was told that its flesh appeared fresh, fat, and perfectly healthy. A very large number of the people of the village ate of the flesh of this hog, partly in a raw and partly in a semi-cooked condition. Not a single person that ate of the flesh escaped infection.

The head of the boar was sent as a present to a family in a neighboring village. It was cooked three times before any of it was eaten. Although quite a number of people partook of it, none of them became sick.

All of those that partook of other portions of the hog remained in a healthy condition until the eruption of the disease made itself evident, which took place in the majority in the second, and by some in the third week. I heard of only one man who was taken with emesis and diarrhœa soon after eating. In this case the phenomena of the disease were very mild. Another ate the meat well cooked, and remained free from any indications of invasion to the end of the fifth week subsequent to the same, and then was not confined to his bed.

The principal phenomena during the third, fourth, and fifth weeks were œdema of the face and extremities, severe muscular pains, more or less fever, and itching over the whole body. The œdema sometimes extended over the whole body. The pain complicated the active muscles, inclusive of those of the lower jaw, the pharynx, and larynx. It was most severe at points where the tendons were inserted upon the extremities. Every movement was painful. The fever seemed to assume a severe type only in the fatal cases. Children suffered less than those of mature years.

The period of convalescence, extending from the fifth week on,

* "Virchow's Archiv," vol. lxxxiii, p. 553.

was very slow, and accompanied by much muscular pain, œdema, and weakness. In some cases distinct relapses were apparent.

The number of persons diseased was:

Males	124
Females	103
Children	35
Total	262

Of these died:

Males	3
Women	3
Total	6

Of those that died, the cause seemed to be the exhaustive nature of the fever, and the constitutional disturbances in the fourth and fifth weeks of the invasion. The last fatal case was that of an elderly woman, in the beginning of the eighth week of the invasion. Some pieces of the musculus biceps brachii from this woman were subjected to microscopic examination and numerous trichinæ found in the same.

This is the first case of the kind reported in medical literature from Oriental countries, and is also of value as showing that the wild hogs of those regions also become trichinous as well as those of Europe.

With reference to the observations of trichiniasis in the dead body:

Dr. Bowditch, of Boston, reported four cases during the years 1842–'44.

Turner says of Scotland, that in five years 1 to 2 per cent of the human cadavers were found trichinous.

Fiedler found 2 to 2·5 per cent at Dresden.

Wagner, 1 to 30 or 40 at Leipsic.

Reports of like nature come from other countries.

Prevention of the Disease in Man.

Aside from the regulations already given for the prevention of the disease among hogs, which, if possible to be carried out, would prevent it in man, there are several which must come into action as public health preventive measures.

There is but one golden rule to prevention: *cook the pork thoroughly!*

Leuckart and other experimenters have shown that a temperature of 140° Fahr., which must extend through a piece of pork, is necessary to the positive death of the parasites.

The direct application of dry heat, by means of a hot table, to specimens under the microscope, demonstrates that a temperature of 50° C.—122° Fahr.—is necessary to kill trichinæ.

The ordinary processes of cooking, salting, and smoking are not always a sure means of killing these parasites.

All hogs should be subjected to microscopic examination by experts, and no hog allowed to be cut up for sale as food until such an examination had been made. Those found invaded should be branded trichinous, and their sale as food forbidden by law under penalty of a heavy fine.

HOG-CHOLERA.

Pneumo-enteritis Suis Contagiosa.

This peculiar infectio-contagious disease of the porcine family has been known to agriculturists and veterinarians for centuries. For years it has been looked upon as a form of anthrax, typhus, erysipelas, etc.; but it has remained for our country to institute the first extensive researches as to its nature, though Klein, in England, anticipated them by doing some good work in this direction. On the Continent of Europe the disease has not as yet been scientifically studied.

I have nothing but praise for the admirable reports of Messrs. Detmers and Law upon the porcine pest, issued by the Agricultural Department at Washington in 1878, and most earnestly recommend it to public consideration.

In 1877 our national commissioner reported a loss to the country of $16,653,428 from contagious animal disease.

Etiology.

As with all forms of infectio-contagious diseases, we find also in hog-cholera, that it was a long time before we gained any accurate knowledge with reference to the nature of the elements causing it. Some have asserted that pigs will not contract the disease when fed on succulent vegetable food; but Law has proved the fallacy of this opinion by direct experiment. Naturally, unfavorable nutritive and hygienic conditions will favor the development of this as well as other diseases, but they are not the direct cause.

Roell says the disease is attributed to hot and sultry weather, uncleanly pens, and offering to the swine of spoiled, moldy food and decomposing material in general.

Harms seems to be the first to have discovered germs in the blood, and to have attributed to them an etiological importance, as he found the blood and other parts of diseased swine, as well as the food, replete with these organisms.

Bollinger also describes micrococci and short cylinder bacteria in the blood, but does not consider the etiological connection with the disease as established.

Roell says further, "The disease has not yet been produced by inoculation."

Spinola wrote a monograph on the "Diseases of Swine," Berlin, 1842, and considers the disease to be of a gastro-bilious character; and says further, it is observed to occur in those swine which have much rest, a surplus of strong feed, especially that which is of a spirituous nature—brewers' grains, etc.—which incline to a surplus production of gall and its accumulation in the system. He also considers the above climatic conditions to exert an influence in the generation of the disease.

It remained, however, for American veterinarians, not indigenous to the country, to establish beyond doubt the true nature of this disease.

The results of the studies of Messrs. Law and Detmers show the disease to be of an infectious and contagious nature, and capable of transmission to other animals as well as swine by inoculation.

They discovered in the blood peculiar elements having a globular or micrococcus form, as well as staff-like bodies—the mature form—to which Detmers gave the name of

Bacillus Suis.

These objects are found invariably in the blood, urine, mucus, exudations, etc., in all pathologically changed tissues and in the excrements of the diseased animals, and constitute, beyond all question, the etiological momenta of the disease. These bacilli undergo several changes, and require a certain length of time to fulfill their development; consequently, if introduced into an animal organism, some time must pass (the incubational or colonization period) before the morbid phenomena become apparent. Three stages of development may be observed—viz., the germ, or micrococcus stage; the bacillus, or rod-bacterial stage; and the proliferating or germ-producing stage.

The micrococci are found in immense numbers in the fluids of the organism, especially in the blood and exudations. If the temperature is not too low, and a sufficiency of oxygen is present, they soon develop, or grow longitudinally, by a sort of budding process —a germ, or micrococcus, under constant microscopic observation, budded and grew to double its length in exactly two hours in a temperature of 70° Fahr., and gradually developed to a true rod. Some of the latter under favorable circumstances commence to grow again in length, until they appear five to six inches long, with a power of 850 diameters. At the same time scission takes place, and they break into two or more segments. These long bacteria appear to be replete with germs; the external envelope disappears, or is dissolved, and the germs become free.

Some of the bacilli move very rapidly, while others appear motionless. The cause of motion seems to be in some way dependent upon the temperature, for they appear motionless if the latter be low, but soon move if the temperature be increased and caused to exert a direct influence upon them.

Another change to be observed is the collection of the germs, or bacteria, in the so-called zooglea clusters, which are often to be met with in the blood and other fluids, and invariably in the exudations in the lungs. In the ulcerous tumors of the intestinal mucosa these clusters are comparatively seldom, but the bacilli are very numerously represented. These tumefactions in the intestinal tracts appear to afford the most favorable conditions for the growth and development of these bacteria.

Whether these zooglea clusters are instrumental in the production of capillary embolism is still an open question, though it appears highly probable. The vitality of the germs, and especially of the bacilli, does not appear to be very great (Detmers) except where they are contained in a medium not very prone to decomposition, such as water which contains a slight amount of organic substances. In the water of streams, brooks, etc., the germs are not very rapidly destroyed. In fluids and substances subject to putrefaction the bacteria lose their vitality very soon, and apparently disappear. They are also destroyed when acted upon by alcohol, carbolic acid, thymol, iodine, etc. With reference to the vitality of the infectious elements, Law says of the

Virulence of Dried Virus.—This was indicated three years ago by Professor Axe, of London, who successfully inoculated pigs with virus that had been dried on ivory points for seventy-six days. Law inoculated three pigs with virulent products that had been dried on quills for one day; one with the same kind of virus that had been dried four days, another with virus that had been dried five days, and another with virus that had been dried for six days. The quills had been sent from New Jersey and North Carolina, without any special protection. Of the six inoculations four gave positive results, while two, in which the quills were subjected to the action of disinfectants, gave negative.

Virulence of Dried Intestine.—Pieces of dried intestine, which had been dried for three and four days each, were used for inoculation, and gave positive results.

Virulence of Moist Morbid Products if secluded from the Air..—In these experiments a pig was inoculated with a piece of intestine sent from Illinois in a tightly corked bottle. The specimen had been three days from the pig, and had a slightly putrid odor. The disease developed on the sixth day.

A second pig was inoculated with blood from a diseased pig that had been kept for eleven days at 100° Fahr. in an isolation apparatus, the outlets of which were plugged with cotton-wool. Illness followed in twenty-four hours.

These experiments go to prove that the exclusion of air, or retarding of putrefaction, probably favors the longer preservation of the inficiens.

Probable Non-Virulence of Morbid Products that have undergone Putrefaction.—This seems to be proved by direct experiment.

Virulence of the Blood.—Law produced positive results by experiments upon two pigs, which is opposed to the single experiment of Klein; but Law does not know but that at certain stages of the disease the blood may be non-virulent.

Infection by means of the air does not seem to be clearly proved.

Transmissions of the disease to other animals than the hog for inoculation seem all to be followed by positive results in sheep, rabbits, and dogs; and Klein succeeded in producing it in rabbits, Guinea-pigs, and mice.

Seasons and Temperatures.

Experience has proved the extension and devastations of this disease to be the most extreme in the late summer and early fall months; but the cold weather of winter does not seem to be able to put that check to its ravages which occurs under the same conditions with other diseases of a somewhat similar nature.

Detmers says: "While, therefore, the very severe weather of the past winter caused a great reduction in the number of animals affected, the disease was not eradicated, nor did its fatality seem to be lessened. The extension of the disease from one herd to another was greatly diminished; but in infected herds where the malady was already prevailing when cold weather set in, there appeared but little difference in the rapidity of the transmission of the disease from one animal to another in the same lot."

Dr. Law confirms this statement, for his experiments proved that "the severe frosts of winter do not destroy the germs of the malady, but simply retard their conveyance from one herd to another."

In another place Dr. Law says: "I have demonstrated that the freezing of the virulent matter does not destroy its activity, and that the virus loses nothing in potency by preservation for one or two months closely packed in dry bran. The same may be inferred of all other situations when it is closely packed, and where the air has imperfect access. These last two points are of immense importance as bearing upon the question of the preservation of the poison in infected pens and yards, alike in winter and in summer, to say nothing of its possible conveyance by means of fodder or other vehicles."

Incubation.

According to the average drawn from a large number of observations, the period of incubation varies from five to fifteen days.

Intra-vital Phenomena.

One of the very earliest symptoms is a marked rise in the temperature of the hog; yet the fact is not without some questionable diagnostic value: first, on account of the variations which seem to exist in the normal temperature of different hogs; and, second, the difficulty which the struggle of the pig throws in the way of the proper application of the thermometer, which may in some cases cause a more or less marked rise in the temperature. Detmers does not consider the thermometer of any great value in the diagnosis or prognosis of this disease. The disease frequently announces itself by a cold shivering on the part of the afflicted swine, lasting from a few moments to several hours, frequent sneezing, and more or less coughing.

These anticipatory symptoms are soon followed by a more or less loss of appetite, a rough and somewhat staring condition of the bristles, a drooping of the ears, loss of vivacity, and in some cases by vomiting; a desire to bury themselves in the bedding and to lie down in dark and quiet corners; a dull and injected condition of the eyes; swelling of the head, eruptions upon the ears and other parts of the body; occasionally bleeding from the nose, and partial or total blindness; dizziness, diarrhœa, and stertorous breathing. The flanks fall in, and the animals rapidly become emaciated, and betray a vitiated appetite for dung, dirt, and saline substances; increased thirst, accumulation of secretions in the canthi of the eyes, and more or less copious nasal discharges. The peculiar offensive and fetid smell of the exhalations and excrements may be looked upon as characteristics of this disease. This odor is so penetrating as to announce the presence of the disease, especially if the herd of swine be a large one, at a distance of half a mile, or even more, if the direction of the wind be favorable. If the animals are inclined to be costive, the fæces are generally grayish or brownish-black in color, and hard; if diarrhœa is present, they are semi-fluid, of a grayish-green color, and in some cases contain an admixture of blood. In a large number of cases the more tender portions of the skin on the lower surface of the body, between the posterior extremities, behind the ears, or even on the nose and neck, exhibit numerous larger or smaller red spots, or sometimes a uniform redness. Toward the fatal termination, this redness frequently changes to a purple color. The physical examination of the thorax reveals, if pleuritis be present, the characteristic crepitation. As the pathological processes progress, the movements of the afflicted animal become weaker and slower, the gait staggering and uncertain; sometimes paretic phenomena appear, especially in the posterior portions of the body. If still standing, the head becomes much depressed, but, as a rule, the diseased animals are found lying down in a dark and secluded corner, with the nose buried in the bedding. An extremely fetid diarrhœa frequently marks the approach of a slow, fatal termination of the disease; the voice becomes very peculiar, faint, and hoarse, the sick animal manifests the greatest indifference to its surroundings; emaciation and general debility increase very fast; the skin is hard, dry, and dirty, the more so according to the duration of the disease; death ensues under convulsions, or very quickly; in some cases a cold, clammy perspiration breaks out over the body. Wherever pigs or hogs have been ringed, the wounds thus made betray a great inclination to ulceration. In those few cases which do not terminate fatally, the symptoms gradually disappear; the cough becomes more frequent but less laborious, the discharge from the nose becomes for a day or two more copious, but soon diminishes, and the offensive odor of the excrements disappears; existing sores or ulcers have a tendency to heal; the animal becomes more lively, and gains slowly in flesh and strength; a short, hacking cough frequently continues for a long time.

Pathological Phenomena.

The morbid processes, though essentially the same, can have their seat in many different organs or parts of the body. The necroscopical aspects of the disease are consequently not always the same.

We almost always find a more or less extensive infiltration of portions of the lungs, as well as serous hæmorrhagic conditions in the pulmonary tissues. In some cases the infiltrated conditions of the lungs are so extensive that they sink when thrown into water. The degree of consolidation is largely dependent upon the duration of the disease. In some lungs these centers of consolidation were circumscribed and rare, while in others they were diffuse, and complicated a large portion of the lung. Where the consolidation was limited, it was principally seated in the anterior lobes. In animals where the disease had progressed slowly, the different stages, or better conditions of consolidation were observable, conforming to the red, brown, or gray hepatization of pathologists—conditions of color dependent on the amount of blood present in the infiltrated pulmonary tissues. The greater the endothelial proliferation, and accumulation of inflammatory products, the greater the pressure exerted upon the capillary loops dipping into the alveoli; hence the variation in color, red, brown, or gray.

The lymphatic and mesenteric glands were invariably found to be enlarged. In some cases they presented a brownish or blackish color, and contained not only disintegrated elements but extravasations which lay between and separated the normal elements of the glands.

The trachea and bronchi were filled with more or less frothy mucus, which contained desquamated epithelium and bacteria. The mucous membrane was more or less tumefied and congested.

Morbid changes were almost invariably present in the pleuræ, mediastinum, and pericardium, as well as slight effusions in the cavities of the chest and abdomen. Pleural adhesions were frequently met with, as well as deposits upon the free surface of the membranes.

The *heart* (myocardium) was found to be complicated in the majority of cases. In some animals it was flabby and dilated, and generally congested. In the majority of cases pathological changes, which may be said to be pathognomonic, were found in the cæcum and colon. These consisted of peculiar growths or ulcerous tumors in the mucosa. (Whether these were limited to the Peyer's patches or not the report does not say.) They varied in size and shape, and were more or less prominent above the general surface of the mucosa. The base of the older ones was frequently more or less pigmented. Their size varied from that of a pin's head to a quarter of a dollar. The smaller ones were generally of a yellowish color, and projected but slightly; the larger ones were of a grayish-brown color, or even blackish, and had usually a slight concavity in the center. The greater part of these growths consisted of connective tissue. In some cases these growths, especially the smaller ones, or those of recent origin, were situated upon the surface of the mucosa, and were easily scraped off, leaving behind an uneven, excoriated surface, having the appearance of granulation tissue. The older and larger tumors penetrated more deeply into the substance of the mucosa—in some cases so deeply that their removal caused perforation of the walls of the intestine. Similar productions were also found in other parts of the intestine.

The contents of the gall-bladder were found, in many cases, to consist of a semi-solid, granular, dirty-brownish substance. In most of them the ductus choledochus appeared to be thickened, so that the semi-solid condition of the bile might be attributed to absorption of its fluid elements, due to retention.

Morbid changes in the skin were frequently met with, consisting of ulcers, purple spots or patches, or diffuse redness.

The blood presented both qualitative and quantitative changes. It was dirt-colored in all cases where death had been caused by extensive pulmonary complications, but was thin and light-colored where pathological changes predominated in other parts of the organism. It invariably coagulated on exposure to the atmosphere. The kidneys exhibited no very marked change.

Microscopic Observations. (Law.)

Skin.—Microscopic sections through the affected portions of the skin showed the various grades of congestion, with blocking of the capillaries, and an excess of lymphoid and large granular cells and pigment granules with extravasations and necrotic centers. With the earlier congestion there is more or less anasarca and consequent separation of the elements of the cutis, while in the later or more severe conditions a fibrinous exudation takes place, and this may even exude upon the free surface and form dark scabs. In no instance was formation of pus in the skin to be seen. One feature, which does not seem to have been hitherto observed, was the implication of the bristle-follicles.

Intestines.—Sections through those portions of the intestines which are merely congested and reddened, but without ulceration, show stagnation and blocking of the capillaries of the mucosa and sub-mucosa, with thickening and softening of the tissues, especially of the epithelium. This last contains a great excess of granules, and aggregations of the same into cell-forms, while the epithelial cells are reduced in size and contain enlarged nuclei. As has been pointed out by Klein, the degeneration is often the greatest around the openings of the crypts of Lieberkuhn, and in their interior, while their cavities are frequently filled with extravasated blood. Aside from the above one frequently finds lymphoid and migrated blood-cells, hæmatine crystals, and micrococci.

The ulcers, with a central slough, present at their base the same characteristics as the congested mucous membrane. The slough is mainly composed of small nucleated cells and granules, and micrococci.

Lymphatic Glands.—The obstruction of the capillaries and extravasation of blood are most common in the cortical portion of the gland; when the medullary portion is complicated, the extravasated blood is oftenest met with in the lymph-channels and inter-stromatous spaces, while the parenchyma seems to escape. The cellular changes are most marked in the protracted cases of the disease.

Organs of Respiration.—The characteristic lesion of the lungs is lobular pneumonia; the exudation being most abundant in the interlobular connective tissues, and is often of a dark color on account of the presence of red blood-cells. A microscopic section transverse to the bronchioli and alveoli reveals the presence of an exudation containing a large number of round lymphoid cells, granules, and in the alveoli similar accumulations.

Kidneys.—Clouded swelling of the cortical, with consequent hyperæmia of the medullary, substance.

Blood.—In most cases no changes were to be observed except the presence of numerous bacteria. No such organisms were to be found in the blood of a healthy pig.

Diagnosis.—From the foregoing detailed description of the phenomena of this disease, it is evident that there is but little difficulty in its correct recognition, especially when appearing in a number of swine at the same time.

Prognosis.—This is always unfavorable, for even though individuals may survive the attack, still the ravages of the disease are such as to almost destroy their value as marketable animals from an economical point of view.

TREATMENT.—On account of its difficulties, medicinal treatment of swine is in general almost useless, and with this disease truly so; the antizymotics are, however, indicated in unison with tonics.

PREVENTION.

As in all infectious diseases, of whatever nature, the aim of modern medicine is prevention. On account of the great liability to extension peculiar to this porcine pest, the regulations of preventive medicine must be fully as much of a general as of a local character.

We shall follow Mr. Law in considering this question. He says: "One farmer may easily eradicate it from his swine, but, so long as it continues to prevail among those of his neighbors, his stock is daily subjected to the danger of renewed infection."

This being the fact with reference to the individual farmer, it is equally the case in every township, county, or State. In our Eastern States the pest is almost invariably due to the importation of diseased stock, and, though from the lack of pigs it never gains wide extension, it illustrates the infectious nature of the disease in the West. To secure a complete or even restricted immunity from its ravages, active measures must be taken over the entire land, and this can only be done under the supervision of one central, controlling power, with the necessary number of local authorities.

The following measures should be adopted:

1. The appointment of local inspectors to carry out the measures necessary to suppress the disease.

2. The injunction on all having the care of or ownership of hogs, and upon all who may be called upon to advise concerning the same, or to treat them, to make known to such local authorities all recognized or suspected cases of the disease, under a penalty for any and every neglect of such duty.

3. The obliging of the local authorities, under the advice of a competent veterinary inspector, to see to the absolute destruction of all pigs suffering from the pest, and all that have been in contact with them, and their burial in some isolated place, and the thorough disinfection of the pens, utensils, and persons around them.

(It will frequently be found most advantageous to the interests of all concerned, to kill and bury the hogs in their pens, and to burn the latter, when of wood, as well as the utensils, and to erect new pens at some place properly distant for any new lot of hogs.)

4. The complete isolation of all domestic animals which have been in contact with the diseased pigs, and in all cases of sheep and rabbits, the destruction of the sick when this shall be deemed necessary.

5. When all the pigs in an infected herd have not been destroyed, the remainder should be placed upon an official register, and subjected to daily inspection by the veterinary inspector, so that the sick may be removed and killed on the first indication of disease.

6. Sheep and rabbits which have been in contact with diseased hogs should be treated likewise, and none should be removed from the flock until after the lapse of a month from the last appearance of disease among them.

7. All animals and birds, wild or tame, and all persons except those employed in the work, must be carefully excluded from the infected premises, and until the same have been pronounced safe, after careful disinfection, etc.

8. The losses sustained by owners from the compulsory slaughter of their hogs should be made good by a valuation to be fixed by a competant board of assessors.

9. Such reimbursement should be forfeited by owners who fail to comply with the law in properly notifying the authorities of the real existence or suspicion of the presence of the pest among their swine.

10. A register should be kept, in prescribed form, of all hogs kept on farms within a certain radius of infected herds—say one mile—and no removal of such animals should be permitted until the disease had been pronounced at an end, unless by special license from the competent authorities, after the veterinary inspector had pronounced the herd in question to be absolutely free from every suspicion of the disease.

11. Railroad and shipping agents of adjoining stations to infected districts should be forbidden to ship pigs, excepting by license of the local authorities, until the plague has been pronounced at an end in such districts.

12. When infected pigs have been conveyed by rail, boat, or other means of transport, measures should be taken to insure the thorough disinfection of such vehicles of transport, as well as the barns, docks, or yards, or other places into which the diseased animals may have been turned.

DISEASES OF CATTLE.

Cattle assume by far the first place among our domestic animals, from an economical point of view. The prosperity of a nation might well be estimated by its wealth in cattle. Of all animals, they supply the greatest proportion of our animal food. Without beef and milk, we could hardly think ourselves capable of existing. Assuming this rank, then, as a source of food, it is self-apparent that the greatest care should be taken in keeping such animals in a hygienic—i. e., healthy—condition.

Animal hygiene differs much from human:

1. The animals must be kept healthy.
2. They must be kept healthy, so that they may yield the greatest possible return to the owner, be it work, flesh, milk, or other products.

To attain this end requires the greatest attention on the part of the owners.

To attain it economically, the owner must pay attention to the different characteristics of each animal, that no food goes to waste. One animal fattens easier than another on the same amount of food. One cow yields more milk, or one ox performs a like amount of work upon food that its neighbor will not thrive upon.

But in many instances, and it is with these we have especially to do, animal hygiene imposes upon the owner a responsibility that has, up to the present time, almost escaped appreciation.

It is the imperative duty of owners, or breeders of animals, to study every influence that may possibly have an injurious effect upon them, when destined to be articles of human consumption, either as flesh or milk.

Thus we see that the interests of public health demand the greatest and most studious care of the water, feeding, and surroundings of such animals.

We are not going too far when we assert that this branch of animal hygiene has been almost entirely neglected, not only by the owner, but by scientists as well.

Tape-worms are not by any means an uncommon occurrence in man, yet how few people realize that one variety is derived from the consumption of improperly cooked beef!

An instance comes to our mind of an M. D., who enjoyed a large practice, that came to us with the segments of a tape-worm, but could not believe it was, because the patient *never* ate any pork.

On being told that man also obtains such a parasite from eating beef, he was completely surprised.

The name which science has given to this parasite is *Tænia medio-canellăta*, or, better, *saginata.*

This parasite exceeds in length that which we have previously described as being obtained from pork. Its sections, or proglottids, are also broader and thicker. *Tænia solium*, or *armata*, derived from pork, has its scolex, or head, armed with hooks, which is not the case with the one we are at present considering. This fact at first led naturalists to think they had before them one and the same tape-worm, the differences in appearance and formation of the heads representing different stages of development, the armed parasite representing a youthful, the unarmed an aged, period in its existence. This has been clearly demonstrated to be a mistake. Proglottids of tænia saginata fed to young swine failed to produce cysticerci, or measles, while the same when fed to calves were followed by positive results—i. e., the development of cysticerci of the unarmed tape-worm in the interfibrillar tissue (Leuckart, Mosler, *et al.*).

As to their presence in cattle, Dr. Thudicum * says:

"The question why the cysticerci of tænia saginata have never been observed in the flesh of cattle, with the exception of those cases in which they have been intentionally reared, is of great interest and importance, from a sanitary point of view. It is possible that these bladder-worms are present in the musculature of cattle in very small numbers only, and consequently do not present any such striking appearance on section of the muscles as is produced by measles in the muscles of swine. For while a pig would devour an entire tape-worm if it came in its way, a calf would refuse to eat it, if it could avoid doing so; hence, only free eggs or single proglottids, adhering to or concealed in the herbs making up the ordinary food of cattle, could be introduced into their systems. Thus, cattle driven along a road or path would be liable to snatch a mouthful of grass, and with it a proglottid of the hookless or five-cupped tape-worm. *The very circumstance of the scarcity of cysticerci in the flesh of cattle facilitates their importation into the human intestines.* The single specimens are not discovered, and consequently not avoided; hence, the tænia derived from them live in almost all countries of our globe, and infest the black and white man, the Mongol, the Malay, and the Indian. I have examined many thousands of specimens of beef from many hundreds of bodies of beeves, and have never yet found a cysticercus of this tænia in the flesh or

* Report to the Privy Council of Great Britain. See seventh report, London, 1865.

any other organ. Probably if calves and heifers were systematically dissected with the same care as human bodies, these cysticerci would appear as frequently as the trichinæ or the cysticercus cellulosæ in man, both which parasites were discovered in the anatomical theatre, and without anatomical dissection would no doubt have eluded the vigilance of science much longer."

As said previously, tænia saginata is found in man in all parts of the world. It seems far to exceed tænia solium in its prevalence among the inhabitants of Austria proper and Lower Germany, while in North Germany tænia solium is more frequently met with. It has been met with in England, and a case of invasion is also reported in an Indian in our own country; but well-ordered statistics in this regard are so out of the general course of events in these two countries, that we are not justified in assuming that the populations of the same are so much favored above their fellow-men in other countries.

With reference to protection from this parasite—

1. We *must* have a well-organized system of inspection of all animals slaughtered, by competently educated men.

2. The people must be educated in a knowledge of these dangers, and also in the means necessary to their prevention.

a. Without the active co-operation of *the people*, we can hope for little successful reform in this country.

3. The consumption of undercooked meat must be looked upon as dangerous to health.

Cattle are also subject to several diseases which threaten the public health, from the fact that they are transmissible to man by means of infectious elements peculiar to each of them.

"Foot-and-mouth disease" is the common name given to a peculiar vesicular eruption which afflicts cattle on the parts indicated by the above name, as well as upon the udder of milch-cows.

This disease has also been observed in sheep, swine, goats, the deer family, occasionally in the horse, and cases have been reported among dogs and turkeys. Further, numerous cases of infection have been reported among human beings.

Fleming says: "It has caused almost as much loss and trouble to the farmers of Britain as has the contagious bovine lung-plague. In 1876–'77 this disease was reported as infecting 11,064 cattle, 4,809 sheep, and 1,904 swine in the kingdom of Prussia. It is needless to say that no statistics exist as to its extension among cattle and other animals in the United States."

The asssertion that animals affected with it have been exported from this country and landed in England, makes it probable that the disease has attained a foothold among our animals. But where?

Veterinary science is in a state so much less than embryonal in this country, that no one knows whence these animals came; whether they were diseased when leaving here, or what portion of them was diseased.

This disease is transmissible to man. So far as my knowledge extends, this has only taken place from diseased cows.

Valentine, of Italy, 1695, noticed the synchronous appearance of a pustulous eruption in the mouths of human beings, and a similar disease among cattle. Sagad, 1764, was the first to notice that human beings acquired the eruption from the consumption of milk from cows affected with the same. Hertwig (of the Veterinary Institute, Berlin, Prussia) first proved the same by direct experiment. He drank daily for four consecutive days a quart of milk taken from cows having the disease. On the second day he observed a mild fever, pains in the limbs, headache, a dry and hot throat, and a peculiar sensation in the hands and fingers. These mild phenomena continued about five days; then the lining of the mouth became swollen, especially the covering of the tongue. In a short time small vesicles began to develop. At the same time that these eruptions appeared in the mouth and on the lips, appeared an eruption of similar character upon the hands and fingers. Two medical practitioners also subjected themselves to the same experiment, and at the same time similar results followed. All three recovered completely. (Bollinger, in Ziemssen's "Handbuch der Pathologie," vol. iii, p. 637.)

The danger from the consumption of the milk of cows afflicted with this eruption is most emphatically demonstrated by the fact that young animals fed upon the same frequently perish in cousequence of gastro-enteritis, i. e., inflammation of stomach and bowels.

For man, milk from such cows, to which ninety per cent normal milk has been added, is still dangerous when consumed. Cooking the milk from such cows completely destroys its infectious qualities.

Bollinger gives the following examples of the eruption of the disease in human beings by indirect infection:

"A boy had a severe aphthous eruption in the mouth after biting the edge of a pail which was polluted with the droolings from the mouth of a diseased cow." "A man accidentally infected himself by putting between his teeth a knife which had been polluted in the same manner." "Another infected himself by chewing a piece of wood which had been used to clean the mouth of a diseased cow." "A veterinarian had a long-continued and painful eruption in the mouth from touching the internal part of the same with his finger after having handled a diseased cow."

In the "Preussische Mittheil. aus. d. thierärztlichen Praxis," 1874–'75, are given three cases of aphthous eruption in the mouths of men who had drunk buttermilk which had been taken from a cow having foot-and-mouth disease.

On account of the paucity of observations from competent medical men, little is known about the disposition of mankind to this disease. Doubtless, as in other infectious and contagious diseases, some persons have a far greater disposition to infection than others. Bollinger says, "Notwithstanding the ruling opinion to the contrary, the disease is much more frequent among human beings than expected."

Numerous observations have been made of the synchronous enzoötic eruptions of this disease among cattle and an eruption in the mouth of human beings.

The outbreak of this disease among human beings is only to be prevented by competently educated and trustworthy veterinary inspectors for all dairies, and by the exact isolation of all diseased animals.

Such milk might be cooked before being offered for sale; but the danger of insufficient or neglected cooking is too great to justify such a procedure, so that its sale should be strictly forbidden, and, if persevered in, as strictly punished.

Such milk, *after being thoroughly cooked*, could be appropriately used for feeding swine. Whether the consumption of butter and cheese made from such milk is dangerous to mankind is an open question requiring more extended and critical observation.

Another subject which has not, as yet, received by any means the attention which it deserves is, the changes produced in milk chemically, and especially microscopically, by the presence of inflammatory conditions of the udder of the cow.

a. The influences of such milk should be critically tested by means of feeding experiments upon young and healthy animals of the same and different species; controlled by feeding young animals from the same mother, or of as nearly as possible like age and constitution, upon the same material.

b. Are there in such milk, from diseased udders or single cisterns of the same, such microscopic changes as to allow their recognition when mixed with milk from perfectly healthy cows?

Fürstenberg * has gone into this subject with no inconsiderable

* "Die Milchdrüsen der Kuh," Leipzig, 1868.

degree of exactness. From his and other researches it is evident that changes in the constitution of the milk *are produced* by so slight a change from normality as a hyperæmic (increase of the quantity of blood) condition of the interstitial and subcutaneous tissues of the udder. A comparison of such milk with normal, or, when but one cistern is complicated, with milk from the other cisterns of the same udder, has shown that the solid elements are greatly augmented at the expense of the fluid; especially are the casein and albumen augmented, while the normal milk contains more milk-sugar, and the so-called "extractives" in greater quantity. The inorganic elements are also considerably increased in the milk from diseased udders.

In other words, such milk assumes characters simulating those of colostrum, containing the well-known colostrum bodies, having a yellowish-white color, is viscid, and coagulates easily. In such a secretion, Fürstenberg found the results of chemical analysis to be as follows:

Water	81·789
Solids	18·211
Total	100·000

The solid elements were:

Fat	5·210
Casein and albumen	8·887
Milk-sugar and extractives	3·070
Salts	1·044
Total	18·211

These 1·044 salts consisted of:

Phosphoric salts and oxide of iron	0·384
Carbonates of lime	0·108
Chloride of sodium (cooking-salt)	0·003
Soda	0·549
Traces of sulphuric acid	0·000
Total	1·044

From the non-diseased parts of the same udder the results of the analysis were as follows:

Water	88·583
Solids	11·417
Total	100·000

The 11·417 solids were:

Fat	3·405
Casein	3·218
Milk-sugar and extractives	4·092
Salts	·702
Total	11·417

The mineral elements were:

Phosphoric earths and oxide of iron	0·317
Carbonates of lime	0·146
Chloride of sodium	0·004
Soda	0·325
Traces of sulphuric acid	0·000
Total	0·702

The same is true, except in degree, of the more excessive grades of inflammation. The important question is, *Is such milk harmful, and to what extent?*

May not the only too frequent cases of so-called "summer-complaint" of children, especially of those brought up on the bottle, be traceable, in a measure, to feeding them upon milk containing these colostrum-like elements?

We know that colostrum exerts a gentle purgative influence. Is it, then, going too far to (in an *a priori* manner) assume that such milk, *when continually given, may produce more serious and lasting effects?*

This can only be proved by direct experiment upon young animals, which can not be done except at some expense to the State. It is, indeed, done by children, at no expense to the State, but at a fearful cost of human life, and all that is needed to close the evidence of this *human vivisection* is the competent veterinary expert at the milk-fountain end of the route, and the exact medical observer at the other. I think there would be little difficulty in establishing the connection between cause and effect, if animal life is not too precious and too tender for sentimental persons who esteem it above human at the present day. While every one is crying out for more economy in reference to State expenses, and while many expenses can doubtless be cut down with great benefit to the people—for instance, the number of representatives might be greatly lessened, with a corresponding increase in quality—might it not be well to call to mind the old adage that "it is not well to hold on to the spile with all one's might, and not look out for the bung."

The work of State boards of health is not surely to be limited to gathering statistics of mortality in man, or inspecting our water-sources alone, but should extend to the investigation of those experiments by which alone the true causes of disease may be discovered. We are too apt to satisfy ourselves with fine-sounding hypotheses with regard to the origin of many so-called strange diseases, which a few exact experiments would soon send to the winds, and which would lead to the discovery, if not of the cause or causes, certainly of means for their prevention.

The real germ of small-pox contagion has never yet been positively isolated, although many fond supporters of the micrococcus-germ theory cherish an idea to the contrary ; yet careful experiment and exact observation, in unison with practical experience, have taught us that exact attention to, and universal application of, vaccination, is an almost infallibly sure means of prevention against its deadly ravages.

With regard to this very milk question, a few facts, gained from actual experiment, are worth thousands of surmises from practicing physicians.

To this end State boards of health should have at their command an experiment station, under the control of a competently educated person as superintendent and observer of the experiments. Such a person should be a veterinarian, and be at the same time a member of the State Board of Health ; the advantage to such boards of such a member is by no means appreciated at the present time, either by the members of such boards or by the people at large.

With reference to the expenses of such a station, the question for legislators, and also for the people, to consider, is not one of immediate outlay, but whether it is cheaper to spend a few thousand dollars yearly for experiments, or to have causes of disease, and sometimes death, existing for years, which it is possible to discover, or at least to find means to prevent their action.

Another most important question to which I desire to call attention is, *Have States or cities done their whole duty when they have appointed inspectors to examine milk after it has left the producer, as it is ready for delivery to the consumer?*

If, as I can but think, experiment will prove that the consumption of milk from cows having diseased udders, so called "garget," is fraught with danger to human health, then *city inspection, or delivery inspection, is next to useless, and the place for the most important inspection is at the stable of the producer.*

All such cows should be isolated by an official veterinary inspector, and the sale of the milk from such isolated cows for human consumption should be punished by most severe penalties.

In fact, the inspection of the milk as it is delivered to the distributors for immediate consumption can only lead to the discovery of dilution—that is, cheating in value—*never to the discovery of an unhealthy or absolutely diseased fountain-head, i. e., cow or cows.*

The unquestionable guaranteeing to the public that the cows producing the milk are healthy is, in my opinion, far more a matter of necessity, from a hygienic point of view, than the discovery of a varying degree of watery dilution, always providing the water itself is pure. In the one case, we have discovered a simple swindle; in the other, what might prove to be the cause of serious constitutional disturbances among the consumers.

It may not be known to many milk-producers that medicine given internally, and many things, such as salves and dressings, especially those used against insects, applied outwardly, are capable of exerting an influence upon milk which is very likely to be disturbing, or even injurious, in a far more serious degree to the consumers.

The following examples, casually gathered in my reading, will sufficiently testify to this remark:

Guenther * found antimony in milk after feeding the tartrate to a cow. Harms observed a hæmorrhagic diarrhœa in two dogs and three young goats, after feeding them with the milk from a cow which had been given a large dose of the above-mentioned tartrate —forty-six grammes—the day before.

Klink † demonstrated the presence of quicksilver in the milk of a woman afflicted with syphilis, that had been subjected to the blue-ointment treatment.

According to Henry and Chevallier, cooking-salt, bicarbonate of soda, sulphate of soda, and iodide of potassium, may be discovered in milk when given to animals.

Twelve cows were so infected by carbolic acid, which had been used in a strong solution to disinfect the stable, that human beings who used the milk, both cooked and uncooked, became sick, but finally recovered. ‡

A large number of persons in Rome were poisoned from the use of goat's milk. ‖ The disease, as it appeared in these people, was strongly characteristic of cholera. Some persons recovered in

* "Jahresbericht d. Thierarzneischule zu Hannover," No. 6, p. 72.

† "Vierteljahrsschrift für Dermatologie u. Syphilis," 1876, p. 207.

‡ Scholtz, "Preussische Mittheil.," 1874–'75, p. 109.

‖ "Med. u. Chirurg. Centralblatt," 1875.

the course of seventy-four hours, but the majority were ill for some four or five days. The violence of the symptoms was in direct proportion to the quantity of milk consumed. The suspected goats were subjected to a careful examination by a veterinarian, but nothing abnormal discovered. Their food was next critically examined, and the following four poisonous plants were found in it: "conium maculatum," "clematis vitalba," "colchicum autumnale," "plumbago Europea." An examination of the milk vomited by the sick people revealed the presence of colchicum, which was looked upon as the cause of the disturbance.

Tuberculosis of Cattle.

This disease of cattle, but especially the milch-cow, is now playing a most sensational *rôle* in the discussions of hygienists, more especially those of Germany.

That the tendency or disposition to this disease is transmissible from parents to offspring has been placed beyond all question by the observation and experience of stock-raisers. This fact is also well enough known, but by far too little appreciated, by human beings with reference to their own race.

Dr. Bowditch, of Boston, has clearly shown the influence which long-continued residence in low, damp, unhealthy localities has upon the generations of the older New England families in extending or keeping alive this disease; but the medical profession has been altogether too silent with regard to hereditary influences.

Mueller * says that, basing his opinion upon 988 cases of personal observation during the course of nine years, in 21·8 per cent of the same the parents had also suffered from tubercular consumption. This percentage increases to 28·6 per cent, if we take into consideration the grandparents, brothers, and sisters. Other observers assume that thirty-eight per cent of the deaths from tubercular consumption in human beings is due to hereditary influence. If, as said, stock-raisers have learned a lesson from costly experience in this regard, and are applying principles of selection or exclusion in their breeding of animals, is it too late to apply like principles to human beings?

Is it not high time that the principles of scientific breeding should be applied by man to his own species? Beauty, form, money, position, should all play their appropriate part in the selection of the partner for life by man or woman; but, as the natural result of marriage, as the result of being made male and female, is

* "Inaugural Dissertation," Berne, 1876.

the production of children, is it not still more imperatively demanded of us to take the health of these products of our lust more frequently than our good sense into earnest consideration by selecting a partner from families in which these tendencies have attained the least possible strength?

Have we any right to condemn children thus to lives of misery and early graves? What stock-raisers do for their pockets, mankind should certainly have sense enough to do for their own offspring.

"'Tis through ignorance they do it."

The blame falls upon the shoulders of an incompetent, avaricious medical profession. Consumptive families bring large fees, help to buy corner-lots, and enable the great doctor to ride comfortably about with *coupé* and coachman.

But to return to our subject. This disease of cattle has been practically known to exist for a long time. Its cause has been sought in all sorts of absurdities, such as acrid or irritable substances in food or water. Even hereditary influences failed for a long time of their due appreciation. In Germany the disease is also known as the "Französenkrankheit," or French disease. It probably received the name when everything evil which befell the German race was only too willingly attributed to their French neighbors as well as conquerors.

The first intimation that some irritating or infectious elements were contained in the milk of cows having this disease is due to Gerlach, the most noted of all German veterinarians, and late director of the Royal Veterinary Institute at Berlin.

The experiments of Villemin, Klebs, Orth, and many others, have amply demonstrated that the elements from tuberculous diseased lungs, lymph-glands, and other organs, contained some peculiar infectious material capable of producing a similar disease when inoculated upon, or in some cases fed to, animals by way of experiment.

With reference to the milk of tuberculous diseased cows, the honor of priority is unquestionably Gerlach's.

Here we have to do with a question of manifold character. Not only is the public health threatened, but both the nation and each individual dairyman, or cow-owner, has to face a question of no secondary economical importance.

If the experimental results obtained by Gerlach and other observers, both German and French, become universally accepted, then governments have no other recourse than to order the most exact supervision of the cattle in their respective countries, by which the disease may be discovered, and their sale as meat at the earliest possible moment of such as are suitable. All others, in which this is found unjustifiable on account of their condition, must be turned over to the knacker.

The loss and expense of such a procedure can be best appreciated by the expert acquainted with the extreme extension which this disease has acquired among cattle, especially milch-cows.

If any government undertakes to stamp out this disease, it will find difficulties by far exceeding those connected with a similar process by any other contagious malady.

The adage, "Touch a man's pocket and you touch his heart," will be more than sufficiently verified.

In Germany, where the majority of the milch-cows are stall-fed, and that, too, in poorly ventilated, ill-arranged stables, this disease has acquired an extension of which we can at present make no appreciation in this country.

The assertion of the infectiousness of the milk from such cows raised a perfect storm of abuse in Germany, which poured down on the asserter's head until he died. The more ignorant, lazy, and indifferent men were, the louder they abused. Many men who were professors at the schools joined in the cry, "Down with him!" without ever making the attempt to prove the assertions wrong by direct experiment. Succeeding experiments have, however, essentially strengthened the assertions of Gerlach.

As these first experiments * with reference to so momentous a question are worthy of all attention, I take the liberty of noticing a very few of them in this place.

Having a cow afflicted with tuberculosis that still gave milk, it was resolved to use the same to test the question "*whether the milk from such a cow is capable of producing a similar disease in young animals when fed upon it.*" †

The cow was seven or eight years old, much emaciated, respiration difficult, and had a rough, weak cough; vesicular respiration perceptible over all parts of the thorax which inclose the lungs, but numerous unnatural, especially dry "râles" were perceptible. *In no place was the percussion deadened.* No fever. Appetite good. Daily milk quantum, 1,500 grammes. After the lapse of three

* It is not our purpose here to go into detail with reference to these experiments, but we will refer those interested to the "Veterinary Journal," London (England), vols. viii, ix, and x, where they will find abundant material.

† Gerlach, "Experiments with Reference to the Milk of Cows having Tuberculosis.' "Jahresbericht d. Thierarzneischule zu Hannover," 1868–'69.

months the cow was killed. The emaciated condition had gradually increased, the milk-secretion likewise decreasing: in the first month the yield of milk decreased 600 grammes; in the second, 500 grammes, and during the last eight days the secretion ceased entirely, although the animal received all the nourishment she could consume.

"*Autopsy.*—The inner thoracic walls, the diaphragm, and the mediastinum were covered with numerous tubercles of variable dimensions; the pulmonary pleura, or covering of the lungs, was far less complicated. The lungs were voluminous, and double their normal weight. Nodules and tubercles were distinctly perceptible on palpation. The bronchial lymph-glands were hypertrophied—enlarged—hard and nodulated. Cross-section of the pulmonary tissues revealed the presence of numerous tubercles and tuberculous devastations; large and small cavities filled with a muco-purulent mass, others with caseous material; numerous miliary tubercles were dispersed over the pulmonary tissue."

With the milk from this cow were fed two calves, two pigs, one sheep, and two rabbits. The first calf died from an accidentally acquired disease.

Calf No. 2. — A healthy, well-nourished calf, eight days old, was fed with milk from the above-mentioned cow, for a period extending over one and two thirds months; at first it received 1,000 and later 300 grammes of milk daily, an average of about 650 grammes per day; in fifty days the whole quantity of milk consumed amounted to from 30 to 32 kilogrammes. Aside from this the calf received other milk; later, diluted milk and oatmeal. Neither phenomena indicating the presence of disease, nor disturbance of the nutritive functions, were observable. The calf was killed one hundred days from the time that the experimental feeding began, and fifty days after the feeding with milk from the tuberculous cow had ceased.

Autopsy.—The pleura of the sharp edges of the right lung was covered with delicate red, filamentous excrescences, which extended as a fringe about a centimetre beyond the edge of the lung. Here and there this neoplastic production formed a connected membrane in which were to be seen miliary tubercles, as refracting points. The costal pleura, the inner lining of the ribs, was also irregularly covered with a membrane of similar character. In the lungs were to be seen tubercles, otherwise the parenchyma was normal; immediately under the pleura were to be seen four small and six miliary tubercles, and eight more were to be seen in the loose interlobular tissue. The smaller tubercles were more transparent, and had a grayish color, having a firm organic character; in the center of one of the larger ones was to be seen caseous material. The bronchial lymph-glands were much enlarged; inwardly disturbed by many purulent and caseous centers; here and there lime-salts were perceptible; the tuberculous centers extended prominently above the cut surface of the gland. The mesenteric and other glands presented a similar character.

The microscopical examinations of the tubercles gave the same characteristics as those of man.

Some of the experiments with the other animals mentioned previously gave negative, while others were followed by positive, results.

These and other more recent experiments prove *that the milk from cows complicated with tuberculosis is not only harmful, but that it also contains elements of a specifically dangerous character; it is capable of generating elements of a similar character: it therefore bears the character termed infectious.*

While I will not go so far as to consider the above-noticed and other experiments as conclusive and unquestionable evidence that the milk from tuberculous cows (and why not human mothers?) *will at all times* produce tuberculosis in young animals fed on the same, yet, such is my confidence in the value of the experiments made by Gerlach and still later by others, *that for myself I have no doubt whatever that the milk from tuberculous cows and mothers will, in the greater number of cases, generate tubercles in young animals when fed with sufficient quantities, and for a sufficient length of time, to produce infection.*

The casual reader might perhaps fail to see the point to which these conclusions necessarily lead us, viz., *that if young animals can be thus infected, what is there to prevent the same taking place in babes brought up on the bottle?* I do not wish to place myself before the public as a visionary alarmist.

Here are facts, however, induced from carefully executed experiments, and by a man noted for his exactness and trustworthiness in other branches of researches.

Bollinger has summed up the feeding experiments upon young animals, with the milk in question, as follows:

"Three pigs—one successfully, two doubtful.

"Three calves—two successfully, one prematurely died.

"One lamb—one successfully.

"Two dogs—two negative results.

"Two cats—two negative results.

"Fourteen rabbits—two positive, six negative results; the other six were fed upon the milk when boiled, and consequently were unaffected."

The excitement which exists with reference to this disease among hygienists, makes it imperative for us to gain all the knowledge we can as to the manner of its extension among animals. The following remarks, bearing as they do immediately upon this point, will, therefore, not be without interest and benefit to the general reader.

That the sputa from people afflicted with tubercular consumption contains elements capable of infection, has been placed beyond all doubt by means of numerous experiments with dogs where the sputa was dispersed by means of a spray-distributor into the air of a small room in which the animals were confined for a time each day, the balance of the time being allowed freedom in the open air. Too many sad cases of death from tubercular consumption have been unquestionably traced to the influence of expired air from persons having the disease, upon nurses and others around them, even in cases where any inherited disposition to the disease could be excluded beyond all question.

Most strikingly, yes, shockingly, illustrating this point, viz., *the infectiousness of the breath of persons afflicted with tuberculosis*, are the cases given by Dr. Reich in the "Berliner klinische Wochenschrift," No. 37, 1878—"Die Tuberculosis eine Infectionskrankheit." In these cases the disease was transmitted to *ten* children by a nurse who had the habit of sucking at, and blowing into the mouths of such little ones as were born asphyctic. Dr. Reich sums up his observations as follows:

"1. In the time which elapsed from the summer of 1875 to the fall of 1876 (July 11th to September 29th), there died at Neuenburg, of meningitis tuberculosa, ten children that were born between April 4, 1875, and May 10, 1876.

"2. There was no ascertainable disposition to tuberculosis in any of the ten children.

"3. All these ten children were brought into the world by the nurse Sanger.

"4. In the practice of the nurse Regisser (in the same town), not one single child died or sickened of tubercular meningitis during the same time.

"5. The nurse Sanger suffered from tubercular consumption at the time. In July, 1875, an examination of her lungs revealed cavities in the same, and she raised purulent ichorous sputa. She died from the disease July 23, 1876.

"6. Nurse Sanger had the habit of removing the mucus from the babes' mouths by means of suction with her own; and of blowing her own breath into the mouths of asphyctic children; and, in general, treated children in a manner which rendered it possible for the expired air from her own lungs to get into theirs, kissing them much, etc.

"7. In three of the cases of tubercular meningitis which came to my personal observation, the sickness began with bronchitis.

"8. Meningitis tuberculosa is not an endemic disease among children at Neuenburg. In the nine years, from 1866–'74, only two deaths are reported from this disease among children under one year old. Of twelve children, under one year old, that died in 1877, only one died from this disease; the parents of this child were both subjects of tubercular consumption."

These cases, and those which follow, that were made by an accomplished veterinarian, in connection with the experimental testimony which we have brought together in a simply suggestive but by no means exhaustive form, should be more than sufficient to call the attention of every reflecting man and woman to the fact that tuberculosis is not only a disease, the disposition to which is transmissible from parent to offspring, both human and animal, but that it is, under certain circumstances, a highly contagious and infectious disease. They tell us in warning words that we must not only be most careful in selecting our partner for life, but in the selection of the nurse, or maid, for children, and, when necessary, *the cow* from which we are to give them milk.

The influence of the expired air from the lungs of cattle afflicted with the disease called tuberculosis upon other animals of the same species confined in the same stable with them.

This question is one of vast practical and economical importance to the farmer and dairyman. I much regret that I am so entirely limited to the observations of foreigners upon cattle in their own countries rather than to observations gathered in our own country; but this fact should stimulate us to more careful consideration of these questions, even though it be late in the day that we begin.

A German veterinarian, Albert, contributes a very thoughtful and interesting paper, detailing personal observations bearing upon this very point, in the "Wochenschrift für Thierheilkunde," Nos. 30 and 31, 1880, under the title "The Tuberculosis of Cattle as an

Infectious Disease." The following is a free translation of the essential points of this paper:

Although heredity is unquestionably a very important cause in the generation of this disease among cattle, still it does not suffice to explain the great extension which the same acquires among them; especially is it insufficient in answering for the eruption of the disease among cattle in stables where no breeding takes place, or where the young animals are brought in from other places. In such stables other causes must be brought into action, and these are the transmission of the disease from one animal to another. I have observed that when there is in a stable one individual which contains in its organism the conditions necessary to the extension of the disease—tubercular process in the lungs—the disease extends to the other animals—cattle—in the same stable which have been there for a sufficient period. This seems to conform to the fact that tuberculosis is a disease peculiar to our domesticated cattle, but not to the wild ones of the plains, and agrees with the experience that certain stables are looked upon as peculiarly favorable to the generation of the disease.

Of the peculiar metamorphoses which tubercles undergo, those of caseous degeneration offer the most favorable conditions for infecting the expired air of a diseased animal.

The following cases will answer to illustrate the point in question:

CASE I.—At the time (1848) that the views of veterinary authors were most crude with regard to the nature of bovine tuberculosis, I had occasion to treat the disease upon a farm where it had prevailed for a long time, and caused much loss to the owner.

Upon the farm were always kept fourteen milch-cows and cattle, a bull, and four calves. Of these, four head were sold each year, and replaced by the same number of calves. The animals sold were not always of the same age each year; in one year the two and three year olds would be sold, in another older cows, and the third some of each, according to the fullness of the owner's purse, so that there were cattle on the farm two, six, and twelve years old. Of these older animals, I found on my first examination two afflicted with a rough, dry cough, and with accelerated respiration. As I was aware of the constancy with which the disease had prevailed among the owner's cattle, it was my advice to get rid of these two as early as possible. This advice was followed. The cattle were fattened, and upon being slaughtered my diagnosis was confirmed.

In the mean time every attention was given to the feeding and general care of the cattle upon the place.

In 1851 I again found two of the cattle that coughed, and gradually became somewhat emaciated. The attempt to fatten them was partially successful in one, but failed in the other. Both were killed, and tuberculosis found in them. Four calves were placed in the spring of 1852 with the cattle in the old stable, and four others placed where they were taken from. All seemed to be healthy to the spring of 1854, when one of the calves, which had become three years old and had been placed in the old stable, began to cough. The cough was at first very slight, but commenced to increase after the heifer had calved. In the following summer it again diminished, to augment very considerably in the fall. This animal was put out to graze in the spring of 1855, and to my surprise became quite fat; but upon being slaughtered the animal was found to be highly tuberculous.

Of the old cattle there still remained a single cow, which we will call "A," that had always stood next to the above-mentioned animal. All the others had been sold and killed, their places having been filled by new ones. This cow had coughed for a long time; but, not suffering in condition, she had been kept, as she was a great favorite with the farmer's wife, especially as I had not then the slightest suspicion of infection by means of the atmosphere. Every animal which during this period had stood beside this cow had begun to cough after a shorter or longer period, and, as the positions of the animals were sometimes changed, it happened that in course of time nearly all of them began to have the same suspicious cough.

The continued buying, rearing, and selling of cattle went on for nine years before I had opportunity to examine the cow "A," which was then sold to a butcher. The examination of the body and its contents resulted in finding it highly tuberculous. The result of all my experience awakened in me the suspicion of the transmission of the disease from animal to animal, an opinion which was then considered ridiculous. I communicated my opinion to the owner, and advised his selling off all his cattle and replacing them with new and healthy ones from parents and places where the disease was not known to exist. My advice was appreciated by the owner calling in a quack to take my place.

Case II.—On another farm were kept from twenty-four to twenty-six head of cattle. In 1864 the owner bought a calf to bring up, the mother of which died a few years later from tuberculosis.

This calf developed very poorly for the first two years of its life; its neck and head were small and long, and its bones very small, so that the whole *habitus* of the animal was cachectic. This animal was killed in the fall of 1869. In the course of the winter of 1869–'70 many of the cattle began to cough, and among them two, "A" and "B," so severely that my services were requested.

I found all the animals in an apparently healthy condition; only the two, A and B, were noticed to cough. By auscultation, I found in A a peculiarly marked bronchial respiration in portions of the left lung. At this time I knew nothing of the breeding, or the phenomena seen in the above-mentioned calf, which had been slaughtered. During this winter and the succeeding summer the two cattle, A and B, besides others, continued to cough. All the animals on the farm coughed during the winter of 1870–'71, except the yearlings and some calves which were kept in another stable. In the spring of 1871 the two cows, A and B, began to emaciate so much that it was considered advisable to kill them. The autopsy revealed the general characteristics of tubercular pneumonia, and tuberculosis of other organs. Basing my opinions upon the previously mentioned experience, I made no hesitation in pronouncing all the cattle in this stable that coughed as afflicted with tuberculosis, and advised the owner to gradually get rid of them all. On account of economical reasons, this was easier said than done, and the owner has never since been free from this disease among his cattle.

During the period from 1864–'71, tuberculosis has been always present among the cattle of this owner, who has lost nineteen head from the disease in that time.

The author gives four other illustrations of similar extension of tuberculosis among cattle upon other farms, and closes his remarks with the following interesting case:

The milk from one of these cows had been used for some time in a *cooked* condition, but the condition of the cow finally became so bad it was decided to give the milk to the hogs, but *uncooked*.

From May of the same year, the farmer's wife noticed that the young pigs (four or five months old) fed upon this milk did not appear to thrive well, and as, in the course of a few weeks three died, I was requested to make an examination of the last one. I found the same much emaciated. I found a tuberculous peritonitis with effusion in the cavity of that organ. The lungs and bronchial glands were normal; the mesenteric glands enlarged—on section of the same, found them filled with a tuberculous mass; tubercles in the liver. In the course of a few weeks the two remaining pigs of the litter also died. I found tuberculosis in one of them, and the owner told me that the other, and another of an older litter which was with them, and fed on the same milk, were also found tuberculous on being examined.

Unfortunately, in this country, there are not at present any statistics with reference to the extension which this disease has attained among our cattle, and the same is almost true with reference to other lands. The following meager statistics may not, however, be without interest to the reader:

Statistics with reference to Tuberculosis among Bavarian Cattle for the Year 1877.

Tuberculous.

Males................ 869. Females.................... 4,107.

1·62 to the 1,000.

64 under one year, or	1·31	per cent.
528 from one to three years, or	10·81	"
1,846 from three to six years, or	37·80	"
2,445 over six years, or	50·07	"

Goring, "Zeitschrift für Thierheilkunde," 4, 286.

From January 1 to December 31, 1874, were killed at Augsburg, Bavaria, 11,331 cattle (calves excluded); of these 134 were *tuberculous*, 1·18 per cent; 42 males (13 bulls and 29 steers); 92 females. Of the whole number slaughtered, about one third were males and two thirds females.

For the year 1876 were killed 13,241 cattle and 25,909 calves. Of these, 250 were found tuberculous; viz., 243 cattle over one year old, one calf three weeks old.

The percentage for 1876 was 1·84; for 1875, 1·40; for 1874, 1·18; for 1873, 1·02; for 1872, 1·27. For 1876, 75 males and 168 females. Of the males, 39 were castrated and 36 were not.

Statistics of Diseases found among Animals slaughtered at Munich in 1874.

Whole number slaughtered at the public shambles:

Cattle	Oxen	231
Cattle	Cows and steers	5,290
	Calves	4,201
	Sheep	1,563
	Swine	303

Of the frequent diseases were observed:

Pulmonary tuberculosis in one goat and	235	cattle.
Perlsucht, or tuberculosis of the serosæ	197	"
Tuberculosis of the liver	29	"
Tuberculosis of the udder	1	"
Tuberculosis of the bones	2	"
Abscess in the lungs	45	"
Pleuro-pneumonia	20	"
Echinococcus of the lungs	44	"
Echinococcus of the liver	10	"
Induration of the liver	264	"
Distoma hepaticum	219	"
Icterus	20	calves.
Nephritis, suppurative	12	cattle.
Abscess in udder and mastitis	8	"
Scabies	242	sheep.
Osteomalacia	9	cattle.
Measles	4	swine.
Slunk veal	57	calves.
Nauseous appearance of flesh in one swine and	25	"

"Department veterinarian Pauli reports* that 12,585 kilogrammes of flesh were officially destroyed at the investigation stations in Berlin from 1877 to 1878. Further, 1,646 cattle, 2,027 swine, 235 calves, and 714 sheep, were killed in the police slaughter-house to determine their hygienic condition. Of these, 213 cattle, 643 swine, 196 calves, and 382 sheep were found unfit for food. Of the 213 cattle, 49 suffered from *general* '*tuberculosis* and initial emaciation,' 46 'from general *tuberculosis* and cachexia,' and 22 'from *tuberculosis*, general hydrops, and cachexia,' and 85 swine were found measly. In 998 cattle, 1,466 swine, 8 calves, and 107 sheep were found single diseased organs, which forbade using the flesh for human food."

There is no subject more urgently requiring the attention of boards of health and the people than this.

However important trichiniasis may be, this far exceeds it. The few experiments which have been made should be repeated by hundreds—yes, thousands, if necessary—by carefully selected men, and at the expense of the State, until this question is forever settled *pro* or *con*.

While this is being done, competent veterinarians (not empirics) should be engaged by the respective State boards of health to gather reliable statistics with reference to the extension of *tuberculosis* among the cattle of each State.

It would be well that the National Board of Health instigate the work.

* "Mittheil. aus d. Thierärzt. Praxis," 1877–'78, p. 99.

As the statistical results of the experiments which have been made unquestionably go to prove *that such milk does contain elements of a specifically infectious character, there is no question that laws should be made, and executed also, so as to prevent the sale of such milk for human consumption, either for itself or mixed with other milk, in no matter how small quantities.*

No such milk should be sold; but such cows should be strictly isolated and fattened, or condemned.

This question of the specific infection of milk from tuberculous cows is no trifling matter; on the contrary, *it is one of life and death.* How many thousand babies are yearly brought up on the bottle with cow's milk!

All the fond parents ask is, *that the milk is from one cow.* This guaranteed, they appear to feel perfectly satisfied. No one seems yet to have thought that a trustworthy and expert *guarantee* of the hygienic condition of the cow giving the milk was necessary. We make great demands, and get terribly excited about the purity of our water-supply. We spend millions of dollars to keep the fountains pure, and to prevent all foreign admixtures on its passage to us. Is it not as much our duty to examine into the purity of the fountains from which comes our milk-supply?

We can not but repeat our assertion that every State board of health should be liberally supplied with funds to be used exclusively for experimental purposes, and in every State there should be a station for such purposes.

I do not know that it has ever yet been proved by direct experiment *how much dilution it is possible to give to milk by means of unduly watery food given to the cow*, or how much the milk can be concentrated, in one and the same cow, by systematically lessening the quantity of fluid given consistent with the health of the animal.

The first form of feeding might be well called dilution of milk within the law, while when the water is added after milking we have dilution under penalty of, or without, the law.

Both forms of dilution are equally a swindle upon the consumer.

An economy which does not recognize the absolute necessity of such experiments as the above is of the "penny-wise but pound-foolish variety," and never in the *true* interests of the public.

INFECTION.

ANTHRAX (*Carbuncle*).

ANTHRAX is *the* disease of all the diseases strictly due to germ-life which is best understood by scientists. Before considering it, however, we desire to introduce some general remarks, and then to consider the subject of germ-infection, though in a very general manner.

The word *infectio* means to pollute.

The subject of infection is one of the most theoretic connected with the study of medicine.

To theorize does not mean to dream of things possible, as the major part of the people and too many professionals seem to think. To be called a theorist, if one is in reality such, is by no means a disgrace; on the contrary, it is the highest honor that can be given. It means, truly, that one is a man capable of reasoning, both by induction and deduction. To be called *a practical man* means that you know nothing but routine practice, or what one has inherited from teachers and fathers, and that we are incapable of reasoning. Theory is the connecting link, the hypothetical bridge of explanation between two known facts.

These facts are, first, that something takes place; second, the phenomena by which you recognize *that* something has taken place. The empiric is satisfied with this knowledge. It is enough for him that a horse has colic, and that certain symptoms indicate it, and that in general a dose of a certain medicine will cure it. This is being practical.

To theorize means to be able to think, and to think logically and well—to be able to trace the connection between cause and effect. If there is any disgrace in this, then those who are called theorists are generally in most honorable company.

The trouble with our profession is and has been that it has *never* yet produced a great thinker. Not one of the men whose names you have been taught to revere as great among veterinarians have ever been great thinkers. Even human medicine has been notoriously wanting in this regard.

Good thinkers are scarce at best. The Bacons, Goethes, Descartes, Humes, and Franklins of this world are always phenomenal. The great practitioners have been numerous; the great thinkers in medicine can be counted upon the fingers of one hand. They are the men who have shaped the course of medicine for years after their death, and frequently during their lives.

Has veterinary medicine ever produced a Bichat or a Virchow? When it does, it will stand scientifically on a level with human medicine, and not till then; for then it will for a time give the direction to all medical research and thought. Good theorists are ever practical in the best sense of the word; for *practical* does not always mean a knowledge of therapeutics alone, as many teach. An erroneous theory, ably defended, is of more benefit to the world than a true one which lacks *earnest* defenders or combaters. It stirs men up, and leads to the discovery of the truth.

Darwinism has been the greatest blessing to natural science that the nineteenth century has produced, even though all its premises should finally be proved incorrect. You have only to think of the immense increase of our knowledge of the lower forms of life, of the physiological functions of both lower and higher animals, to realize this.

Some of our very best veterinarians are getting by far too conceited, and this conceit is unfortunately becoming inoculated into the rising generation.

There is no such thing in existence as veterinary science.

We speak of veterinary pathologists, when in reality we have never had a single one. Pathologists and pathological anatomists are entirely different things, though occasionally united in one person.

Bichat and Virchow were pathologists, because they were good thinkers. Pathology is the philosophy of disease. They were or are pathological anatomists, because they could correctly read, that is, describe the results of disease. From these *results* they theorized; that is, from facts they thought; that is, they tried to tell us how the results took place, for no man has yet seen the processes of disease.

What we see upon the dissection-table, or under the microscope, is not the processes of disease, but the results.

If we are practical in the world's sense, these results will be of no value to us; if we are theorists, they may be very instructive, and we can become truly practical.

I have said that Virchow and Bichat were pathologists, and that veterinary medicine had never produced a pathologist.

This is a fact, contradict it who may. But if we have not produced pathologists, we have pathological anatomists, some say.

Again I say, all wrong. A pathological anatomist is a man who correctly describes the results of disease, of which Rokitansky is a striking example.

Have we produced such a man? Do our text-books tell us much of the results of disease in our animals? Some may quote to me the names of Gerlach, Roell, Williams, Leisering, Bouley, Chauveau, Toussaint, and others, not one of whom deserves to be named with a Rokitansky, a Virchow, or a Bichat.

They have done some good experimental work, in a very limited field, and, like one solitary star shining out from a dark and clouded heaven, loom up all too conspicuously—thankful, as we are, that they have done something to make veterinary medicine worthy of notice. But where is our pathological anatomy? What is Roell, the best of German works on special pathology? Has it any original pathological anatomy? It is Rokitansky from beginning to end; that is, human results transferred, without criticism, to animal conditions. Brückmüller's "Pathological Zoötomy," the only work on pathological anatomy of our animals, is another abortion, born too early to have anything in it but adapted Rokitanskyism.

What do we know about the microscopic pathological anatomy of the brain, the kidneys, or any single organ of our animals? The macroscopical conditions are fairly described; the microscopical have been scarcely thought of, but borrowed from human medicine.

Have we a single contagious disease, the pathological conditions of which have been carefully studied and described by veterinarians? No!

Do we know the pathological condition of the lungs, in direct progress from beginning to end, in pleuro-pneumonia?

Are our methods of investigation, urine analysis, microscopic technic and examination, any of them, the result of veterinary genius? No—all, all borrowed!

Then why speak of veterinary science? These things are not written to discourage, but rather to stimulate, for I, for one, believe the day will come when veterinary medicine will have its pathologists who shall give the key-note to medical thought, and veterinary pathological anatomists equal to any that human medicine has had, or will ever produce.

In that day we shall not grope in darkness, but shall see things as they really are. We must learn to observe well, and, above all, to think well, and next to that to be able to express ourselves well. Medicine has its language, and the exact and logical use of language is the best characteristic of an educated man.

I will illustrate my meaning by a few of the incongruities of medical literature. We frequently read of collapsed conditions of the lungs, by which is meant the dark-blue, airless spots which lie somewhat beneath the general level of the pleura. This is reality atelectasis pulmonum, that is, airless. The structural changes of the lung by which this condition and true collapse are produced are absolutely different. In atelectasis we have a shutting off of the supply of air, a gradual absorption of that which was present, and a consequent retraction of the pulmonary tissue, by which the blood-vessels come nearer together; a non-oxidation of the blood in the same, hence the darker color; *but the lung-tissue retracts, it retains its elasticity. In collapsus pulmonum the lung-tissue has lost its elasticity*, an entirely different condition. Such a lung has lost all the springy characteristics of normal lung-tissue; it is dead, doughy to the touch, which is *never* the case in atelectasis. Again, clinicians speak of hepatization, instead of solidification or infiltration of the lung. Hepatization means, indeed, solidified (liver-like), *but only to the touch.* The observation and language of the dissection-table have been transferred to the bedside, where they do not belong. Each place has its appropriate language.

We speak of apoplexia cerebri, as if there were no other form of apoplexy, whereas the word means *to strike down*, to cease acting suddenly; hence we may also have apoplexia cordis, pulmonum, laryngia, medulla oblongata, all organs the continual action of which, or of parts of them, are absolutely necessary to the continuance of life. We here again mix up cause and effect. Apoplexy is the cessation of function, not the cause. The hæmorrhages in the brain are that and nothing more; but because in some cases apoplexy accompanies them, they are not always apoplectic centers. The part complicated, or the amount extravasated, causes the clinical expression apoplexy.

While these things have, as it were, become sanctified by usage, they are not in accordance with the logical use of language.

Concussion of the brain, by which life ceases, may be supposed to take place without hæmorrhage, yet is essentially apoplexia cerebri, though we never hear it spoken of as such.

With reference to some of the infectious, or, better, contagious diseases, we find medical writers falling into the same error when they speak of the elements by which the disease is transmitted to human beings as "animal poisons." There are animal poisons, such as come from reptiles; but the infectious elements of the contagious diseases are not, logically speaking, poisons.

A poison is something which in well-defined quantities causes specific effects. Unless this quantity of a given poison is introduced into the system, this effect does not follow.

In contagious diseases the quantity necessary to infection can not be measured. The elements of infection in contagious disease multiply within the organisms into which they are introduced. Poisons do not thus multiply of themselves.

The quantity of poison remains the same, unless a second introduction takes place.

Infectious or contagious diseases have their period of incubation—that is, a period elapses before the infected organism shows to us that anything has taken place. Even in inoculation the action is not immediately visible. In some diseases, as rabies, this period may extend over weeks or months, while in others only a few days elapse.

By poisons the action is immediate, provided the quantity introduced is sufficient.

Infectious diseases have their cycles, or stages. They have the above period of incubation, their period of full development, and that of reconvalescence, their "stadium accrementi and decrementi," while poisons have no such course.

The diseases which are known as contagious, or infectious, do not by any means belong to a single class or group.

We have the group of acute exanthemata, such as the variolæ, measles, scarlatina, certain forms of mange, the foot-and-mouth disease, the *maladie du coit*, and the pustulous eruption upon the genitals of our domestic animals. These diseases are frequently accompanied by catarrhal conditions of the respiratory or digestive tracts, with cerebral, hepatic, or splenic disturbances; but these latter do not constitute the essentials of the disease. They are also generally accompanied by fever, which of itself is nothing specific, fever being a general phenomenon accompanying all serious constitutional disturbances.

There is no such thing as specific fevers. Of specific causes there are many.

We have also a group of infectious diseases known as the acute intestinal, that tract being the chief seat of the same, though, as with the above, other parts or organs do not escape complication. Such are abdominal typhus, cholera, dysentery, and rinderpest.

Then we have those of the respiratory tract, the influenzas—a collective name—pharyngitis et laryngitis diphtheritica, tussis convulsiva, pleuro-pneumonia, and the malarial influenza, or pneumo-pleuro-enteritis of the horse. Also the group of septic diseases, which embraces those classed under the general names of septicæmia or pyæmia, erysipelas, gangrena septica, phlegmonia, puerperal fever, etc.

Another group embraces the so-called essential or malarial fevers, such as febris recurrens, flava, and the Texas cattle-fever; and, finally, the zoönoses, or contagio-infectious animal diseases, rabies, glanders, anthrax, as well as those peculiar to one species or another, as syphilis of man.

After these general remarks we will now consider what are at present looked upon as the elements of infection, in one form or another, of all these different groups—viz.:

The Bacteria.

What are bacteria?

"Cells deprived of chlorophyl, of globular, oblong, or cylindrical form, sometimes sinuous and twisted, reproducing themselves exclusively by transverse division, scissiparity, also by spores, bacillus subtilis, living isolated or in groups, and having affinities to the algæ."

Owing to their microscopic minuteness, it is not to be wondered at that most varying views have been held as to their real nature and place among living things.

That they constitute veritably a *contagium vivum*, that is, are living things, there is at present no doubt, various as have been the opinions as to what the true meaning of such a term should be.

A living contagium is such by which the infectious elements have the principal characteristics of life; that is, they live and die, and are capable of reproducing themselves: whether the reproduction takes places within or without the animal organism is non-essential to our definition.

Even very ancient writers seem to have arrived at some vague idea of the existence of a *contagium vivum*. We find the same in the writings of the Roman fathers of agricultural and veterinary literature of the fourth century, A. D. Varo and Columella, who asserted that many malarial fevers were caused by the penetration of lower organisms into the body. Even before the discovery of the microscope, animal organisms were supposed to have an etiological connection with the pest.

Leeuwenhoek, the father of microscopy, is said to have been the first observer who described anything like true bacteria. This occurred in 1675, while examining some water, in which he describes minute globules as crossing the objective field. The following year he recognized similar objects in fæces, and the tartar from the teeth, and gives such descriptions that we are warranted in assuming that they were bacteria, vibrios, and leptothrix.

An author of the seventeenth century attributed the epizoötics which prevailed at that time to the action of some sort of grass-hopper or locust, and recommended that the inhabitants make large fires to drive away or kill them, in order to prevent the diseases.

Later, we find various absurd ideas being supported, and cholera, variola, syphilitic and other animals described by authors as being the specific cause of such diseases.

Such absurdities led to the ridicule of the idea of living infectious elements, which found its counterpart in the idea of infectious gases, a theory which has been of late abandoned, owing to the great advances in microscopy and the technicalities of scientific research during the last ten years.

The Classification of Bacteria.

As early as 1773 O. F. Müller made an attempt to classify these objects; others followed, among them the noted German naturalist Ehrenberg in 1838, and the Frenchmen Dujardin (1841) and Davaine.

Ehrenberg speaks of—

1. Bacteria, as filaments linear and inflexible, and gives three species.
2. Vibrios: filaments linear, flexible; nine species.
3. Spirillum: filaments spiral, inflexible; three species.
4. Spirochæte: filaments spiral, flexible; one species.

Dujardin (1841) classed them as—

1. Bacterium: filaments rigid, with vacillating movement.
2. Vibrio: filaments flexible, with undulatory movement.
3. Spirillum; filaments spiral, with rotary movement.

Up to this time the bacteria had been looked upon as animals, and placed at the foot of that kingdom. Later, the idea that they belonged to the vegetable kingdom has been gradually gaining ground, and is at present almost universally accepted; although the renowned German naturalist Haeckel places them in his intermediate class or kingdom of protista. Davaine (1859) was the first to clearly demonstrate the vegetable nature of the vibrios, and their near relation to the algæ.

Davaine's classification was as follows: Filaments straight or bent, but not spiral, moving spontaneously. When rigid, bacterium; when flexible, vibrio; when motionless, bacteridium; when the filaments were spiral, spirillum.

From this time on we find the study of these objects assuming a new and more exact character, thanks to the work of Pasteur, Davaine, Haller, Cohn, Koch, and others.

The absence of chlorophyl distinguishes them from the algæ, and places them among the fungi; a view which is supported by nearly all the best botanists of our day. The generally accepted classification is at present that of Cohn, and is—

1. Spherobacteria, or globular bacteria.
2. Micro or rod bacteria.
3. Desmo or filamentous bacteria.
4. Spiro or spiral bacteria.

In 1874 Billroth, the noted surgeon and author on surgical pathology, published a large work upon disease-germs—viz., upon coccobacteria septica—and arrived at very different conclusions from those of Cohn, which have not, however, gained any general acceptance. Billroth claims that there is but one single original species of bacteria, and that all others are derived from it, viz., coccobacteria septica. This vegetable organism may present itself in two forms: the globular *coccus*, and that of rods, *bacteria*. These two forms may reproduce by elongation and transverse division, or may pass from one to the other.

According to the variation in size, Billroth speaks of micrococcus, microbacteria; mesococcus, mesobacteria; megacoccus, megabacteria. And, according to their relations to one another, as monococcus, monobacteria; diplococcus (in pairs), diplobacteria; streptococcus (in chains), streptobacteria; gliococcus, gliobacteria; petalococcus (foot or base), petalobacteria.

We have said that the most generally accepted classification was that of Cohn, but, before considering it more particularly, we feel obliged to notice that of another noted German author, which is based upon the action of these germs.

Nägeli speaks—

1. Of mucorini, or mold-fungi.
2. Saccharomycetes, or budding fungi, which produce the fermentation of wine, beer, yeast, etc.
3. Schizomycetes, or fission-fungi, which produce putrefactive processes. This group embraces the micrococci and bacteria.

I. Spherobacteria.—Spherical bacteria are defined by their name. They are round or oval bodies of very small size. They are sometimes found isolated, often appearing in pairs—diplococcus; or again we meet with them in the form of chains, or articulations—streptococcus; or united together by a sort of homogeneous material—zoögleaform. When in this condition they are young and in process of active proliferation. Sometimes they form a coating upon the surface of liquids. When we speak of a mycoderma, they have no independent movements, but simply display the well-known molecular trepidation.

The function of spherical bacteria has been determined to be zymotic; that is, ferment-producing. According to Cohn, they do not take part in the production of putrefying processes.

While the above includes a distinct form of germ-life, there is no question that the spores of some other forms of germ-life, viz., bacillus, give no distinguishing means by which to separate them from spherobacteria, except the results of experimental cultivation; as the Bible says of men, "By their fruits shall ye know them."

There is but one genus of the spherobacteria, viz., "micrococcus." They are described as cells, colorless or scarcely colored, very small, globular or oval, forming by transverse division, filaments of two or several articulations in the form of a chaplet, or united in numerous cellular families, or in glutinous masses, all motionless. This genus is divided into three groups:

Micrococcus chromogenes.
Micrococcus zymogenes.
Micrococcus pathogenes.

The first groups are again distinguished as to the solubility or insolubility of the coloring-matter, and are found upon vegetables, milk, etc.

The second group contains but one variety of special interest to us, viz., *M. ureæ*, found in urine, where it transforms the urea into carbonate of ammonia (Pasteur).

The pathogenetic micrococci are of so much more importance that we must give them particular attention.

They are spherical bacteria, which are found in affections of a contagio-infectious nature, such as *M. vaccinæ*, being very small, appearing isolated or in pairs in recent vaccine virus, and in the pus of variola-pustules. They are looked upon as the active principle of vaccine virus.

M. diphtheriticus.—Granular ovoid cells, isolated, or more frequently united in pairs, or in a chaplet of four to six cells, sometimes multiplying in colonies, and extending themselves in all the complicated tissues, decomposing and destroying them.

M. septicus.—Little round, motionless cells, crowded in masses or united in chaplets; found in the secretions of wounds in cases of septicæmia, as zoöglæa in callous ulcers, as isolated cells, united *in pairs*, or chaplets, in the serum of epidemic puerperal fever, and in all tissues, vessels, etc., in pyæmia and septicæmia.

Many others have been found and given specific names, especially by Hallier, Zurn, etc., as in scarlatina, epidemic diarrhœa, typhus, glanders, rinderpest, syphilis, gonorrhœa.

II. The Second Group of Cohn, the Microbacteria.—We have here the single genus bacterium. Cells cylindrical or elliptical, free, or united in pairs during their division, rarely in fours, never in chains, sometimes in zoöglæa, having spontaneous movement, oscillatory and very active, especially in media rich in alimentary material and in the presence of oxygen.

As with the spherobacteria, we might divide the rod-bacteria into three groups: first, those of putrefaction, *B. termo, lineola;* second, those of lactic acetic fermentation; third, the pigment-bacteria of colored milk and pus.

B. termo is the most common of all varieties. They are cylindrical cells, slightly swollen in the middle, isolated, sometimes united in pairs, two to five times as long as wide. Movements oscillatory. They can easily be produced in all infusions of animal and vegetable substances. This bacterium is said to have cilia or hair-like projections from each end of the rod.

It is the veritable agent and first cause of putrefaction, and hence is to be found in all cadavers where this process has commenced.

B. lineola is larger and found in various animal and vegetable infusions, but is not definitely known to cause a specific fermentation.

The other forms of lactic and acetic fermentation are not of especial pathogenetic interest.

III. Desmobacteria.—This group of Cohn's is of especial interest, as it contains the specific germ of anthrax, that germ upon which the germ-infection theory of disease largely depends for support.

They are filiform bacteria, composed of elongated articulations, isolated, or in chains more or less extended, and resulting from transverse division. (In this form they correspond to leptothrix, but differ from torula in that the filaments are not constricted at the point of articulation.) They may be motionless or not, dependent upon the presence or absence of oxygen, the reaction of the medium which contains them, and other unknown conditions. Some forms *never* exhibit movement.

We have here but one germ to consider—bacillus.

The bacilli are characterized as slender filaments, straight, short, or of moderate length, rigid or flexible, and as being with and without movement. One species is a pigment bacteria.

Bacillus subtilis.—Very slender elongated filaments formed of a single cell, or of two, three, or more segments. Thickness unmeasurable; well-defined flexible movement of an active or passive character. Reproduction is by fission and by globular or oval spores, which develop in the interior of the articulations. They are to be found in stagnant waters.

This bacillus plays an important part in butyric fermentation. It exists in rennet, and can support a temperature of 105° C. and live in a medium deprived of pure oxygen, in which case it takes a peculiar form and contains persistent spores which when set free give rise to other rods.

Bacillus anthracis is a species very similar to the preceding, but generally longer, and always motionless; length four, twelve, and even fifty micrometers; thickness scarcely measurable.

Bacillus anthracis is developed in charbon—carbuncle—of cattle, man, sheep, horse, rabbit, rat, etc.; never in dogs, the cat, birds, and cold-blooded animals. It is found, above all, in the capillary vessels. When cultivated in suitable media, such as the aqueous humor of the eye of the ox, and the different cultivation fluids, this bacillus develops spores in the interior of its segments which may germinate and develop rods.

The other bacilli of this group are without any special interest.

The only form of special interest is the "spirochæton hermeieri," found in the blood of persons suffering from recurrent fever (chills and fever), but only during the access, never during the intermissions of the disease.

Distinction of Bacteria from Inorganic Substances.

No one has ever questioned the living nature of bacteria, except with reference to the most invisible varieties. These smaller forms may be often confounded with various matters, such as organic particles, molecular granules, fat-globules, or fatty *detritus*. To distinguish them from micrococci is almost impossible, unless the greatest circumspection is taken by the observer.

The *detritus*, or the amorphous powder, or precipitated molecules, of inorganic substances, though they equally well exhibit the noted Brownian movement, are to be distinguished from micrococci by such optical signs as their angular or irregular form, their lesser refraction, and their action toward certain chemical agents.

The case is quite different if the molecules are of an organic nature. They enjoy, in common with micrococci, a round form, movement, and refraction. However, their form is wanting in the regularity proper to germs; they vary in color, and their refractive power is always less. Warming the slides, the action of ether and other known reagents will enable one to distinguish them.

The most difficult of all objects to distinguish from micrococci are fat-globules, or so-called fatty *detritus*. The difference in refraction is very small, and in mucilaginous solutions the action of reagents is not always to be depended upon. Cultivation is the only secure course to employ in cases of grave doubt.

Only such globules as have the power of multiplication are vital bodies: when this does not take place, we may assure ourselves that we are having to do with some form of pseudobacteria.

Nägeli says there are but three diagnostic signs by which we are enabled to recognize, to any degree of certainty, that molecules under our observation are organisms—spontaneous movement, proliferation, and equality in dimensions, united with regularity of form.

The most certain characteristic is movement in a straight or curved line—a phenomenon never to be seen in inorganic molecules.

Multiplication is a character of less importance, because of the liability to adhesion of inorganic or other molecules. Granules, of varying size and of a more or less irregular form, ought not to be considered as belonging to the segmented fungi.

As to chemical reagents, concentrated acetic acid, which causes all animal tissues to clarify, is without influence on bacteria. Many coloring-stuffs used in microscopic technics are of assistance in diagnosing bacteria; among the best of these are hamatoxylin, fuchsine, and Bismarck brown.

The Development of Bacteria.

Of all living organisms known to natural science the bacteria are the most widely dispersed: they may, in fact, be said to be everywhere—in the air, water, upon and in solid animal and vegetable bodies.

Origin.—The origin of all inferior organisms has ever been a question open to most variable and vital discussion; but, in general, three ways have been assumed for this most important function:

1. By *heterogenesis;* that is, by direct production from mineral or organic substances (spontaneous generation).

2. On the rule that "like begets like" it has been asserted that all bacteria must come from others of the same kind, by one of the recognized forms of generation: fission, spores, etc.

3. Others assume that, while they derive their origin from

organisms already in existence, they represent nothing more than different stages or forms of development of known species. This latter hypothesis is known as polymorphism.

THE DISSEMINATION OF BACTERIA IN DIFFERENT MEDIA—AIR AND WATER.

The experiments of Pasteur, Tyndall, and others, have clearly demonstrated the presence of vegetable germs in the air which has been allowed to pass through apertures into vessels prepared for the purpose. These germs generally have the micrococcus or microbe form, and are present in lesser numbers in winter than in summer and fall, which fact finds its explanation in the greater degree of vegetable decomposition and telluric evaporation which takes place during the warm months in comparison with the cold.

The experiments of Cohn and others have demonstrated that the atmosphere contains very few adult bacteria ; in fact, they are rarely found therein in a complete state, but rather as bright, refracting points, very difficult if not impossible to distinguish from one another. These points probably represent the latent or permanent spore-condition of bacterium life, capable of generating into true bacteria under favorable conditions. These spores may form the point from which epidemics take their origin, and in this condition are capable of wide dispersion.

NUTRITION AND RESPIRATION OF BACTERIA.

As bacteria have some of the essential characteristics of organized beings—a cell-membrane and protoplasmic contents—they must naturally receive nourishment and respire in the same way as all colorless vegetables and inferior animals which have no special apparatus for such purposes ; that is, by endosmotic absorption.

It matters not in what medium they may be met with, they require—in order to live—water, nitrogen, carbon, and oxygen, as well as certain salts from the mineral world, which enter in very minute quantities into their organism.

Water is indispensable to the activity and development of bacteria. Desiccation, drying out, completely arrests the movement of those that are mobile, and the functional activity of all bacteria. Desiccation does not, however, kill them, unless it is too prolonged, as is proved by the activity retained by the various kinds of virus used for inoculation. In the condition of permanent spores they retain their vitality a long while. It is a surprising fact that the great chemical difference existing between salt and fresh water appears to exert little or no influence upon the development of bacteria.

NITROGEN.—The experiments of Pasteur have demonstrated that an albuminoid nitrogenous substance is not necessary to the life of bacteria, but that other nitrogenous substances, as ammonia, will answer the same purposes.

Pasteur's cultivating solution is as follows:

Distilled water	100 parts.
Sugar-candy	10 "
Tartrate of ammonia	1 "
Ashes of one gramme of yeast	0·075.

Cohn's fluid is designed to counteract the development of mold due to the cane-sugar in the above solution, and is as follows:

Distilled water	100 parts.
Tartrate of ammonia	1 "
Ashes of yeast	1 "

Mayer gives us another fluid which does away with the ashes of yeast, viz.:

Phosphate of potash	0·1 gramme.
Sulphate of magnesia	0·1 "
Tribasic phosphate of lime	0·1 "
Distilled water	20 c. c.

CARBON.—Aside from other sources, bacteria can obtain this important element to their life from organic acids.

OXYGEN.—Numerous controversies have taken place among *savants* as to the *rôle* this element plays in bacterial life.

It seems, *a priori*, that, like other living things, oxygen must be necessary to germ-life. Pasteur has demonstrated that it is not so, however, with all forms of bacteria. In putrefying processes he has demonstrated that, after certain species have developed *B. termo*, which depend upon the presence of oxygen, and come to the surface, forming a coating upon it, the fluid beneath is free from this gas, and yet other forms of bacteria come to development in it.

The first of these organisms—that is, those dependent on oxygen for life—he has styled aërobic fungi, and the others anaërobic. Other observers do not agree with this theory. Hoffmann, a very able German *savant*, says: "These little beings can not live without air—that is, without oxygen. If this gas is wanting, they cease to move and to proliferate. If a drop of liquid full of bacteria is placed upon a glass slide and covered, the active bacteria will all gradually approach the margin of the cover, and at the end of several days will be found alive, while those situated toward the center will be dead."

Toussaint, the ablest veterinary student of this subject, has recently published the following results with reference to *B. anthracis:*

"The bacteria which occupy the central portion of Ranvier's moist chamber, and which by reason of their situation receive very little oxygen from the groove, are soon arrested in their development, while those which occupy the borders are long and collect in immense numbers. Those in the center remain small, formed of two, four, or five articulations, which are easily separated. They soon cease to grow, and are not transformed into spores."

Cohn, an unquestionable authority, also says that "the complete development of bacillus, and, above all, the generation of spores, only take place under the free access of air."

Reproduction of Bacteria.

We have already mentioned that bacteria reproduce either by scissiparity—fission—or by the endogenous production of spores, which are again capable of developing into bacteria. We have also frequently mentioned that these spores are so wanting in specific characteristics that it is impossible to assert whether each variety of bacteria has its own specific spore or germinal form, although this theory is mostly supported; while able authors also hold to a metagenetic theory—that is, that a metamorphosis between the different forms of fungi is possible, the same being due to the influence of the different media in which they may be cultivated or live.

When proliferation takes place by fission, or transverse division of the cell, we see the cell gradually yet rapidly increases in length, the protoplasma in the middle becoming clearer, and a partition forms in the middle of the cell, separating the protoplasma into two distinct portions. The partition is at first very delicate, but soon thickens, and the cell divides in two.

This phenomenon takes place more or less rapidly, dependent upon the richness in nutritive material of the media in which it is, on the temperature, moisture, etc.

In some cases a constriction takes place in the middle of the cell, the two ends having a figure-8 or bulb-like form.

Reproduction by Spores.

Until recently multiplication by fission was the only form of bacterial reproduction admitted by naturalists.

The formation of spores has been observed in bacillus subtilis (Cohn), bacillus anthracis (Koch), and in bacillus amylobacter by another observer.

In cultivation experiments made with hay-infusion we may see, at a certain moment, in the homogeneous filaments of the bacilli, very refractive corpuscles making their appearance. Each of these corpuscles becomes a spore, oblong, or in the form of a short filament, highly refractive, and having well-defined outlines. We find the spores arranged in a simple series in the filaments. So soon as the formation of spores has terminated, the filaments can no longer be distinguished, and one would say that the spores were completely free in the mucus; but their linear arrangement shows that they are produced in the interior of the filaments. These dissolve slowly, and the spores, being reduced to a fine powder, settle to the bottom of the liquid, where they may be found in great quantity.

The germination of spores does not apparently follow in the same medium; but, if we remove them to a new cultivating fluid, we may observe the spore to swell up and elongate, resembling a bacterium with a head. Soon the head, the most refractive portion of the object, disappears, and the tube stretches into a short rod-bacillus, commences to display motion, and becomes jointed by transverse division.

The Action of Bacteria with Reference to Contagious and Virulent Diseases.

One of the peculiarities of all life is the struggle for existence. Both animal and vegetable life is encompassed by this fact. Individuals of the same kind and those of a different kind all live at the expense of one another. Many perish in the conflict.

Life is a constant struggle with death. Even the individual cells of which the organs of our body are composed undergo this constant struggle; the stronger overcome the weaker. So it is with disease.

The germs of infectious diseases on entering the animal organism at once begin a conflict with the elements of the same for nutritious material. If the elements of our bodies are the stronger, they finally overpower these disease-producing enemies, and we live; if the latter are the more powerful, we die.

While many forms of fungus-life are known to have an economical value, which we make practical use of in the production of wine, beer, vinegar, yeast, etc., it is still more important to us, and of no less practical value, that we should know the nature of the action of those which produce disease, either in ourselves or in our domestic animals. In both instances we have to do with questions of natural economy, though the directions in which we pursue our investigations are so manifestly different.

While much has been written upon the action of bacteria as regards their etiological relation to disease, still we are forced to admit that the subject is yet buried in the greatest obscurity. We find it a hard task to distinguish the essential from the unessential in our studies.

The task we have before us is, then, to discuss the *rôle* which bacteria play in the generation of disease in the animal kingdom.

The diseases which have been attributed to germinal action are very numerous; in fact, the list includes all the infectious and contagious diseases, and many of a questionable character. Some enthusiasts (Hallier, Zurn, and others) have even professed to discover the specific germ in every case, and we have in their writings most explicit descriptions of the peculiar fungi of glanders, cholera, hay-fever, rinderpest, and numerous other diseases, observations which the most exact experiments of other equally proficient authorities have failed to confirm.

While our knowledge of specific disease-producing bacteria is thus limited, we can safely assert that, with increasing years and consequent improvement in the means and methods of investigation, it will be constantly extended and augmented.

It is well known that there are forms of fungus-life which live upon plants. A peculiar fungus—*ustilago maidis*—is the specific cause of the rust of grain. It is also known that during one period or form of its existence, this fungus lives upon the leaves of the barberry-bush; and practical experience, based on this knowledge, has proved that with the removal of these bushes in certain districts the sequential disease of corn has ceased to appear.

A very important question is, Are the infectious elements of disease of a gaseous nature, or are they organisms?

We know from experimental experience that a very small quantity of infectious material is necessary to produce certain diseases. We also know that, when in case of a certain disease (anthrax) we introduce the smallest quantity of material into the organism, a multiplication of this material takes place.

We know that the disease-producing germs are capable of suspension in the air, thereby impregnating it with the property of infection.

If we place healthy cattle in the same stable with others afflicted with contagious pleuro-pneumonia, we know that they will probably acquire that disease, even though none of the healthy may be placed in direct relation with the diseased ones. The same has often been found to result when healthy cattle were placed in a stable where the disease had been, and the sick and all others in it at the time had been removed and some attempts at disinfection taken place. I shall relate circumstances which will sufficiently prove that cattle in the same stable with others having tuberculosis have acquired the disease, and that by means of the aspired air.

Of our own species we know that it is only necessary for a susceptible person to be in a room for a few moments with an individual afflicted with the measles, scarlatina, variola, exanthematous typhus, to acquire these diseases, or to live for a short time in a certain malarial district, to acquire either the yellow fever or intermittent fever.

These examples sufficiently demonstrate the infectious nature of the atmosphere at certain times and in certain localities. While this is a fact, still the most contradictory views are entertained, both by the medical profession and the public, as to the real nature of the infectious elements. We find our medical writings constantly mentioning "volatile contagiums," or "gaseous miasmas"—things which do not exist, and are entirely in contradiction with the results of modern research.

We can speak of the infectious elements as fixed, or movable; that is, such as must be attached to some vehicle, be it a living organism or something polluted with the excretions of the same, or such as are easily taken up by the air and transported to some distance from the place of generation. But neither of these definitions corresponds to our ideas of a gas.

A poisonous gas when suspended in the air is more or less widely dispersed, and soon loses its activity. If it enters the body, it must enter in certain quantities, or no evil action follows. We know of no means by which it can multiply itself within an organism. On account of their liability to dispersion, it is almost impossible for an organism to inhale enough of a poisonous gas to cause serious disturbance in the open air. The gas and person must be confined in a room, and a given quantity inhaled, before evil consequences result. Even though a person may inhale a considerable quantity of such gas, removal from it soon relieves its effects.

As many of you may have read, in the Catacombs of Rome and other such places carbonic-acid gas is generally very abundant in the lower strata of air in the passages, and while it is impossible for dogs or cats to follow their owners in such places, yet the latter, on account of the greater elevation of their respiratory apparatus, can walk along in perfect safety. We know also how quickly unpleasant odors are dispersed by the atmosphere.

A poisonous gas must be very soon so dispersed as to lose its specific characteristics.

Were the generation of cholera dependent on infectious gases, we should find it rapidly extending over every part of a city or district, instead of being confined, as is frequently the case, to certain streets or districts. So in the case of rinderpest. If the infectious elements were of a gaseous nature, our endeavors at stamping out would be utterly futile; yet we know we can frequently confine it to a single stable in a village where many cattle are kept. Were the infectious elements gases, all individuals with any disposition to infection would contract given diseases, as they would be far more likely to take up a correspondingly equal amount of infectious material than if they were of an organized nature.

Again, if they were gases, the infectious elements would soon be so widely dispersed as to lose their activity.

While we know the minuteness of many forms of bacterial life, so minute that our strongest powers give us but the most inadequate idea of their nature, may we not safely assume that there are many forms which still escape our observation?

Are the elements of infection formless, or are they organic individuals—that is, objects having form and life?

We have two possibilities to consider: either they enter an organism in such quantities as to cause immediate action, or they enter in very small quantity, and have the power of multiplying within the organism.

By poisoning the first takes place. A given quantity of a known poison causes direct and specific action. This never takes place by infection.

Specific poisons have no period of latency.

The most poisonous of substances act only in this manner. Minus a given quantity, no poisonous action, though we may have what is known as a physiological or medicinal action which we make use of in many of them. If we carry these medicinal doses beyond a certain limit, a poisonous action frequently results, which is known as the cumulative action of drugs—as with strychnine.

While a given, appreciable quantity of poison is necessary to specific action, we find in infectious diseases the contrary to be the case. We can not appreciate the minuteness of the quantity of infectious element necessary to produce an infectious disease.

A single bacterium, in a condition of active proliferation, can lead to the development of anthrax, if inoculated into a susceptible organism.

Who would have temerity enough to introduce under his skin even the smallest part of the point of the finest needle which had been dipped in the saliva of a rabid dog? Yet we can neither weigh nor otherwise appreciate the quantity of the inficieus introduced.

You need no further proof of the impossibility of unformed elements causing infection. Unformed elements have not the power of self-multiplication.

We are, then, naturally driven to the assumption of organized elements, as the etiological momenta in infection.

The elements of infection must have the faculty of multiplication. They must have the faculty of taking up soluble nutriment from their surroundings.

What, then, must be the real nature of these elements? Our studies and experiments have clearly shown that, of all organic life, but one form has the characteristics which conform to these conditions. That is the bacteria; or, more particularly, the schizomycetes, or fission, spore-producing fungi.

These fungi correspond in every particular with our theories. They are small enough to be taken up in numbers, under favorable conditions, and widely dispersed by the atmospheric currents. They possess the ability to multiply to an incredible degree, doubling their numbers, under suitable conditions, in a few minutes. Their tenacity of life exceeds that of any known objects.

While the essential characteristics of the bacteria in question so fully conform to our hypothesis, our practical experiences are not so full of assurance.

While, in some few diseases—diphtheria, intermittent fever, anthrax, and emphysema infectiosum—we find the fission-fungi or spores present in great numbers, in other hypothetic germ-diseases they are frequently wanting, or very seldom met with.

While we must admit the meagerness of our knowledge as to the manner of life of these bacteria, yet we may assume that their deleterious action extends itself in three directions.

While the infectious elements act in the smallest quantities in the purely contagious diseases, when introduced into a suitable organism, experience seems to justify us in assuming that much greater quantities are necessary with regard to the so-called malarial diseases.

Miasmas are not transportable in the sense of the infectious elements of purely contagious diseases.

We can not acquire intermittent fever at any time or place, but must be in localities where it is generated.

In septic diseases, we have, fortunately, still another condition.

The continued introduction of infectious material is necessary to produce septicæmia; for experience has taught us that if, by disinfection of the wound, we can shut off the supply, even though the wound continues, we may prevent the general disease. We know, further, that we can introduce, subcutaneously, no inconsiderable amount of septic material into a rabbit, without causing fatal results; but, if we continue the supply, the general disease, blood-poisoning, follows.

We do not know why it is that one individual of a given species is susceptible to infection by a contagious disease, and another not; or why at one time an individual may become infected and at another not; or why at one time we may go to a locality where intermittent fever or yellow fever prevails and not become diseased, while at another time we may acquire either of them.

In fact, when we come to the earnest study of the causes of contagious infections, as well as malarial diseases, we become more and more convinced that our ignorance far surpasses any knowledge that we may possess.

Dispersion of Bacteria, and their Entrance into the Animal Organism.

The deeper we seek to penetrate into the life and functions of the bacteria, the more do we feel ourselves as lost wanderers upon an unknown sea. We find very few known facts to cling to, as rocks of refuge to the storm-tossed mariner. There are but few beacon-lights along this coast.

There are no more important questions in connection with bacterial life than as to the means by which they become separated and dispersed from the original places of generation; and, again, how they enter from these into the animal organism.

Notwithstanding our poverty of knowledge, we have still some points of practical value at command to aid us on our way.

We have all-sufficiently established the non-gaseous nature of the elements causing contagio-infectious diseases—a fact which will become still more apparent as we pursue our studies.

In all strictly contagious diseases, you will remember, the elements of infection are always generated within the diseased organism, aud pass off with the excretions, or are attached to them.

In miasmas they are always generated outside of any animal organism. This distinction must never be lost sight of.

It is true we have infectious diseases, in which, originally, the etiological elements are generated outside the organism, and which have a certain degree of contagiousness by means of their excretions. This is the group of infectio-contagious diseases of which febris flava and anthrax are examples.

Wherever infectious germs are produced, their generation is based upon the presence of moisture, either as a watery fluid or some substance containing moisture sufficient to the purpose.

We find no difficulty in comprehending the dispersion of infectious elements when they are still contained within or upon the materials where they have been generated; that is, by means of streams, or of solids or fluids impregnated with them. Distribution or dispersion of infectious stuff in this way is by no means the rule; in fact, it is seldom that it takes place to any distance, unless artificial means come into play. Glanders, variola, and syphilis can only be acquired by direct contact with an infected organism, or with a vehicle which has been polluted with the specific elements of either of these diseases.

Only the infectious elements—*inficientia*—of purely contagious diseases are capable of any wide dispersion, and this can only take place through the moving of diseased individuals or the transport of derivatives from the same—clothing, excretions, hides, horns, hair, etc.—or through accidental substances which may have become impregnated with excretions from them. Elements of infection can only be dispersed in two ways:

1. By means of water or fluids, or moist substances containing them.

2. By the air, or in some desiccated vehicle or condition.

Infectious elements do not long retain their original condition and activity in water. The nature of the nutriment found in such media exerts a corresponding influence upon the nature and activities of germs. Metamorphosis into non-malignant forms is frequently said to take place.

In pure spring or rain water they soon demonstrate changes for want of sufficiency of nutriment. They retain their specific characteristics longest in those media in which they are originally generated.

The excretions of purely contagious diseases conform more to this condition than external media; but when these are exposed to the action of an excess of moisture, decomposition of the media and germinal changes soon follow, which are opposed to further contagion.

We are justified in asserting that contagions which are supported in moisture not their natural media soon lose their activity. Such disturbance takes place more rapidly in a warm than in a cool temperature.

The more water a given medium contains, the poorer its nutritious qualities, and the quicker destruction or change takes place upon germs suspended in it.

In a frozen condition media as well as germs suffer but little change. Distribution of infectious elements in a desiccated or dried condition takes place either by means of the atmosphere, or upon the surface of or within desiccated vehicles.

The elements of infection retain their vitality longer in a desiccated condition than when in or upon media of a moist nature, or when the desiccation takes place with sufficient rapidity to prevent decomposition or changes in the media, or the germs in or upon it.

If the processes of desiccation take place with such a rapidity and to such a degree as to remove *all* moisture, the germs perish. Some degree of moisture is necessary to their vitality. Germs retain their activity longer in a cool, moist atmosphere than in a warm and dry, and less long when suspended in a dry atmosphere than when contained in a dry substance, where they are protected in some measure from further desiccation. We know that the transportation of infectious elements to any great distance by means of the atmosphere does not take place, but that they may be transported a long distance by means of diseased individuals or infected vehicles. From what has been said you must infer that infectious elements are largely transported by means of the air or desiccated objects, and that these are the chief sources whence to gain entrance to the animal organism.

Infectious elements must be generated in media containing moisture. They are not volatile—gaseous—and must first become desiccated and reduced to powder before they can be taken up and transported by the atmosphere.

Some authorities have mistakenly asserted that the germs are, as it were, torn away from their moist media with the molecules of water which pass off with evaporation. That this is false is proved by the evaporation of salt water. The salts remain; the volume is less, but the quantity of salts is the same. Where we find salts suspended in the air, there has been sufficient mechanical action not to remove molecules of water, but to take it up in drops, as in a storm at sea. With the cessation of the storm the salts drop of their own weight; but evaporation does not cease. Bacteria can not be removed by simple processes of evaporation; small as they are, they are larger and heavier than the molecules of salt dissolved in water. Infectious elements can only be taken up and transported by the atmosphere when in a dried or dust form.

Two important adjunct circumstances come also into consideration in this regard:

1. The degree of adhesion with which such elements cling to their place of birth or lodgment.

2. The mechanical means to which they are subjected.

With reference to the latter, the most simple case is where the dried mass, or the remnants of an evaporated fluid, are disturbed or ground to a powder by some mechanical means which renders it easy for the atmosphere to remove them.

The formation of dust in our streets, which may frequently contain bacteria, and its removal by the wind, is a fitting example.

To this end it is essential that the material which contains the germs does not contain anything of a mucilaginous or adhesive nature, and that the particles of the same are sufficiently small.

The dissemination of a gas takes place very rapidly in the atmosphere. Even though the movements of the latter be imperceptible, a bad-smelling gas soon disappears if the supply be cut off.

The distribution of dust is dependent on its fineness and the violence or force with which the air moves; but in no case is it capable of very extended dispersion. In a motionless atmosphere dust molecules or germs soon fall to the ground. The smaller they are, and the more rapid the movement of the air, the longer they are kept in suspension.

So many circumstances are necessary to the dispersion of infectious elements by means of the atmosphere, it is evident that they may be confined for a long time to an individual, a house, street, or locality.

An organism is, therefore, so much the more exposed to a given infection, the more it is confined to a locality where infectious elements are or have been generated, or the more the air-currents come from such a place.

Infectious elements do not all possess the same degree of dispersion; so that, under otherwise similar circumstances, one disease may attack a far greater number of individuals than another.

The Infection of the Animal Organism.

Here, again, we find ourselves mostly upon a hypothetical foundation.

All is not gold that glitters; so it will be with many of the existing theories of fungi-infection; but out of all we shall finally winnow many facts.

The penetration of germs into the body by means of an intact outer cuticle may be looked upon as impossible.

Whether they can also penetrate through the mucosa, and walls of the capillaries of the intestinal or respiratory tracts, is also very questionable.

In anthracis pulmonum, a condition of the lungs due to the presence of coal-dust in the finest form, we find it accumulates in the alveolæ, but we find no proof of its gaining access to the circulation; the same is true in the so-called "grinder's pneumonia," which is due to the presence of stone-dust in the lungs.

In the intestinal canal we know, from our physiological studies, that even the finest qualities of solid fats are incapable of absorption; the action of the gall and pancreatic fluids is first necessary, by which they are reduced to an emulsion.

We are not, then, justified in assuming that bacteria gain access to the living organism, either on account of their minuteness, or in any passive way. Action on the part of the bacteria themselves must play no secondary part in this phenomenon.

To a passive entrance, or in fact to any entrance into the living organism, the respiratory tract offers by far the most favorable opportunity.

As may be known to many, the capillaries of the lungs are of an extremely delicate nature; they also dip into the alveolæ; that large number of bacteria are taken up with the aspired air seems very probable; that very few, even in a profusely impregnated atmosphere, gain access to the air-cells of the lungs, must be also true; for the mucosa of the respiratory tract extends from the entrance of the nostrils to the beginning of the infundibula, or conglomerate of air-cells. The alveolæ themselves have no mucosa. The viscid nature of the covering of this membrane is of such a quality as to warrant our assuming that the major part of such germs are caught by it, and gradually find their way back to the pharynx by means of the ciliary movement of the tracheal and bronchial epithelium.

We know that the fission-fungi have a boring movement, and that this is apparently in a forward direction; the question is, Is it strong enough to penetrate these fine capillaries?

The answer is, We do not know!

Again, some authorities have described openings, or vacancies, between the individual epithelium cells lining the alveoli, and have looked upon them as the endings of the pulmonary lymph system.

If such stomata or openings really exist, they offer a natural and favorable atrium to the penetration of bacteria into the system by means of the lungs.

As we have said, but a very small number can certainly penetrate so deeply as the alveoli; but we know that, on account of the wonderful degree of proliferation, a very small number is sufficient to produce infection.

The blood, from its chemical composition, and the presence of oxygen, united with the temperature of the body, offers the most favorable condition for the multiplication of bacteria.

As to the intestinal tract, we have already said that the nature of the mucosa is such that we do not believe it possible for the bacteria to penetrate its different membranes.

The acidity of the stomach offers very unfavorable conditions to the life or multiplication of germs.

Some have assumed, and among them the ablest of mycologists, that an abrasion (wounding) of an intact surface is necessary to the entrance of bacteria into the system. When we reflect on the minuteness of these objects, and how frequently results of this nature may take place, both in the respiratory, and particularly the digestive tract, we find good grounds for accepting this hypothesis as the one favoring the general way in which infection takes place.

Slight abrasions of the mucosa of the nostrils, pharynx, cheeks, etc., or even that of the œsophagus, stomach, and intestines, are very common with our own species: how much more so in our domestic and other animals which seek their food in a natural manner, or receive it from the none too careful hands of man!

An unhealthy mucosa is of itself seldom intact; abrasions of its epithelial covering are very common, even though they do not occasion such disturbances as to lead one to suspect any very serious trouble. The proneness of the ruminantia to take up all sorts of foreign objects—nails, hair-pins, broken glass, and even knives and forks—is well known to many.

Traumatic inflammation of the stomach and heart are no uncommon diseases in our cows, especially such as are grazed on road-sides and house-yards.

Traumata, wounds in the cutis, are very common among our animals, and much more so among grazing animals, especially on the feet and legs and around the hoofs; and as these parts are frequently in places where germs would be abundant (marshes, etc.), they offer the most favorable atria to the penetration of germs.

How do germs act?

By depriving the body of nutritive material, by obstruction, capillary embolism, and by the products which either of themselves, or by the disease-processes, are induced by them.

That they require large quantities of oxygen has been made apparent; and it is self-evident that, on their entrance into the body, there must be a constant struggle with the red blood-cells for this necessary gas. Whether they produce carbonic-acid gas (CO_2), and thus add to its accumulation in the system, is still an open question.

That capillary embolism is possible has been too frequently observed to be questioned. This condition would be but another way by which parts, not the whole, of the system, are shut off from oxygen and other nutritive material.

Infectious diseases do not seem to last long enough to cause necrosis, or necrobiosis (death), in parts thus shut off from the circulation; at least, never in my reading have I met with any description of phenomena similar to those we meet with in ordinary embolism.

When an organism withstands the invasion of an infectious disease, we may assume that it offers no longer a favorable condition to the bacteria; they die, suffer some sort of a dissolution, and are passed off as an effete material.

Disinfection.

The birth of crude empiricism may be asserted to have been coeval with the first realization of pain or suffering on the part of man. The aim of modern medicine is prevention. We are earnestly endeavoring to make practical the old saying, "An ounce of prevention is worth a pound of cure."

The men who boast of their "cures" are slowly becoming less numerous among the true practitioners of medicine.

As observers slowly came to the idea that one disease, and then another, was due to some inficiens; that many such diseases were strictly or partly contagious—that is, passing directly from one animal organism to another—they began first to take means to prevent them: hence restrictions of commerce, not only with regard to human beings, but animals and their products. This restrictive, preventive medicine, if we may be allowed the term, has been rewarded by the grandest results, though it at first paid little or no attention to the primary causes of the diseases it sought to prevent. The causes it recognized were those of intercourse and commerce. It sought to regulate these with reference to the contagious diseases, and the result has been that the black-death and bubo-pest have become entire strangers to Western Europe; Asiatic cholera is no longer the terror of the civilized world. Aside from the benefits of vaccination, the variolæ no more carry horror into the human family. The cattle-owner of Europe does not awaken on any morning and find the rinderpest devastating his herd. The lung-plague of cattle is kept within restricted limits, and so of other diseases of like nature.

These remarks have no relation to diseases of a purely malarial character, which are based on locality. Here we have to do with questions of drainage, tillage, and the like, which we will not discuss at present.

While this work of modern medicine is of no secondary importance, the results of the observations and experiments of recent years have opened still another path to the workers in preventive medicine.

They have discovered the causes of some diseases, and gained knowledge that justifies us in assuming that the causes of all infectious and contagious diseases are of a similar nature. This cause is the schizomycetes or fission-fungi, and their germs, which bear the general name of micrococci or microbes.

Having discovered these objects, the next step has been to study their mode of life, how they live and multiply, what elements favor these processes, and what are opposed to them.

Our conceptions in this regard are still far from clear, and too frequently our action is based on mistaken reasoning.

We too often think that, when we have removed the odor from an offensive place or substance, we have destroyed its disease-producing qualities, a hope which is only too soon negatived by experience.

The resistibility of germs is such that we may look upon it as very nearly fallacious to disinfect the atmosphere by adding to it chlorine-gas, or sulphur, or any similar disinfectants. Such disinfection is more or less an idea inherited from the earlier days of preventive medicine, and not in conformity with our present knowledge.

In considering the question of disinfection we must ever bear in mind that the fission-fungi, or their spores, always occur in one of two conditions; that is, moist or dry. This fact should always be settled before we decide as to our disinfecting procedures. When in a moist medium, bacteria are much more easily destroyed than when united with a dry.

If we meet with them in a fluid, a boiling-heat is necessary to their destruction. Temperatures of 77° to 104° Fahr. are in general favorable to bacterial life. The most advantageous has been found to be 95° Fahr. The resistibility to high temperatures varies in the different bacteria. A temperature of 113° to 122° Fahr. has been found sufficient to kill bacteria thermo, while bacilli have been found to resist 176° Fahr. Extreme degrees of cold are far less effective to their destruction than heat. We have too often assumed that when our antiparasitics, or, better, antiseptics, have prevented the fermentative processes, the germs have been destroyed also. While heat is the most effective of all the disinfectants, we shall make no mistake in adding to it those chemicals which are at enmity with bacterial life.

Nägeli sums up his remarks on disinfection as follows:

1. The infectious elements can not be securely destroyed when in an absolutely dry condition.

2. Boiling-heat can only surely kill them when they are in a moist or fluid medium.

3. The antiseptics which have gained acceptance are not positively death to them; they only place them in an inactive condition, that is, consume them. (This argument is open to the objection that, in disinfection, the disinfectants have been, or have to be, used in too diluted a condition, or in such a way as not to come either directly or in sufficient volume in contact with the bacteria. This last must nearly always be the case in spray or smoke disinfection, which we believe to be an illusion.)

4. They are changed, not destroyed, by decomposition of media, by means of a surplus of water or heat, so that they lose their infectious properties.

5. They are harmless when removed in a moist condition.

The true value of the internal application of the antiseptics is of a very questionable nature; for these materials exert fully as poisonous an influence upon the autositic as the parasitic organism.

In some cases, as in intermittent fever, it would seem as if we could bring the organism so under the influence of quinine as to act against the proliferation of the spirillum. That this bacterium disappears in the intervals of the fever has been mentioned. Where it comes from again during the paroxysms is an open question.

While this may be true, in a measure, of quinine, boracic acid, and some other materials, the internal use of the stronger antiseptica in sufficient volume is too dangerous to be tried.

A special study of the antiseptics would lead us too much into details for our present purpose, and I must refer my readers to the works upon that subject; among the disinfectants are the corrosive acids, carbol, thymol, boracic acid, hypermanganate of potash, the coal-tar preparations, and the long list of antiputrids.

Anthrax and Anthracoid Diseases.

The word *anthrax* is of Greek origin, and means *a coal.* The name was not originally given to a single disease, but to a group of diseases which were characterized by a black, tarry appearance of the blood. In any form, the blood is essentially complicated, while all the organs of the body are more or less affected.

Modern research has led to the isolation of one disease from this group as anthrax.

The others may be called anthracoid (i. e., anthrax-like) diseases.

They are all germ-diseases; but the germ which has led to the isolation of one disease as anthrax has singular characteristics in its mature or bacterial form which enable us to distinguish it from other almost similar bacteria.

The disease is also known as charbon (carbuncle), Milzbrand, etc.

History.

Of all the pests, or infectio-contagious animal diseases, anthrax seems to be the one of which we have the earliest historical record. Moses has apparently described it as one of the plagues by which Jehovah punished the Egyptians. The early Greek and Roman writers mention it under the names of sacer ignis; gutta robea; also by its present name, and it is also mentioned by Arabic writers as "Al humrah" or "Persian fire."

Charbert was the first author to enter into any clear and critical study of the various diseases of this group, and published a work, "Description et Traitement du Charbon," Paris, 1780, which even at the present day exerts more or less influence, especially in France.

Although the observations of the eighteenth century led many authors to declare for the contagiousness of anthrax, still others declared it to be non-contagious. Kausch, an author early in this century, gave a good description of the pathological changes of this disease, and looked upon it chiefly as a paralysis of the pulmonary nerves, but declared himself for the infection of man and animals by means of the blood, flesh, etc.

Delafond, 1843, studied the disease among sheep ("Maladie de Sang"), and looked upon the abomasum and intestines as the chief seats of the disease, and declared it to be an acute enteritis by which the blood was also complicated. He denied the infectious character of the disease, and sought its etiology in hyper-nourishment, and in abnormal chemical changes in the earth. Gerlach, 1845, looked upon this disease of sheep as identical with anthrax, and proved its infectiousness by direct experiment, and considered the contagium to be volatile and having great tenacity.

Heusinger, in his noted historical work upon "Animal Plagues," looked upon the disease as a malarial neurosis, and assumed that the infectious elements acted chiefly upon the ganglionic nerve-centers. The primary changes consisted of a paralysis of the blood-vessels of the spleen and the consequential death of its tissues, hence its German name, "Milzbrand"; following this, the disease is characterized by vascular paralysis, blood-stasis, extravasations, and necrosis in different organs. Contagious elements are developed by the disease, which lead to its extension. These elements are taken up by the lymph and blood-vessels, chiefly the latter, from the parts primarily complicated. The apparent divergence with which the disease manifests itself in different animals is not essential, as the essentials of the disease are nearly the same in all. The disease develops primarily in grazing animals, solipeds, ruminants, and swine. All animals are open to infection.

In 1855 Virchow followed Heusinger in declaring for the malarial nature of the disease; he emphasized its septic character, and looked upon the cause as a specific ferment. Wald, 1862, laid special emphasis upon the nature of the soil in the generation of anthrax.

In 1856 Pollender broke the ground which has gradually led to our modern views of the true nature of anthrax, and its isolation from kindred diseases; so early as 1849 he had found peculiar staff-like bodies in the blood of anthrax-diseased animals. Entirely independent from the observations of Pollender, Brauell, professor at Dorpat, Russia, found (1857) the same microscopic elements in the blood of men, sheep, and horses that had perished from the disease. He looked upon them as vibrios, and as he found them *intra vitam* (during life) in the blood of such animals, considered them to have *diagnostic value*, while Pollender declared their importance to be still an open question.

The discovery of these two observers gradually drew the attention of scientists to the study of this disease, and it may be truly asserted that no single disease has enjoyed so much observation in modern or ancient days.

By means of a succession of experiments Brauell came to the knowledge that the peculiar staff-like bodies appeared from one, two, or three, and in some cases eight to ten hours before the death of the diseased organism, and when the course of the disease was very acute, but a few moments before its fatal termination, while they were not to be seen in the blood of convalesents, He credited these objects with a prognostic and diagnostic value, but denied to them any etiological importance, as the disease could be produced with blood which did not contain them, a fact which will find its explanation later on.

These peculiar bodies were not looked upon in the same light by different observers, some considering them as coagaluted fibrin (Brückmüller, "Zoötomie Pathologique"), fragments of broken-down tissues, blood-crystals, while Delafond looked upon them as a species of leptothrix. In 1860 the last-named author adopted the views of Brauell.

In 1863 Davaine declared these bodies to be bacteria, and, in order to distinguish them from the motory bacteria of putrefaction, gave them the name of *bacteridiæ*. As the blood without them was not infectious, he declared them to be the specific cause of this disease. The bacteridiæ are destroyed by putrefaction, but may be preserved for a long time in a desiccated condition.

After this time, there followed a period of the greatest divérgence in the views of different observers as to the true nature and place of these objects: all sorts of things—blood-crystals, the bacteria of putrefaction, the cent-like rolls of the blood-cells, etc.—were declared to be the same as the bacteridiæ. Davaine's work, more than that of any other author, gradually led to the production of order out of this chaos.

He found the bacteria to be present in the majority of cases of anthrax, and that they frequently appeared before the outbreak of the symptoms of diseases; when they disappeared, by putrefaction or otherwise, the infectiousness of the blood ceased. The number of bacilli in a single drop of blood was estimated by Davaine at eight to ten millions; and he claimed that a drop of blood diluted to a million times its volume by water was still competent to produce infection.

The modern workers in this field of mycology are sufficiently known through our general study of the bacteria.

Etiology.

Our studies have led us to the conclusion that anthrax is an acute infectious disease due to the action of specific germs called bacteria. The disease very frequently assumes an enzoötic or epizoötic form, although it is frequently sporadic in its appearance and occurs mostly in grazing animals and swine, but is also transmissible to man.

The nature of the earth plays no unimportant part in enzoötic outbreaks of the disease. The disease is found most frequently in localities where the earth contains much moisture, and in regions where the rivers, brooks, or swamps are subject to drying out; in fact, in just such districts where intermittent fever prevails among men.

In many regions, such places become generally known as infected districts, and are either fenced off or the animals kept from grazing upon them, or they have been turned to cultivation, which has led to the manifest decrease of the disease. Such regions are especially frequent in the Bavarian Alps, where I studied the disease under the guidance of Professor Feser, of the Munich Veterinary School. One is surprised that such infected localities are often to be found at the very tops of the mountains or upon highly situated levels.

An undue degree of moisture in the earth seems to favor the development of the bacteria.

While there is much similarity in the telluric nature of regions where anthrax and intermittent fever prevail, it is not in accordance with practical experience that both diseases should prevail in them, for we find the one where the other does not appear, and *vice versa.* While anthrax is a disease, the generation of which seems so largely dependent on the nature of the ground, it is by no means a malarial disease. It never prevails to any such extent as intermittent fever, even in regions where it appears, and which offer every condition favorable to its development.

The presence of the peculiar infectious elements is always necessary to the generation of the disease, no matter how favorable the telluric conditions may appear to their development.

My friend Dr. Oemler reduced an annual loss of twenty-one per cent among the sheep of his district in Germany to two per cent by energetic opposition to the burial of all cadavers of animals that had died from the disease. Similar results have followed a like procedure on the part of numerous other competent observers.

A Russian commission, appointed to look into the causes of anthrax, *reported the chief cause of the epizoötic outbreaks of the disease to be the incomplete burial and removal of the cadavers of horses which had perished from it.*

Every animal diseased with anthrax, or its cadaver, or any portion of the same, must be looked upon as a dangerous center from which infection may proceed.

The physical conditions of the earth, viz., its amount of water, chemical constituents, and temperature, must always be looked upon in considering the generation of anthrax.

Practical experience goes to prove that extreme drying out or draining of a suspected or known district is unfavorable to the development of its infectious elements. In such cases, rains following great heat and drought are generally characterized either by the reappearance of the disease or its greater prevalence. On the contrary, drought and heat favor its appearance in very moist districts. The disease is generally most prevalent in such districts when the temperature of the earth has reached its highest maximum. This is generally in our latitude in the months of August and September.

A question of importance in the generation of this disease is, Is an impregnation of the earth with the infectious elements necessary to the development of the disease, or are they capable of independent development in such earth by the metamorphosis from some other kind of fungi already present?

The previously mentioned practical observations of the careful removal of cadavers, instead of burial, would seem to favor the first of these views.

The chief, if not the only, cause of anthrax must be sought in infection, in general, not direct, but by means of some vehicle, the infectious elements being extremely tenacious of life and easily transported, as has been painfully illustrated by cases in man due to dried hides brought from a distance, curled hair, or other animal derivatives.

The most frequent carriers of infection are either diseased animals, their excretions, or their products—hides, horns, hoofs, etc. Again, healthy animals, or even men, flies, gnats, etc., may serve as vehicles to infection. Gerlach reports numerous cases among sheep due to the bite of the dogs used to tend them, where the latter have been fed or have fed themselves upon the cadavers of sheep that had perished from the disease.

Davaine frequently produced the disease by inoculations with the probosces or feet of flies which had first been permitted to pollute themselves with the blood from animals that had died from the disease.

Bollinger reports finding the specific bacteria of anthrax in the blood of flies which were caught upon the cadavers of such animals, and to have produced the disease in rabbits by inoculating with the same.

As further vehicles of infection we may mention the harness, stable-utensils, straw, and hay, etc., which have been in contact with diseased animals.

Articles of food—beets, turnips, carrots—which have been raised upon lands where cadavers from anthrax-diseased animals have been buried, have been asserted to have caused this disease when fed to cattle.

The fluids of the stable—urine, etc.—seem to be less dangerous, as putrefaction is known to be in opposition with the life of these germs.

The respiratory tract, the external cutis, and digestive tract, are the chief atria of the infectious elements, though the flesh of such animals has often been consumed with impunity; still, feeding experiments upon animals susceptible to the disease have sufficiently proved the infectiousness of such meat. The susceptibility to infection is greater in the ruminants—tame and wild—than in the solipeds, less in the omnivora, and still less in the carnivora; the cat, however, more so than the dog.

Nature of the Infectious Elements.

While we have already noticed this subject in our general consideration of the bacteria, it is of such great importance that we may be warranted in treating it still more in detail.

The fact that authrax could be generated in an experimental way, with blood in which the bacteridiæ could not be discovered, has led many authors to deny to them any etiological importance. This fact remained incontrovertible until observers had advanced in the study of the life of these parasites.

First their minuteness, and again the very small quantity necessary to infection, may have led authors to this mistaken conclusion; but, above all, it was the ignorance of the earlier observers of the spore of the schizomycetic fungi which led them into this error.

An interesting fact with reference to the intra-organismal life of the bacteria of anthrax is, that the placenta offers a natural filtration apparatus, which prevents them passing from the blood of the mother to that of the fœtus. Inoculation experiments have demonstrated not only the presence of the bacteria in the blood of the mother, and their absence in that of the fœtus, but also that, while the blood of the mother was highly infectious, that of the fœtus was wanting in this quality.

This only goes to prove that in this case, even if the micrococci, or germ condition of the bacteria, be present in the mother, it is not so in the fœtus; but does not militate against the proved fact that blood from anthrax-diseased animals without bacteria is still infectious.

Feser has made some interesting experiments with regard to the filtering ability of the milk-glands in sheep. He has inoculated ewes with lambs by their side, and proved that infection had taken place, both by examination of the blood and by experiments with the same upon other animals; but the lambs did not become infected from the mother's milk, although isolated bacteria were to be seen in the same. Inoculations made with such milk, however, produced the disease in other animals.

The presence of the bacteria in the milk, and its infectiousness on inoculation, while the lambs feeding upon it were not infected, go to support a theory of infection we have already considered in our general remarks, viz., that a wounded or abraded surface is necessary to the infection of an organism. In lambs feeding upon milk alone such is surely impossible in the course of the digestive tract.

The fact that bacteria pass the membranes of the milk-glands and not those of the placenta, may be explained by the mechanical action and minor lesions, which can result to the milk-glands from the sucking and butting of the lambs.

As we have frequently mentioned, this disease is now known to be due to a specific cause—a schizophyte, or vegetable parasite, bacillus anthracis—a staff-shaped bacterium which multiplies by spores.

An English observer, Ewart, of University College, London, gives a very clear description of the life of these germs, which may not be out of place here, notwithstanding all we have previously considered:

"At first the bacilli were absolutely motionless—they had been taken from the spleen of a mouse—but in some cultivations, after keeping them in a temperature of 33° C. for a few hours, a great number of them began to move actively about the field. While at rest they were not altogether without change, for clear lines across them indicated that they were in the process of division into segments. Sometimes a number of rods ceased moving, and, previous to lengthening out into filaments, arranged themselves into patches of zoöglea.

"The division into two or more segments is not always a very rapid process. A rod, which was watched until it divided, was made up of three segments, and one of them from the beginning looked as if it might separate itself from the others; but after six hours of almost constant endeavor, it was still connected by a very delicate thread, and before final separation, which took place after seven hours' observation, it was divided into two segments in a comparatively short time, so that, when it did escape from the other apparently inactive pieces, it moved about the field of the microscope like two freely movable links of a chain.

"After assuming this motile phase for some time, the rods lengthened out into *spore*-bearing filaments.

"The lengthening of the rods into filaments is an extremely rapid process, and is apparently affected by the temperature. In five hours, at a temperature of 32° C., a rod may have increased so as to be from eighty to one hundred times its original length, and in twenty-four hours the filament may be full of spores. If the temperature be kept at about 28° C., the spore may not appear until the thirty-sixth or fortieth hour. When the spores have once appeared, all the other changes go on at an ordinary temperature of from 12° to 18° C., but not nearly so rapidly, even when the preparation is kept in the sun for a few hours daily, as when artificial heat is employed. On the other hand, a high temperature, 37°–40° C., at once checks all development.

"The filaments, when first formed, are perfectly hyaline, but soon the central protoplasmic contents can be distinguished from the gelatinous-looking sheath. The protoplasma next divides into numerous short pieces about the size of the original rod out of which the filament was formed. These contract, leaving clear empty spaces between them, and often again divide to form still shorter masses of protoplasm.

"At each side of this transverse line of division minute clear specks appear—the first indication of spores. These gradually increase in size and luster, and as they increase the protoplasma disappears; in fact, the spores seem to be developed from the protoplasm. Soon after the appearance of the spores the filaments seem to be made up of numerous segments, each segment containing one spore, the spores lying at the adjacent ends of the segments. The spores now begin to escape. The filament gradually disappears, and the spores appear surrounded by a mass of gelatinous material. The spores, when free, according to previous observers, develop into rods. My own observations lead me to believe that the spores do not always at once grow into rods, but that they may divide into four sporules, in which the envelope as well as the spores take part. The spore then elongates, becomes dumb-bell shaped, and finally develops into rods."

The action of the bacteria within the autosite is, as we have said, the consumption of oxygen, for which they have a great affinity, and the production of CO_2. This fact, the absorption of O and accumulation of CO_2, would seem to account for those cases of sudden death by anthrax, and for the symptoms by which the disease manifests itself—such as dyspnœa, cyanosis, clonic spasms, distended pupil, falling of the temperature, and asphyxia—which all correspond with the phenomena of poisoning with CO_2. The necroscopical results correspond to the same: congestion of the venous system, a dark, tar-like condition of the blood, extravasations, cyanotic coloring of different parts.

A peculiar diagnostic characteristic of bacillus anthracis is the abruptness with which each segment terminates: the ends are square, as if cut off, a condition which has not as yet been observed in any other bacteria, not even *B. subtilis*, which resembles it very closely in every other particular.

The tenacity of *B. anthracis* is very great. They may retain their virulence in a desiccated condition for months or even years. $\frac{1}{10000}$ of a drop of blood has been found sufficient to cause infection. Davaine has caused infection with blood that had been kept in a dried condition for twenty-two months.

Bollinger sums up his conclusions as to the nature of anthrax as follows:

"It is an acute infectious disease. The infectious elements constitute a vegetable parasite, which generates (endogenous) within the infected organism, and perhaps externally (ectogenous), that is, in the earth, when it finds conditions favorable thereto; that is, when the earth has been first impregnated. The disease is not contagious in the general acceptance of the word, as infection from animal to animal directly seldom takes place; but it is highly transportable by means of vehicles, from the peculiar characteristics of its etiological elements.

Appearance and Extension.

Anthrax occurs in all countries and climates, though to what extent it appears among the animals of this country we have no definite knowledge.

In making a diagnosis as to whether a given disease is anthrax or not, it must always be borne in mind that no bacillus anthracis, no anthrax; when, in doubtful cases, you can not decide, inoculation experiments will always give you the key to a correct diagnosis.

In 1864, 72,000 horses died in Russia alone from the disease. In the province of Novgorod (Russia), from 1867–'70, over 56,000 horses, cattle, and sheep, and 528 men, perished.

Phenomena of the Disease.

The disease, in general, presents itself under one of three forms:

1. The apoplectic form (anthrax acutissimus), the duration of which varies from a few minutes to several hours.

2. The acute form (anthrax acutus), the duration of which varies from a few hours to some days.

3. The subacute form (anthrax subacutus), which includes all cases of longer duration.

Great divergence exists among the various authors as to the duration of the period of incubation in anthrax. In some cases the appearance of the symptoms of the disease seems to follow immediately on the introduction of the inficieus. Fever has been observed within two hours subsequent to inoculation. Among cattle the incubation may continue for four or five days; in small animals, rabbits, etc., twenty-four, thirty-six, or forty-eight hours; seldom three or four days. On account of the variance in form with which the disease appears, it is difficult to give any concise description of its phenomena.

In the so-called apoplectic form the infected animals frequently drop, almost as if struck by lightning; they fall into convulsions, dyspnœa, cyanosis, and in a few minutes death results. Frequently, these violent symptoms are wanting in all prodromic phenomena, the animals eating and appearing apparently as well as ever. It is not unfrequent to find animals in the morning dead in the stall which were apparently perfectly healthy the evening before. The acute form of the disease appears about as follows in horses and cattle: Animals apparently healthy suddenly develop a loss of appetite; in cows, the milk secretion is restricted, or ceases altogether. The animals begin to tremble, and frequently chills may be seen to be present; the superficial parts of the body become cold. This cold stage passes into a febrile, after a longer or shorter period. Peculiar contractions and clonic spasms of the extremities are quite frequent. During the remissions the animals appear weak and depressed, or they may be apparently quite well and ruminate, and take to feeding.

The pulse is increased to double its normal rapidity; the temperature rises from 41° to 41·7° C. The excrements are frequently tinged with dark blood, or are bloody and diarrhœa-like.

These symptoms are not constant, but are interrupted by remissions, which may continue from six to twenty-four hours, during which the animals often appear as if quite well again.

Aside from the apoplectic and acute forms of the disease, we have a subacute and exanthematic form, in which we meet with a carbunculous and erysipelatous tumefaction distributed over different parts of the organism, especially on the posterior extremities. These tumefactions are generally hot, and more or less painful. The general habitus of the animal seems to suffer but little change. Resorption of the exudations soon begins, and it is not very frequent that we meet with excoriation and ulceration.

From sixty to seventy per cent of the cases of anthrax in horses and cattle end fatally, and are characterized by the above-mentioned phenomena—dyspnœa, cyanotic condition of the different mucosæ, opisthotonic condition of a variable intensity, spasms of the musculi palpebrarum, so that we can only see the whites of the eyes; the animals become extremely weak and are unable to stand; the temperature falls below normal; the extremities become cold, the pupils distended, and death appears, under the phenomena of asphyxia, in from twenty-four to forty hours from the first appearance of the disease.

In favorable cases, the recovery is very rapid. The carbuncular formations in the cutis are much less frequently met with in cattle than horses; otherwise, the symptoms of the disease among horses offer no essential differentiation from cattle.

The intra-vital phenomena of anthrax in the smaller domestic animals are far less distinctly marked; however, we meet with convulsive phenomena, dyspnœa, and mydriasis.

Pathological Anatomy.

The pathological anatomy of anthrax shows no essential differentiation among the bovine or equine species. In cattle which have perished during or of the disease in its acute or apoplectic form, we find the blood of a black-red color, thick and tar-like, and without the ability to coagulate. The blood has the same character during the intra-vital progress of the disease; the entire venous system is congested; the ingesta are frequently mixed with extravasated blood;

the intestinal parietes, especially of the jejunum, are more or less infiltrated with a sero-hæmorrhagic mass. Similar gelatino-hæmorrhagic infiltrations may be seen in the omentum, mesenterium, in the capsula adiposa of the kidneys, the connective tissue of the inferior parts of the neck and mediastinum. A sero-hæmorrhagic effusion is frequently to be met with in the abdominal and pleural cavities, particularly the former.

Ecchymoses of variable dimensions are frequently to be met with in the muscles of the heart, also extravasations of variable extent under the endocardium and epicardium, particularly about the auricles. Hæmorrhagic effusions are frequently to be met with in the sexual organs of females. Genuine carbuncular eruptions are seldom met with along the intestinal canal of cattle. The rigor mortis is not of a very severe grade; a frothy, blood-stained fluid is frequently to be seen issuing from the natural apertures of the body; the abdomen is frequently distended with gases. If animals are slaughtered early in the disease, it is frequently impossible to conjecture its nature, if they have been allowed to bleed freely, and the intestines, etc., have been carefully removed. This is an important fact from a public-health point of view.

The chief patho-anatomic variation in horses is that we meet this gelatino-hæmorrhagic infiltration to a far greater extent than in cattle. This peculiar yellow, serous, blackish infiltration is difficult to describe; but, after having once been seen, it does not easily pass from remembrance, and, aside from anything else, even the frequently asserted pathognomonic tumefaction of the spleen, is one of the most characteristic pathological phenomena of anthrax. These infiltrations may be met with wherever we have normally loose connective tissue, the retro-pharyngeal and laryngeal region, along the trachea and large blood-vessels and nerves, in the mediastinum and mesenterium, the organs of the pelvis, and fatty capsule of the kidneys.

The disease is not so marked along the intestinal tract in horses as in cattle; but we find carbuncular eruptions and erosions to a greater extent than in the latter.

The large glands of the body—kidneys, liver, spleen—are generally tumefied, the parenchyma clouded, and the vessels filled with blood. The lymph-glands also show signs of hypertrophy, and many bacteria are to be found in them.

Aside from the characteristic bacteria, we find the white or colorless blood-cells numerically increased, sometimes immensely.

Leucocytosis.—This condition is a transient numerical increase of the white or colorless blood-cells in proportion to the red, while leucæmia is a permanent increase of the former over the latter. This increase is to be traced to the hyperplastic condition of the lymph-glands and spleen.

The red blood-cells seem to suffer some changes; they are less firm in their contours, and have a greater degree of adhesiveness than is common to them.

Bacteria are, naturally, to be discovered only by the use of the microscope in the entire capillary system, many of them being virtually the seat of embolic bacterial obstruction. The parasites are also plentiful in all the effusions and extravasations, and frequently among the tissues.

In the smaller animals the necroscopical phenomena of anthrax are far less characteristic: the spleen is but little enlarged; the sero-hæmorrhagic infiltrations are by no means so numerous, as well as the extravasations.

A special tendency to rapid cadaveric changes does not seem so common to cattle, sheep, and goats, as to horses. The *rigor mortis* often fails, or is present to a minor degree.

Prognosis.

The prognosis in anthrax is to be considered as exceedingly unfavorable, sixty to seventy per cent of the cases ending fatally among the larger animals. In the acute and apoplectic forms recovery seldom takes place, and in the sub-acute the mortality is very great.

Diagnosis.

The diagnosis is often very difficult *intra vitam*, especially without recourse to the microscope, in sporadic cases in localities where the previous occurrence of the disease does not give cause for suspicion.

During the intermissions of the disease, the microscopic examination of the blood is often followed by negative results, as well as inoculative experiments. However, these should ever be resorted to, and, when taken in unison with the above detailed necroscopic phenomena, one need seldom make a mistake.

The bacteria may, however, generally be found in the blood soon after death. It must not be forgotten that putrefaction is opposed to the life of the bacteria.

On account of the extreme degree of infectiousness possessed by this disease, the practitioner must ever remember that, in a certain sense, he takes his life in his hands in making autopsies upon animals which have died or are suspected to have perished from it. With wounded hands, or even the slightest abrasions of the cutis, no one should make such an autopsy. Great care must be taken not to wound one's self with the knife, or upon sharp edges of broken bones, for death is almost sure to follow.

While a student in Virchow's laboratory at Berlin, the body of a tanner who had died from anthrax was brought in; the patient had simply removed the scab from a razor-scratch on his neck with the edge of a raw South American hide—sun-dried, however—which he was carrying. This case also illustrates the extreme tenacity of the germs of anthrax when dried.

Prophylaxis.

Notwithstanding the prevalence of the idea that the prevention of the enzoötic or sporadic outbreak of anthrax in regions where it has constantly appeared is a task of great difficulty, we must say that this does not accord with practical experience, as we have proven by examples taken from the observations of persons of undoubted ability.

Although it is beyond question that such soils or districts are highly infectious, yet we know that the thorough disinfection, and other removal of cadavers than by burying, also a similar care with reference to the excretions from such animals, have tended greatly to diminish the annual losses from the disease in notorious districts.

Diseased animals, as well as their cadavers, must be thoroughly protected from the attacks of flies, by keeping the stables dark, blankets, etc.

As an excess of moisture, or drying out of the ground-water, are both known, under certain previously mentioned conditions, to favor the development of the bacteria, and consequent infection of animals exposed thereto, and as practical experience has proved that thorough draining of such districts has been of beneficial effect, this procedure should always be resorted to.

Animals should never be allowed to graze upon known anthrax districts or suspected pastures. Such places should be fenced off and used for agricultural purposes after careful drainage.

While these remarks upon the soil as an infectious medium should by no means be disregarded, still there are numerous observations and experiences on the part of unquestionably competent men which seem to stand in open contradiction to the theory of the infection of the earth by means of the cadavers of anthrax-diseased animals.

While so high an authority as Pasteur asserts that the soil takes up the bacteria and preserves them, and acts as a medium of culture for them—also claiming to have found the common earthworm impregnated with them, and looking upon the latter as a vehicle aiding in their dispersion—we KNOW that putrefaction is opposed to their life and proliferation. All cadavers have to undergo the processes of putrefaction and chemical decomposition.

Collin buried anthrax victims within a limited district, and used every means known to be favorable to the life of the bacteria, yet he fed thirty-five animals with plants in every condition grown upon such soil without producing any evil effects.

Professor Feser buried a very large number of animals which had perished from inoculated anthrax, and from which repeated successful intra-vital and *post-mortem* experiments were made, in the grounds around the government experiment station at Lenggries, in Upper Bavaria, yet during the ensuing summer, when I was assistant with him, we were unable to produce a single successful inoculation, not only from the soil, but from the remnants of the cadavers. The same results followed like experiments made with material taken from a very large number of places where anthrax-diseased animals had been buried in the mountains.

Roloff, the present director of the Berlin school, is, however, a strong partisan for the infectiousness of such places.

Therapeutics.

The administration of the antiseptics has been extensively tried, and, in general, found unavailable in the treatment of this disease; although large doses, as large as safe, of carbolic acid, are said to give favorable results to some practitioners.

Immunity.

The question of the immunity to infection on the part of individuals of the same species of animal life, as well as the immunity against certain diseases of other species which exist all through the animal kingdom, is one of the most hidden subjects in connection with the study of disease.

The consideration of this subject belongs, rightly, in our general remarks upon bacteria; but for special reasons we have placed it here.

We know that one condition to infection is expressed by the practical though scientifically blind remark, want of susceptibility. In what this consists we know not. Not every person exposed to variola acquires the disease; the same is true even of syphilis, gonorrhœa, diphtheria, and all the contagious diseases of man. It is equally true with regard to pleuro-pneumonia, anthrax, rinderpest, etc., of our animals, though the individual immunity to infection is far less in some diseases than others.

Again, syphilis can not be transmitted to our domestic animals; the glanders to the bovine family; pleuro-pneumonia to man, or most other animals, and so on of numerous other diseases; while rabies is the most generally infectious of all contagious diseases, passing to nearly all warm-blooded animals. Foot-and-mouth disease is, again, very general in its ability to infect the various species. Man has a far greater receptivity to the contagious diseases of animals than they have to those of man.

The carnivora possess a very slight degree of receptivity to anthrax, while birds and fowls are said not to possess any in a natural condition. Pasteur has endeavored to show, and has, in fact, apparently experimentally proved, that it is the high temperature of fowls, 42° C., which is the cause of this immunity to anthrax infection. Normally the bacteria do not develop in their organisms, but, when he cooled their bodies off artificially, they did develop, and the fowls died.

I can not accept these conclusions, and think the immunity of fowls must rest upon something else than their high temperatures, for we know that a temperature of 42° C. is not at enmity with the life of bacteria.

At the time that the above-mentioned experiments of Pasteur came out, I was myself busy in the experimental study of bacteria, particularly bacillus anthrax. In the disease itself in cattle, sheep, horses, and rabbits, the temperature frequently rises above 42° C.; then why do not the bacteria cease to develop, and the animals recover?

I have frequently inoculated sheep that had a normal temperature of 42° C., yet the bacteria developed and the animals died. Successful reinoculations were also made from them. I have inoculated horses suffering from influenza and pneumonia that would surely have ultimately recovered, with a temperature of 42° C. or more, yet the animals died from anthrax, and a plentiful development of bacteria took place.

The above condition is what is called "natural immunity."

We have also what is known as "acquired immunity."

A person who has once had the measles, whooping-cough, scarlatina, variola, etc., seldom has the disease a second time. Exceptions do not contradict the validity of a rule, though they would a law of nature. The same is true of pleuro-pneumonia.

Another form of acquired immunity is that produced by inoculation, as in variola, pleuro-pneumonia, and, according to Pasteur, in chicken-cholera and anthrax. By this procedure the artificial production of a mild form of the disease is able to prevent natural infection. According to Pasteur, we have a still more striking phenomenon in anthrax.

His experiments led him to affirm that the inoculation of animals with a virus which has been attended by a certain series of artificial cultivation, made in a peculiar manner, was capable of preventing the eruption of the diseases when inoculated with blood of a most virulent character.

He says: "Fifty sheep were placed at my disposition for inoculation. Twenty-five of them were inoculated with a known virulent material, and twenty-five were vaccinated with a prepared attenuated virus. The first twenty-five all died. Two weeks subsequent to the vaccination the other twenty-five were reinoculated with a virus of known malignancy: they all resisted infection. (This subject is of the greatest importance, but governmental support is necessary before we can thus advance the science of preventive medicine in this country.)

Again, there is a species of acquired immunity of another kind. It is known that syphilis is slowly becoming less virulent among the people of the civilized world. We are less open to infection, and the disease is not so malignant. People acquire a certain degree of immunity against the poisonous action of certain drugs, by gradually increasing the amount taken, as illustrated both by the sick-bed and by acquired habits in the use of opium, arsenic, or even those luxuries tobacco and alcohol.

The first cigar makes us sick, but finally we can smoke all day. So it is with alcohol: we can gradually adapt ourselves to larger and larger quantities.

To my mind there is but one explanation to all this, and that of a very philosophical (i. e., theoretical) nature, although we have observations and experiences in the natural world which serve to confirm our theory.

The two great forces which Darwin claims have exerted an influence upon the changes that centuries have produced in the forms and characters of any species of animals, are—

1. The struggle for existence.
2. The gradual adaptation to natural conditions and surround-

ings, by which are meant food, air, water, temperature, climate, etc.

These two influences have tended to fasten upon a given species certain characteristics which become transmissible or hereditary.

The struggle for existence leads to the survival of the fittest.

We have already said that in all life this struggle existed. It exists not only between all members of the same species, inclusive of man, but also between the cells which make up our organs. In the battle for nourishment, only those cells which are best adapted, from their chemical and physical characteristics, to their specific work, survive; the others perish. The worn-out are continually replaced by the new. It is so in all life.

By contagious or infectious diseases we have learned, to our satisfaction, that a living organism enters the animal body. Being a living organism, it must naturally seek for the necessary constitueuts to its nourishment within the organism, or else it must die. Where it does not find it, it causes no infection; with its inability to procure it, the disease caused by it must cease.

We have learned that the life of the foreign organism is dependent on most of the elements of nourishment upon which the life of the animal organism, as a whole, or its individual parts, the cells, depends. The red blood-cells enter into a struggle for existence with the bacteria for that life-gas, oxygen; the various other cells of the body for the different chemical constituents necessary to their life, the sum total of which constitutes the life of the infected organism.

In this struggle, one or the other must win. If the cells are the stronger, the bacteria perish, and the animal or individual infected lives. If the bacteria are stronger; if, added to their parasitic nature, they also produce chemical stuffs at enmity with autositic life, they are in a measure supported by an ally in their struggle with the cells of the body, and the autosite dies.

But, with reference to the immunity acquired, we have but one reasonable explanation, which is that, in some unknown way, the cells are enabled to withstand the influences of their parasitic enemies; they gradually acquire a nature which renders them insusceptible to further attacks—i. e., they adapt themselves to the influence exerted by the above-named poisons.

Like the habitual drinker or smoker, the cells are the same as the individual of which they are the component units: they become accustomed to the alcoholic poison.

So it must be in those cases where immunity follows vaccination or inoculation. The cells become accustomed to the material introduced in such small quantities, or it becomes so changed that it is robbed of sufficient of its deleterious characteristics, so that, while accustoming themselves to its action, they are still able to overcome it in the struggle for existence.

The continual infection of the human race with syphilitic germs for centuries has hardened the cells of the organism, so that they can better resist their attacks on exposure to infection. In the natural world, this acquired adaptability to circumstances exerts such an influence as to become strongly hereditary: may it not be so, in a less degree, with regard to some diseases? There seems to be no other reasonable hypothesis by which we can explain both the natural and acquired immunity which the animal species possess against certain forms of infectious diseases and poisons.

Summed up: Either the cells are strong enough to win in this struggle for life; or, in the struggle, they become, as it were, accustomed to such influences, and are no more open to the attacks of the germs; or they are overcome in the struggle, and the autositic or infected organism dies.

Anthrax in Man.

Pustula Maligna, Carbunculus Contagiosa.

The fact that this disease is transmissible to human beings should be known to every one. On account of the liability to infection of those having the care of anthrax-diseased animals, it is essential that the veterinarian, as well as the public, should have some knowledge of its deportment in the human organism.

Until recent years the disease has been looked upon by most medical writers as belonging exclusively to the surgical branch of medicine.

That the disease occurs in human beings was known to very early medical writers.

Etiology.

The idiopathic or spontaneous eruption of the disease must be strongly contradicted, especially as we have conclusively shown that such is not the case among animals.

There are no sufficient proofs that show that the disease ever occurs in man, except by direct inoculation from diseased animals, or their products.

Medical writings do not give any evidence that the disease ever occurs among human beings from the mere residence in notorious anthrax districts.

Man acquires the disease—

1. *By direct inoculation.* That is, persons acquire the disease whose occupations bring them in direct relation either with anthrax-diseased animals or their products.

The most dangerous procedures are phlebotomy, slaughtering, and skinning diseased animals. The infection is in general external, and we can generally find some wound or excoriation which made the atrium to infection.

2. *By the consumption of the flesh of diseased animals.* Excoriations or wounds along the whole extent of the digestive tract may be atria of the disease.

This form of infection is very rare, but a sufficient number of well-constituted cases have been recorded, many of them terminating fatally, to make the consumption of such flesh a forbidden article of food.

3. *By means of flies and insects.* Cases of this kind of infection have been far more numerous than the former.

4. Infection from man to man has been observed, but few cases have been recorded, however.

Those parts of the body upon which infection has primarily taken place are generally the uncovered (84 per cent, Virchow), such as the face, lower arm, hands and fingers, and neck; or, in other words, infection takes place most frequently in those parts naturally exposed to contact with infected material.

Summed up, we may say: Anthrax occurs most frequently in man in those places where it prevails to the greatest extent among animals, and among those whose manner of life brings them more or less intimately into relation with the diseased animals or their products—such as those employed at tanneries, wool-pulling establishments, and horse-hair factories.

The susceptibility to infection is less in man than in the larger domestic animals.

Man enjoys no immunity to secondary infection from having once had the disease.

(This seems to stand in more or less direct contradiction to the experimental results obtained by Pasteur and others.)

Symptoms and Course.

We will not go into detail, but shall simply consider the chief primary symptoms, such as we should observe in a groom, or a person in whom infection would be likely to take place, for the treatment of the disease is such that an accomplished veterinarian might sometimes be the means of saving either his own life or that of others by immediate action, in cases where the delay in procuring a doctor would be fraught with great danger to the infected person.

The period of incubation is seldom less than from four to seven days (though shorter periods have been affirmed), and never longer than from twelve to fourteen days. The first indications of infection are sensations of burning and itching, similar to the sting of an insect, upon the parts where infection took place. Such places appear as small, reddish flea-bite spots, with a blackish center. The spot at first swells, but rapidly becomes an itching nodule, upon the apex of which appears a reddish or bluish vesicle, which soon bursts and presents a dark-red base. The patient frequently destroys these vesicles by scratching before they come to maturity. The excoriated places become dry, brownish, or red, and scab over; a red or violet circle surrounds them, upon which small vesicles soon develop. These secondary vesicles contain a yellowish, reddish, or blackish fluid. The circle sometimes fails, but in general extends, becomes more and more tumefied, and the surroundings œdematous and very extensive.

It is not necessary to our purpose to extend these remarks further, but the detailed account of the symptoms of anthrax can be studied in any good work on human medicine.

The disease generally runs its course in fatal cases in from five to eight days.

The first phenomena of the disease after the consumption of the flesh of diseased animals generally appear very quickly: in six to eight hours. The patients complain of shivering, weakness, headache, or general sickness. Death frequently results in two or three days. Peculiar pustulous or carbunculous centers are frequently to be met with in the digestive tracts; transudations in the cavities of the body, sero-hæmorrhagic infiltrations of the loose connective tissues, glands, etc., in which as well as the carbuncles the characteristic bacteria may be found, as well as in all the capillaries of the body.

Beautiful microscopic specimens showing the bacteria may be prepared from the skin, kidneys, or other organs.

The diagnosis is comparatively easy where reasons for infection exist. The examination of the blood with the microscope should never be neglected, particularly of blood obtained from suspicious wounds or pustules, as the bacteria remain much longer locally confined than in animals.

Therapeutics.

The chief aim is prevention of infection, much of which depends upon the veterinarian instructing those exposed to the danger of infection as to the care of their persons and of animals that may have the disease. The danger which may arise from the bites of flies, and the necessity of keeping cadavers covered, and of care in handling them, should ever be especially emphasized.

The chief therapeutic interference consists in the thorough destruction of the local centers where infection has taken place with concentrated carbolic acid, or nitric or sulphuric acid. If the carbuncle is fully developed, it should be at once cut out and the wound thoroughly cauterized.

In inward infection by means of the digestive tract, appropriate doses of carbolic acid and quinine should be resorted to in unison with iron, wine, and other tonics.

Anthracoid Diseases.

This name has been given to a group of diseases in which the necroscopic phenomena are more or less allied to those of anthrax. They are unquestionably germ or infectious diseases, but differ from anthrax in wanting the specific bacteria of that disease in their course, and the clinical or intra-vital phenomena. These facts should ever be borne in mind in the nomenclature or classification of diseases.

In veterinary medicine we have never yet arrived at an individual independence, and our pathological anatomy is far more human than zoötomic. But, what is still more absurd, clinicians, and especially the authors of our books, both past and present, have given names to diseases of our animals because of some fancied relation in the clinical phenomena to human diseases. They have forgotten that the *cause* of a disease should ever have much to do with its nomenclature or classification.

What real relation have the diseases called measles or scarlatina of our animals to the diseases of that name in man? Not only are they pathologically different, but their cause is different.

The measles of the hog is the cystic form of an animal parasite. It is an invasive not an infectious disease.

To speak of scarlatina, or typhus, of the horse or any animal is equally absurd. There are peculiar infectious diseases of man due to specific causes which have never yet been known to exert any influence on animals. You might fill a stable with horses and with children having scarlet fever, but no infection would take place; or strew its floor with the alvine dejections of typhus patients, without causing infection of the horses.

Who ever saw the characteristic lesions of the Peyer's patches of human abdominal typhus in the horse or any animal?

The diseases which we will consider under the head of anthracoid are the so-called emphysema infectiosum (black quarter) of cattle, splenic or Texas fever, and the hog-cholera.

The disease which Roell calls typhus equina (purpura of Williams), and which he looks upon as *anthrax* or nearly akin to it, bears far more relation in its clinical phenomena to anthrax in man than to genuine anthrax in the horse, though it is unquestionably an infectious disease and not a consequential complication of the infectious pneumo-enteritis—influenza—of the horse, or strangles, as some veterinarians claim. It occurs as frequently idiopathically as it follows either of these diseases. In such cases they simply act as a purveyor or preparer of the equine organism to the action of a new inficieus.

Emphysema Infectiosum.

This disease, which is known to us as black quarter, from the peculiar color of sections of the muscles, or as Rauschbrand to the Germans, from the peculiar rustling which follows stroking the skin or cutting through the flesh of such animals, has quite a number of pathological phenomena in common with anthrax, and frequently occurs in the same localities. In its clinical appearances it is very different.

It is peculiarly a bovine disease; but I have had a case in a horse in Boston during the past year. I saw numerous cases of the disease among cattle during my studies of anthrax in the Bavarian mountains in 1878.

In the following remarks I shall mainly follow the description of the disease as given by Professor Feser, who with Bollinger has been the only one that has given any special study to it.

This disease of cattle has undoubtedly been known for a long time, but has always been looked upon as an abortive form or peculiar symptom of anthrax, no independent study of it having ever taken place until the two observers named paid especial attention to it. It occurs everywhere, but the Bavarian Alps are especially visited by it. It is not so much found in the hot months as anthrax, but in general occurs at about the same period. It is neither anthrax nor any form of anthrax.

Etiology.

Like anthrax, it is also due to specific infectious elements belonging to the same class of bacteria—the fission fungi. The bacteria of this disease are shorter and finer than those of anthrax, and do not end with the abruptness which is the characteristic of bacillus anthracis. They are also movable bacteria, while those of anthrax do not in general betray any motion. They multiply by spores.

Feser gives the following necroscopical description: "Distinct *rigor mortis* of the well-fattened cadaver. Visible mucosæ dark red. The left over-arm, the left shoulder and a part of the right, and the middle portion of both posterior limbs were much tumefied, and a distinct crepitation—rustling—was both to be felt and heard on passing the hand heavily over these parts. The axillary and inguinal lymph-glands were to be distinctly felt as hard nodes under the skin. The subcutis and tendinous aponeuroses were filled with a yellow, gelatinous infiltration in those places which were tumefied. The connective tissue in the vicinity of the large vessels was much thickened and infiltrated with a mass similar in appearance to the above. The muscles appeared in many places of a dark-red color—red infiltration—rich in blood, softened, emphysematous, crepitating, and of a peculiar sweetish, sickly odor. (This odor of the flesh in this disease is very striking, but can not be well described.) The blood which oozed out of the vessels was black, viscid, and tar-like.

"The above-mentioned lymph-glands were swollen, soft, and full of blood.

"The abdominal cavity contained a reddish-black, peculiar-smelling exudation. Peritoneum clean, lustrous, and smooth. In the vicinity of the kidneys was a tumefaction filled with a yellow, gelatino-hæmorrhagic infiltration. Omentum infiltrated here and there as above. The contents of the rumen soft, the epithelium, or rather the mucous membrane, frequently peeling off and attached to the ingesta. Reticulum filled with soft ingesta; epithelium intact, without injection of the vessels. Contents of the omasum firm. Abomasum filled with a reddish-brown fluid, the contents having a fetid odor; epithelium adherent; mucosa swollen, dotted with ecchymoses and hæmorrhagic infiltrations, or rather diffuse hæmorrhagic centers. At the beginning of the ileum was to be seen a very much contracted portion one decimetre long, of a diffuse dark-red color; the walls were thickened; the epithelium desquamated, and the underlying sinuses exposed. This portion of the intestine was filled with a blackish coagulum. Many other portions of the intestine were the seat of diffuse red infiltration and ecchymoses. The epithelium was loose and easily detached; the contents of the intestines in general of a yellowish-red color, creamy, and full of gas-globules. Nothing particular to be remarked in the large intestines. Rectum stained dark red in many places; fæces watery and green in color.

"The spleen was enlarged from two to two and a half times its normal size; of a dark-brown color outwardly; inwardly almost black, soft, and disorganized. Liver dark red in color, swollen, and full of blood. The blood was coagulated in the large hepatic vessels; kidneys, bladder, and testicles offered nothing very abnormal.

"The thoracic cavity contained a small amount of a sero-hæmorrhagic exudation. The left costal pleura presented ingested vessels, circumscribed red infiltrations and ecchymoses. Both lungs filled with blood, but contained air in all parts; here and there dark-red spots. The pericardial sac contained a small amount of clear serum (the normal quantity is somewhat less than a tablespoonful, about ten grammes); the muscles of the heart of a dark-red color, with here and there dark striations. The ventricles contained a considerable quantity of a dark, black-red fluid and some coagulum; yellow sero-hæmorrhagic infiltrations into retro-pharyngeal and laryngeal spaces.

"Microscopic examination:

"*a.* The blood from the heart contained, aside from the blood-cells, numerous micrococci and long, straight, and delicate *movable* bacteria, from 0·005 to 0·01 millimetre in length.

"*b.* The spleen contained the same parasitic objects in addition to its usual elements; also the ingesta.

"*c.* These bacteria were also numerously represented in the sero-hæmorrhagic infiltrations and the dark stained parts of the muscles."

Feser gives the following *résumé* with reference to his observations and experiments:

The disease known as Rauschbrand presents similar phenomena wherever it appears. The animals look as if the cutis had been blown up, and crepitation may be heard and felt on passing the hand over any such parts. The gas from these emphysematous tumefactions burns with a pale-greenish color.

The disease is confined to localities, and appears with varying constancy each year, causing with anthrax the chief losses of herdsmen. The disease appears especially in the summer and fall months.

Young animals are far more susceptible to it than old ones. In the latter it is a very rare occurrence.

The microscópic examination of the blood, flesh, etc., of the diseased animals allows us a view of the nature of the disease, for everywhere we find the same characteristic—movable, delicate bacilli and micrococci.

The disease, in all probability, must be looked upon as an acute putrid infection. Numerous facts seem to strengthen this view. Aside from the resemblance of the bacteria to those frequently found in putrid masses, we have the acute course, the complication of the lymph-glands and spleen, the textural decomposition, the development of gases, and its transmission to other animals by injection of its fluids into their organisms.

The necroscopical results following experiments with purely septic fluids are the same in general as those obtained in this disease.

The fact that similar bacteria are to be found in the surroundings of the animals—swamps, stable-fluids—makes it almost sure that this is due to infection from outward and the multiplication of the germs in the infected organism.

The disease is neither contagious nor is it of a transportable nature, and thus is strongly distinguished from true animal pests. Infection from animal to animal, or by means of vehicles, has never been proved. The diseased animals come as isolated cases in the midst of numerous others, both in the fields and stables. Sometimes several cases may occur among a herd; but then they have been exposed to the same external causes, and of the herd are those in which the inner condition renders them susceptible to infection.

This predisposition to the disease must be especially emphasized, otherwise we are utterly unable to explain why it should only occur in young animals, and of these the best developed and conditioned are in general the ones to become affected, while the remainder of the herd are subjected to the same feed, and exposed to like external conditions. The flesh from such animals has and retains an alkaline reaction, while normal flesh soon acquires an acid reaction.

The therapeutic treatment of animals having this disease has so far been entirely useless. Carbolic acid, and external cleansing and disinfection of the animals, should be tried, however.

Experience has proved that the meat from such animals *can* be eaten, if well cooked, with but little danger to the consumer; whether it is justifiable or not, is another question. If it is to be so used, the animals should be killed when first attacked, and the flesh cooked and eaten as soon as possible, as the meat soon suffers putrefaction.

Bollinger gives the following conclusions with reference to his study of the disease :

1. The disease is neither a form of anthrax nor of septic or putrid infection, but—
2. It may be considered as a mycosis of a most dangerous kind, which invariably terminates fatally.
3. The infectious elements may be either endogenous or ectogenous.
4. The disease, like anthrax, belongs to those forms which may be transmitted by the soil. It is not contagious.
5. The infectious elements are active when introduced into the subcutaneous tissues, but also when introduced into the digestive tract.
6. The disease can be experimentally transmitted to cattle, sheep, goats, rats, and mice, though cattle become *only* infected in a natural way upon enzoötic outbreaks.
7. Bollinger gave it the name of "emphysema infectiosum."

We have now come to the consideration of a disease of the bovine family which seems to be essentially American in its nationality, the—

TEXAS, SPANISH, OR SPLENIC FEVER.

I wish it were possible for me to refer to a really reliable report or description of this disease. My own studies have been made upon the report of John Gamgee to the Commissioner of Agriculture of the United States, on animal diseases, and published in 1871.

I wish it were possible for me to say one single word in favor of this report. It is a disgrace to the veterinary profession, to the man who wrote it, and to the Government which published it. It is a miserably arranged, illogical, and erroneous production. Symptoms, definition, and periods, are mixed up, and there is no connection between the parts. The pathological anatomy is simply abominable, and one which I should be ashamed to have a student produce.

History.

An attempt at the history of the disease is made by another than Gamgee, but is of such a quality that we do not need to refer to it.

Definition or Nature of the Disease.

Gamgee says, "It is a disease peculiar to the bovine species, which has never been described as attacking Southern cattle, and which occurs in a more or less latent form among them."

I admit my inability to comprehend the above language. Even though a disease appears among a certain species of animals in a "latent" form, it still attacks them, and we know that it does attack the cattle of Texas, or it would not have received its name of Texas fever.

Texas fever should be described as a peculiar infectious disease of cattle, due to some unknown inficieus, undoubtedly of a bacterial nature, which for its primary generation is dependent upon special localities, climatic and telluric conditions.

With reference to its "latent" or mild character among the cattle native to the localities where it originates, it exactly corresponds to the rinderpest of Europe, which appears in just such a form among the cattle which graze upon the places where it is said to originate, viz., the vast steppes of Russia. It also bears some resemblance to this disease in its clinical phenomena, as well as pathological, but differs from it in not being strictly contagious, that is, passing from animal to animal.

I have been unable to find anything in this report regarding the influence of the infected localities upon new stock imported from other places to them.

It is like anthrax or black-quarter in that it is confined to locality, and some pathological phenomena, viz., the enlarged spleen.

Gamgee says further: "It is, so far as we have ascertained, incapable of communication by simple contact of sick with healthy animals; and, in the strictest sense of the terms, *is neither contagious nor infectious.*"

That it is not contagious, there seems to be unquestionable evidence, for we read that when Texan cattle are put in a pasture, and merely *separated* by a fence from other cattle native to these places, that the latter do not acquire the disease. But that it is not an infectious disease is quite another question.

That it is not an infectious disease as a contagious disease is, we freely admit; but that it is an *infectious disease of a very malignant type we positively assert.*

In this regard it is very interesting to note that it exactly corresponds with an infectious disease of man, which is bound on nearly the same localities—viz., yellow fever.

While the nature of this disease is still a matter of grave discussion, all authors unite in looking upon it as malignantly infectious, still the greater majority deny that it is also a contagious disease.

Like Texas fever, the yellow fever is confined to localities, upon moist regions, and a hot climate for its generation. By south and west winds its ravages extend, while the cooler winds of the north and east seem to check them; and in a northern climate it does not prevail, or dies out of itself. The same is the case with regard to Texas fever: the famous "northers" of the Texas plains having the influence of checking or putting an end to its ravages, and it dies a natural death in a northern climate.

The yellow fever, again, takes a milder or latent form among people indigenous, acclimatized to the climate and telluric influence, as does Texas fever among cattle; some races, as the negro, are said to be almost exempt from its ravages.

Naturalized persons, once having had the yellow fever, acquire a certain degree of immunity from a second attack, which they lose, however, if they leave such regions for a time and then return to them.

Our "report" does not tell us whether Texan or naturalized cattle acquire such an immunity from second attacks of the Texas pest. Provided susceptibility to infection exists, the inficieus of yellow fever enters the human organism and causes the disease. They are said *not* to reproduce themselves (?) in the infected organism, but to act directly; they do not pass from one organism to another—contagion.

They retain, however, their infecting power a long time, when once infesting a vehicle, and are highly transportable, either by means of the sick, or ships, etc.

Our National Board of Health has given a great deal of attention to this disease, and reports that it is a locally-generated infection, and looks upon the inficieus as some at present unknown form of bacterial life, which it hopes yet to discover, and then to be able to prevent its action.

This Texas fever exactly corresponds to the above, and it is no less the duty of our Government to spend time and money in searching for its cause, than it is to study the same with regard to yellow fever.

Gamgee says the disease "*is not infectious, in the strictest sense of the term.*" We assert the contrary, and will quote his own testimony in proof of our assertion, and to show the utter fallacy of his words, which will sufficiently indicate the weakness of his report. On page 87 he says: "Nevertheless, there are important data which indicate that, from the period of arrival of a Texan herd on any distant or any defined pasture, *five to six weeks elapse before the disease appears in the indigenous stock, grazing with or after Southern cattle.* It is proved that animals may simply pass leisurely over a road or prairie, feeding as they move along, and, without remaining for any length of time on any portion of the ground they traverse, *leave behind them a poison sufficient to destroy all, or nearly all, the cattle which continue to feed upon it.*"

He then goes on to give cases illustrating this statement.

On page 88, he says: "At Tolono the largest body of Texan cattle arrived toward the end of May, and the disease broke out (in the native stock) on the 27th of July. One gentleman of Tolono gave accommodations one night to three hundred Texan steers, on the 25th of June, and the disease appeared among his own stock on the 28th of July. In Champaign County, Texan cattle were placed on the prairie on the 15th of June, *and the indigenous stock began to die* on the 3d of August, twenty out of thirty-eight head dying in four days."

"*Thus we see that thirty to forty days elapse between the placing of Texan stock on a pasture, and the manifestation of the disease to the stock-owners of the neighborhood.*"

If this is not being "infectious" in the extremest sense of the term, and to the full letter of the law, then I admit my utter ignorance of the philosophical use of language, and logical connection between cause and effect.

Still further, page 109, Gamgee says: "Near Homer, where there were 4,527 Texan steers, which had been driven to Broadlands, *and had communicated disease not only to cattle feeding on their trail, but also to a herd of Illinois cattle with which they mixed in reaching their destination.*"

Page 110: "That they" (the Texan cattle) "communicated the disease to a very serious extent is beyond all doubt. . . . At the time of my visit the mortality (among native cattle infected by Texans) was raging at its highest point, and men were busy from sunrise to sunset, skinning, digging graves, and burying."

The whole report is replete with such testimony. Further comment on our part is unnecessary.

If Professor John Gamgee does not consider the disease infectious, the people of many of our Western States seem to have come to quite the contrary opinion, for, in the renowned Scotchman's own words, page 124, "stringent laws have failed to avert the most disastrous and wide-spread losses, and while, on the one hand, persons interested in the Texan trade have justified their inattention to legal restrictions by declaring them one and all unconstitutional, instances have not been wanting of mob-law adopting its own expedients. Dealers and farmers who owned Southern (Texan) cattle have been threatened; they have been pounced on in the dead of night, that they might surely be found in their homes, and there and then they have been requested to attend meetings of indignant and impoverished neighbors."

What more can I say? Surely mankind never makes restrictive laws, especially in this country, to prevent traffic in a harmless disease, nor do men go about tearing people from their beds on account of a "strictly non-infectious disease."

Etiology.

The cause of Texas fever has yet to be discovered. Gamgee says, "It is an enzoötic disorder" (another contradiction, for *enzoötic* itself implies some general cause, of an infectious or invasive nature), "due to the food upon which Southern cattle subsist, whereby their systems become charged with deleterious principles, that are afterward dispersed by the excreta of apparently healthy as well as obviously sick animals."

This is a very nice way of using many words to say nothing. Modern infection knows nothing of any such "deleterious principles" which work in this way. "Deleterious principles" means nothing. They might be chemical in their nature, which would be utterly incompatible with all our present ideas of infection. They might be gases, although modern observers do not accept gases as infecting material; gases they should be, to conform with the gassy nature of the report.

Stages of the Disease.

Gamgee speaks of four stages or periods of the disease, and yet he says it is not an infectious disease.

Pathology teaches that *only* infectious or contagious diseases deport themselves in this manner.

He speaks of—

1. The incubative stage.
2. The invasive stage (an infectious is not an invasive disease, this term being used with reference to the action of animal parasites; hence we should say the period of active infection).
3. The congestive or bleeding stage.
4. Termination.

I would classify the disease as follows:

1. Stadium incubationis.
2. Stadium accrementi.
3. Stadium decrementi.
4. Stadium lethalis; although I do not see the necessity of a fourth stage, as it is always but the final determination of the disease.

1. Stadium incubationis. The period of exact latency or incubation has not been accurately determined; it is not so well marked as in many other infectious diseases, but may be said to be from thirty to forty days.

2. Stadium accrementi. The period of active infection—i. e., the progressive stage of the disease—is first indicated by a rise in temperature. The temperature varies from 102° to 107·8° Fahr. This period extends to from four to seven days, and should also include the hæmorrhagic stage of Gamgee, which, according to him, lasts from two to six days longer.

3. The stadium decrementi is of indefinite length, but begins with the cessation of the progressive or active symptoms.

Intra-vital Phenomena.

The ears of the animal droop, its movements become sluggish, and the secretions retarded, especially in milch-cows. The appetite at first continues as well as rumination; a disposition to lie down soon makes itself apparent, and, wherever pools exist, the sick animals apparently seek them out to lie in.

Some observers assert that a cough appears early in the disease, but this does not accord with Mr. Gamgee's experience. Depression of the head, drooping ears, arched back, hollow flanks, with a tendency to draw the hind-legs under the body, and knuckling over in the hind fetlocks, are early and very marked phenomena. The skin appears dry and attached; the fæces are not materially affected, but in some cases clots of blood are attached to them. The urine is at first clear. Many cases do not attract notice until the animals are suffering from hæmaturia, but the urine retains its natural color in some ten to fifteen per cent of the cases.

The visible mucosæ are somewhat anæmic, but a hyperæmic condition may sometimes be observed, accompanied with a viscid discharge; the mucosa of the rectum is frequently congested.

The pulse is frequent; in the early stages hard and thin; it gradually becomes more feeble, and in the later stages, as death approaches, it is impossible to feel it. It varies from sixty to one hundred and twenty beats in frequency.

The thermometer is an invaluable aid in the diagnosis of this disease. The temperature is high at the commencement, but becomes reduced with the approach of death and hæmaturia. The temperature of the external parts of the body varies. Frequently the poll, ears, and extremities are very hot in the active stage of the disease. At other times they are cold, particularly the posterior extremities.

The respirations frequently rise as high as one hundred per minute; but in the comatose condition they are slow, deep, and labored.

The nervous phenomena are very marked. Trembling of the muscles of the posterior parts is very frequent, as well as of the neck. Weakness of the limbs, particularly the posterior, is very common, so that many animals are unable to rise, or, if they get up, walk with a feeble and tottering gait.

Listlessness and stupor indicate the approach of the end.

The state of the secretions is usually indicatory of the course of the disease. Perspiration is much restricted; œdema of the cutis is quite frequently met with.

The urine naturally contains albumen in large quantities when hæmaturia is present. The milk secretion is almost if not entirely suspended.

Termination.—In most cases the depression increases; the pulse becomes more feeble and accelerated, the respiration labored, and the temperature falls to 100° or 98° Fahr., and the patient becomes outstretched upon the ground and dies without a struggle.

In rare cases the febrile symptoms subside, the secretions again become active, the urine clearer, and the patient recovers in a few weeks.

Gamgee has seen animals apparently recovering, and again the febrile symptoms with diarrhœa have appeared, and they have died within thirty-six to forty-eight hours.

Post-Mortal Phenomena.

"That form of splenic fever which is most latent and seen among Southern cattle is not recognizable after death by the condition of the skin, muscles, or in many cases even by the mucosæ, with the exception of that of the stomach."

The spleens and livers are enlarged to a more or less degree.

On removal of the skin, hæmorrhages and serous infiltrations are sometimes found beneath the lower jaw and neck.

The muscular system is normal (?).

The organs of respiration are in many cases healthy.

The mouth, pharynx, and œsophagus are always healthy. The rumen is generally found full of food and its coats healthy.

The reticulum has often been found the seat of red imbibitions.

The omasum is almost invariably in a healthy condition.

The abomasum, on the contrary, is almost always the seat of distinct and pathognomonic changes. It is often found of a pink or dark-red color. The pyloric end is more commonly of a natural color. Minute ecchymoses are frequently to be seen studding its surface. Erosions of the epithelium are common. The duodenum is often of a deep-red color; sometimes its mucosa is deeply tinged with bile; ecchymoses are frequently met with.

The jejunum is frequently reddened, and circumscribed hæmorrhagic centres are often to be seen. The cæcum is often the seat of extensive ecchymoses; in the colon the same. The rectum is often the seat of extensive hæmorrhages; the liver of fatty degeneration, congested, and heavy.

(I will here state the gall-ducts are filled with gall, and that the microscopic examination of the liver often reveals a most beautiful condition of natural injection of the gall-capillaries, though no microscopical examination of tissues or organs seems to have been made in this report.)

The gall-bladder is usually found distended and filled with a viscid fluid.

The spleen is uniformly enlarged, and weighs from two to ten pounds. Its pulp is soft and degenerated, and oozes over the cut surface. The kidneys are perfectly healthy (?), but are most commonly of a dark brown-red color from intense congestion.

In the majority of cases the bladder is found filled with bloody urine.

No marked changes are found in the nervous system, except in those cases where paresis exists, when hæmorrhages may be seen in the cord of the lumbar region of varying extent. The dura and pia are sometimes the seat of ecchymoses of variable extent.

Microscopic Examination.

As we have said, no microscopical examination of the tissues or organs appears to have been made. Neither germs nor anything abnormal seems to have been found in the blood; but I am entirely dissatisfied with this part of the report.

Treatment appears to be useless, yet quinine in large doses and carbolic acid in appropriate doses should be tried in case of valuable cattle, and purgatives are certainly indicated in certain conditions of the disease.

Prophylaxis.

In reference to Texas, or wherever this disease originally appeared, we are as yet in such ignorance of its true cause that we can not well speak of successful means of prevention.

It would seem that the same rules which are applicable to anthrax and kindred diseases—as to draining the land, etc.—should be of value here.

The trade in Texas cattle should be regulated by national laws, so that no contact between them and natives could possibly take place.

The disinfection of rail-cars, stock-yards, the proper isolation of pastures on which such cattle had been grazed or unloaded for a period of at least two months from the time the last Texans were upon them—all these measures are indicated by the report which we have just considered; and, lastly, our present knowledge is as yet so imperfect with regard to this disease, and the losses the country yearly incurs from it so extensive, it is surely indicated that our Government should institute further researches in regard to it.

THE DOG.

WE have previously considered some of the most direful influences exerted by certain diseases of swine and cattle, or their products, upon the human race, and have now to consider some of the dangers to which we are subjected by that faithful companion of man, not to be less highly prized but more carefully watched—*the dog.* It is very doubtful if mankind truly appreciate these dangers, threatening not only their health but their lives in too many instances; and especially is this true of the dog. One of the most disturbing forms of parasitic invasion is derived in some unknown way from the dog.

Tænia echinococcus is the name which has been given to the smallest tape-worm yet found infesting animal life, being about four millimetres long, and consisting of but three sections or proglottids. The scolex, or head, is marked by a prominent rostellum, or crown, and armed with from thirty to fifty hooks, placed in two rows around the base of the rostellum. This parasite, in its mature form, makes its home in the superior (anterior) part of the intestinal canal of the dog, where it is sometimes met with in such numbers that one could hardly believe the mass before him was made up of countless examples of this tænia. They frequently give rise to most severe disturbance to the canine organism, the animal demonstrating such furious phenomena that they have been mistaken for those of rabies. This tænia, or rather its cysticerc (embryo) form, gains access to the human organism, as well as that of many animals, as the horse, cattle, sheep, and swine, and gives rise to the development of enormous cysts or sacs, sometimes multilocular or compound, seriously disturbing the invaded organ.

Examples of invasion among human beings have been met with among the inhabitants of nearly all countries, but most notably among those of Iceland, where, according to Thorstensen, every seventh inhabitant serves as an autosite (host) for these pests.

These cysts have been found in nearly all organs. Bollinger gives the following percentage of invasions among the different organs of the human body, taken from 252 cases:

In the liver	176 times.
" " kidneys	3 "
" " spleen	2 "
" " abdominal cavity	54 "
" " lungs	7 "
" " head	4 "
" " mammæ (breasts)	1 "
" other places	8 "

Of 9,703 autopsies, made at different pathological institutes, echinococcus cysts were found as follows:*

Berlin	from	4,770	autopsies,	33	cases.
Dresden	"	1,939	"	7	"
Göttingen	"	639	"	2	"
Erlangen	"	1,755	"	2	"
Zurich	"	400	"	0	"
Rouen	"	200	"	6	"
Total		9,703	"	51	"

Naturally, the great aim with reference to this parasite, as of all others, *is prevention. This consists entirely in keeping dogs in their proper places*—in absolutely disdaining all those disgusting familiarities which are only too frequently indulged in by lovers of ca-

* Bollinger, "Zeitschrift für Thiermedicin," vol. iii, p. 44.

nine pets, such as sharing bits of cake, bread, or other articles of food, drinking from a common glass, allowing them to lap one's face, or those of children.

Rabies of the Dog.

It would be fortunate indeed for the human race were this parasitic disease the only one to which they were liable from their canine friends.

Of all the diseases, however, to which our poor humanity is liable, there is not one which so calls upon our deepest sympathies as that derived *from the bite of a rabid dog*, known as lyssa, rabies, hydrophobia. (This last name should be dropped, as it is based upon the misleading and erroneous opinion *that rabid dogs are afraid of and shun water. Numerous observations have been, however, recorded*, by competent observers, *of rabid dogs crossing streams of water, and attacking animals upon an opposite shore.*)

The disease in man has been known since the early days of the Christian era. It does not seem to have been known to Aristotle, for he says: "Dogs are subject to rabies; it makes them mad; all animals that they bite also become mad, with the exception of man." The validity of this last passage has been questioned. The disease in man can be said to have been unknown, at least undescribed, before Aristotle. It is doubtful if Hippocrates described it in the dog. Up to the time of Celsus, A. D. 200, we still find no description of it: it is in his writings that we find the word "hydrophobia" first appearing. The views of the writers of the third and fourth centuries (Plutarch, Pliny, Cælius Aurelius, and others) were adhered to, and but little enlarged upon, by medical authors as late as the sixteenth century.

As nearly every one knows, and as every one should know, rabies of man *is a disease which owes its genesis solely to the bite of a rabid animal, more especially the dog, and is an acute infectious disease, having an invariably fatal termination.* The disease in man has been artificially communicated to animals by inoculation, but transmission from man to man has never yet unquestionably taken place.

As said, mankind in general owes its infection to being bitten by a rabid dog: it has been statistically estimated that 90 per cent of the cases of human rabies are due to this source, while from other animals it has been estimated that 4 per cent have been due to bites from rabid cats, 4 per cent from wolves, and 2 per cent from foxes.

"Of 796 human beings that died from rabies in France, Würtemberg, and Milan, 716 owed their infection to the bite of rabid dogs, 30 to that from cats, 31 of wolves, 19 of foxes, and 1 to that from a cow."

As regards that part of the human organism which has been most frequently bitten, Bollinger further says that, in 495 cases, 263 = 53 per cent, were bitten upon the superior extremities, hands and arms; 110 = 22 per cent, upon the head and face; and 14 = 3 per cent, upon the lower extremities. The bites upon the face appear to be accompanied with a greater percentage of mortality than those of other parts of the human body. An interesting yet horrifying example of the devastations and suffering which may be caused by a single rabid dog is given by the German veterinarians Oemler and Guenther:

"In December, 1871, the dog of a butcher showed indications of being rabid. It was confined in a stable, where it tore in pieces a goat and two geese, and finally freed itself by gnawing through the stable-door. Before morning, it had bitten several dogs in the village, and then commenced roaming over the country, passing through villages, and in thirty hours encompassed some thirteen German or fifty-two English miles before it was shot. On its way it bit many living things. The people of the villages became terribly frightened, from the fearful tendency to bite shown by the infuriated beast. Nine persons coming out of a church were sprung upon and terribly bitten, one of them, a woman, to such a degree as to necessitate conveying her home in a wagon. In all, fifteen persons were bitten by this dog, mostly upon the head and face; of these eleven died of rabies." (Bollinger, *loc. cit.*, p. 574.)

It is highly probable that dogs can communicate this disease in the earliest stages of its incubation, even before any very striking phenomena of illness may betray themselves. This seems amply sufficient to explain those cases of rabies in man which have followed the bites of dogs in which no suspicious phenomena had been observed, and which has led to the erroneous opinion that, if a dog afterward "goes mad," the person bitten by it will also "follow suit," and which has also led to the serious mistake of the immediate killing of the dog. In this regard I once knew of a singular case of superstition. A coachman in one of our leading families of Boston kept quite a number of bull-terriers, and indulged in fighting them: he was engaged one day in the so-called "training" of one of them, when the dog accidentally bit the man's hand. Like most of this class of persons, the man was strongly superstitious with reference to the bite from a dog: he had heard that a sure means to prevent himself from ever becoming mad was to cut the heart out of the living dog and bind it, split open, upon the bitten part. The dog was muzzled, triced up, and the heart cut out and applied as described. As the man had not become "mad" at last accounts, he probably thinks that his "cure" was effectual.

A few cases have been recorded of persons becoming infected from non-suspected but already infected dogs licking parts of their persons which were wounded, or where veterinarians have been made victims of their devotions to their studies, at a time when they had abrasions upon their hands, by making autopsies of dogs dying of rabies. About 50 per cent of the persons bitten by rabid dogs die from this horrible disease. Of 855 cases, 399 died. If we take, however, the bites which have resulted from suspected animals, and add them to the above, the percentage is reduced to about 8 per cent. Of 1,362 bitten by rabid and suspected dogs, 105 died.

The importance of the value of cauterization of wounds caused by the bite of a suspected or rabid dog is well shown by statistics given by Bollinger, page 618:

"Of 195 deaths from rabies in France between 1850–'62, 111 were not cauterized at all, 45 too late, and 39 insufficiently. Of 200 human beings bitten by rabid dogs, 134 were thoroughly cauterized; of these 92, 69 per cent, remained healthy, and 42, 31 per cent, died from rabies. By non-cauterization of the wounds in 66 cases, the mortality was 55, 84 per cent. *Consequently, while after cauterization of the wounds made by the bites from rabid dogs, scarcely two sixths (31 per cent) of the persons bitten die, by the neglect of this simple process five sixths (84 per cent) have terminated with death.*"

With relation to bites of clad or unclad parts of the body, we find the percentage of mortality for the face and head as 90 per cent; for the hands, 63 per cent; for the body, 63 per cent; for the lower limbs, 28 per cent; for the superior, 20 per cent. As to sex, we find 60 per cent ascribed to males, and 40 per cent to females.

The consumption of the flesh and milk from rabid animals has been found to be without harm to human beings.

The percentage which the disease attains among human beings is dependent upon its extension among animals, especially among dogs. In Prussia, we find that the average deaths for fifteen years, 1820–'34, amounted to 71 yearly; in Austria, for eighteen years, 1830–'47, 58; in France, for twelve years, 1850–'62, 24–25 cases; in Bavaria, for five years, 1863–'67, 13·8 yearly; for the seven years between 1868 and 1875, 18 per year; in the district of Upper Bavaria, in 1875, 8 persons died of rabies. (Bollinger, *loc. cit.*, page 600.)

"Dr. Hermann, of St. Petersburg, gives quite an interesting paper on the 'Nature of Hydrophobia and its Treatment,' in the 'St. Petersburg medicinische Zeitschrift' for 1875. From it we learn that rabies is on the increase among the dogs of Russia, and consequently among human beings. From tables given by him it may be observed that, in 1863, the reported cases of rabid dogs were 8, suspected 7, while the number of people who perished from hydrophobia was only 3. From that year up to 1874 there has been a varying increase, until, in that year, 49 people were bitten by rabid dogs, 12 by suspected dogs, 74 by diseased dogs, and 268 by healthy dogs, while the number of people who died from hydrophobia was 8. Altogether, in twelve years, 2,724 people were reported as having been bitten by dogs, of which 1,895 were healthy, 103 suspected, 198 rabid, and 528 affected with various diseases. In St. Petersburg during that period, 25 people perished from hydrophobia, and 22 in the Oberhoft Hospital." *

The Registrar-General's report, of Great Britain, gives 74 deaths as taking place in England in 1874 from the bites of rabid dogs.†

Hydrophobia caused the death of 47 persons in England in 1875. The "Lancet" remarks: "It is an undoubted fact that hydrophobia has been increasingly fatal in England in recent years. The annual death-rate from this disease, to a million living, which, according to the Registrar-General's report, did not exceed 0·3 in the five years 1860–'65, rose successively to 0·9 and 1·8 in the two succeeding quinquennials, and further increased to 2 per million in 1875. In London six deaths from hydrophobia were registered, both in 1875 and 1876; and in the first twenty-nine weeks of 1877, ending July 21st, nine cases had already been recorded." ‡

Hydrophobia in France.

"It is one of the duties of a French prefect to give information of the particulars of every case of hydrophobia in his department; but, as may be supposed, these political servants very often neglect a matter which has so little party interest. For eight years, 1869–'77, only thirty-five out of eighty-six departments returned replies to the official inquiries. Of these, however, Dr. Proust, in his own name, and that of Professor Bouley, has recently issued an interesting report. Their statements show that only one half of the persons bitten by

* "Veterinary Journal," vol. ii, p. 216. † "Veterinary Journal," vol. iv.
‡ *Loc. cit.*, vol. v, p. 385.

rabid dogs, or other animals, escape hydrophobia. The number of deaths from this cause during a period of twenty-six years, according to their notes, was 740, or little less than 28 per annum. More men than women were bitten, but sex made very little difference in the mortality. The liability to be bitten by young persons of from five to fifteen years of age was found to be greater than that of their seniors, though the fatality of the bite was not so great, not more than one fourth, while among aged people, from sixty to seventy, it amounted to two thirds, and above that age to three fourths. Children, therefore, seem to be less readily infected by the poison, though their chances of meeting with the accident are greater.

"The animals reported as causing the bites during the twenty-six years were: Dogs, 707; wolves, 38; cats, 23; fox, 1; cow, 1; and the disease was pretty equally distributed over all seasons. Observations on the incubation of the disease show that in a large proportion of cases it declares itself within the first sixty days of the inoculation. Thus, out of 221 attacks, 139 occurred within three months of the bite, 54 between sixty and one hundred days, 21 between one hundred and one hundred and eighty days, and 3 at later periods. The disease lasted from one to fifteen days, the greater number of cases holding out about four days.

"Cauterization, either by actual burning or with butter of antimony, is generally resorted to by French surgeons. This remedy seems to have a great influence with reference to the effects of the poison. In a given number of cases duly operated upon, the mortality was only 35·7 per cent; while, out of 117 persons left to themselves, 96, or 82 per cent, died. Facts like these prove that the great evil is not the number of deaths, but the terror and anxiety caused to persons bitten by a strange dog.

"The moral is, somebody ought to be made responsible for every dog in the country." *

It would have afforded me much pleasure to give some statistics with reference to the extension of this disease among our own people for a period of years; but, unfortunately, we have not yet arrived at that stage of civilization when authentic statistics are critically gathered by the various State authorities, and in many States there are no State boards of health. Some day (may it come soon!) we shall have such, and the results acquired by the respective State boards will be published in a compact form by the National Board, in unison with the devastations caused by contagious and infectious animal diseases.

* "Veterinary Journal," vol. viii, p. 217.

Numerous cases have undoubtedly been reported in the various medical journals; but the time at my disposal has been so limited and interrupted by other calls upon it, that it has been impossible for me to pass them in review.

As has been repeatedly emphasized, rabies occurs especially in the dog, then in the wolf, cat, and fox; also in the jackal, hyena, badger, as well as in the horse, sheep, goat, swine, deer, antelope, and rabbit; but it is originally a canine disease. It is not definitely known when man first came to a realization of this disease among animals. Aristotle, 322 B. C., makes the first undoubted mention of the disease among dogs. Xenophon, Democritus, and others, also mention it. Hippocrates, 460 B. C., has not left anything in the writings which have come down to us to render it certain that he knew of the disease. Later authors, however—as Virgil, Horace, Ovid, Plutarch—seem to have been well acquainted with it. Celsus says: "When a wound resulting from a bite is not at once energetically treated, then follows *hydrophobia*, a most terrible evil, that permits of neither hope nor salvation for the person bitten. We should seek to withdraw the poison by means of dry-cupping, and, when possible, by firing, and, when that is impossible, by corrosion and bleeding."

Galen, 131–201 A. D., describes the disease as the most fearful known to man. As a prophylactic he mentions cutting out the wound.

From this time on, notwithstanding much was written upon the subject, little new was added to the knowledge of the ancient authors until the latter part of the last century and the first of this. There is still room for much work upon the subject.

This disease, like many others, seems to be wanting in characteristic pathological phenomena, while its clinical or intra-vital phenomena are so striking that he who sees them once in well-developed form will scarcely ever forget them.

The most important workers in this important field have been Chabert, John Hunter, Meynell, Youatt, Hertwig, Magendie, Bruckmüller, Bouley, Virchow, and many other eminent scientists.

The best work accessible to the American reader is undoubtedly the compilation of the English veterinary author, Mr. George Fleming, "Rabies and Hydrophobia," London, 1872.

Whatever may have been the historic origin of this disease, it like many other contagious diseases does not originate spontaneously, but in our day owes its origin to the bite of the rabid animal, especially the dog, and owes its extension to this means alone. It deserves repeating: *rabies does not arise spontaneously, it does not originate from nothing.*

All sorts of theories have been adopted and found numerous defenders, to sink again into oblivion. Among them may be mentioned the influences of extreme heat, extreme cold, want of water, domestication, training, confinement, too much ease and petting, but, most absurd of all, and consequently held to with religious respect, *non-satisfaction of the sexual desires.*

What has not been laid to this last cause by an absurdly ignorant and superstitious humanity?

Every form of mental or nervous excitement, superabundance of spirits, depression of spirits, poor appetite, a good appetite, too much desire for sleep, want of sleep, good spirits, evil spirits, ill temper, and about every ill which could be hypothetically connected with the sexual organs, has been attributed to abuse or non-exercise of their functions.

I by no means wish it to be understood that there is not a most intimate connection between the sexual organs and many nervous centres, but I must affirm that many of the things attributed to their influence is most absurd nonsense.

The medical profession seem not only too willing to support and favor this unfounded superstition, which has been nourished by man since history's beginning.

Man's selfishness has been fostered at the cost of woman's happiness and health, and the medical profession has done its part to support it.

One would think the science of comparative physiology did not exist, or that its teachings were a myth.

Blind fools seeking to lead an equally blind humanity! "Pluck the mote out of thine own eye before thou seekest to remove the beam from thy brother's eye."

Some day, when what Haeckel calls "physiogenie," or what I would prefer to call functio-genesis, or the genesis of the physiological functions, becomes a naked and cold-blooded part of comparative physiology, and is taught in our medical and public schools and described in our text-books, the world will learn and know that no functions are given to contribute to man's pleasure or selfishness; but that, when pleasure is united with the exercise of the physiological functions, it is for the proper action of those functions, and not for the sensual gratification of a conceited member of the animal creation. It may be axiomatically asserted, and it is time that mankind should learn it, *that man has no functions which he enjoys in common with the remainder of the animal world for any other purpose than they are made to fulfill in the lower animals.*

The doctrine, or rather the belief, in the superior position of man has been altogether too much extended. The pleasure united with the enjoyment of functions is an attribute, as I have said, to their physiologic action, and is no special gift to man.

Whoever heard of a person taking pleasure in eating with a severe toothache or a sore-throat?

The *pleasure of taste* is united to the functions of mastication, not that man *may enjoy* the blessings which the Lord has given him, but that the food may remain so long in the mouth that it may be made small, and the starch in it so much changed into dextrin and sugar as to fit it in part for absorption by the organs for that purpose situated deeper down.

This fact is not stated in any physiology written by man. The chemical changes are, of course, carefully delineated, but the "*words* between the lines" seem to have entirely escaped physiologists and medical men. Were this not so, did mankind and the ruminants and some other animals not take pleasure in mastication, they would bolt their food like a dog. Some men do!

A second axiom is, that where functions do not exist, or are rudimentary, either in individuals or species, certain anatomical, structural differences exist in such organs which, while we may not be able at present to demonstrate their existence, will surely not escape the observation of scientists in the future.

In this regard I hold that the organs of taste are either not developed or very rudimentary in the dog, which bolts its food, the sensation of emptiness (hunger) being uppermost.

It would be extremely interesting to ascertain if the organs upon which taste depends slowly atrophy and become rudimentary in human beings who have acquired this natural attribute of the canine family—that is, bolting their food.

To return to our subject.

Radi and Bourgelat subjected dogs to starvation in order to see if rabies would develop itself; but their experiments were followed only by negative results. Ménecier received similar results from subjecting dogs for a long-continued period to poor food and care. Pillwax, of Vienna, observed that a larger percentage of rabid dogs came from the homes of wealthy or well-to-do owners. As to the influence which has been hypothetically attributed to sex, the difference falls away when we consider for a moment the great disparity which exists between the number of male and female dogs. The same is true with reference to the supposed *favorable influences of castration.*

Schraeder gives the proportion of 267 cases of canine rabies at Hamburg, in the years 1852–'53, as 256 males, 10 females, and 1 castrated dog.

When we take into consideration the exceedingly high stage of development which is enjoyed by the nervous system of the canine race, and the great want of scientific knowledge with reference to the psychical diseases of the same, it does not appear strange that many diseases, the true cause of which must be sought in disturbances of nervous centres, have been, and still are, mistaken for rabies. Nearly every uneducated and casual observer would be excused, considering the want of knowledge on these points, if he mistook a series of epileptic attacks, or the phenomena caused by inflammatory processes in the brain or its meninges (the membranes inclosing the brain), for rabies. In the last case, the phenomena displayed would be sufficient to warrant the educated veterinarian to isolate and securely confine a dog in which they were present, so little is our knowledge upon this subject.

We will again repeat that rabies, like all other known contagious diseases, never generates spontaneously, *but through infection; that is, the inoculation or transmission of an infectious element from a diseased organism to a healthy one is absolutely necessary to the production of the disease.*

All theories with regard to the influences exerted by the seasons fall to the ground in the face of the facts collected by exact observation. Epizoötics of rabies are recorded from the icy fields of Greenland as well as from the sunburned sands and arid tracts bordering on the Mediterranean Sea. Scarcely a land seems exempt from its devastations; but it does not appear, as yet, to have extended to Australia, New Zealand, and some portions of Africa, Germany, France, Holland, Northern Italy, and of late England especially.

Bollinger gives some interesting statistics with reference to several eruptions of canine rabies on the Continent:

"An epizoötic reigned at Hamburg, from 1851 to 1856; during this period 600 cases of rabid dogs were reported, while for twenty-three years previous not a single case had been reported. In Saxony, from 1853 to 1867, 807 cases have been recorded; an average of 160 per year. In a total of 275,000 dogs in Bavaria, for a period of five years (1863–'67), an average of 800 cases of suspected and genuine rabies were reported. For 1873, the total number of dogs reported in Bavaria was 292,000, and 821 cases of suspected and genuine rabies were recorded. In Vienna, from November, 1873, to August, 1875, 332 cases of canine rabies were reported.

While I have been unable to find any statistics of a similar trustworthy character for our own country, it is not without interest to know that "in 1860 we had 112,000 dogs *recorded* in Massachusetts; and further, that for the year ending May 1, 1875, 11,489 were reported as having killed sheep valued at $10,584.53." (Flint, "Massachusetts Agricultural Report," 1878.)

Notwithstanding the repeated publication of the phenomenology of canine rabies, still the subject is of such vital importance to every dog-owner, and to every citizen as well, that the more frequently it is repeated the better it is for the community at large.

Phenomena of Rabies Canina.

The wound occasioned by the bite of the rabid dog heals in general very quickly, leaving little or no indications of its presence behind, unless it has been quite an extensive laceration.

The smallest abrasion of the epidermis is sufficient for infection. This fact, in unison with the rapid healing of such wounds, sufficiently explains those cases which have been frequently quoted in proof of the spontaneous generation of this disease, where rabid dogs have died or been killed, and then been most carefully shaved, and not the slightest indications of a wound of the cutis could be found.

The period of incubation—that is, the time which elapses between the bite and the appearance of the first suspicious phenomena—extends, in general, to from three to five weeks; sometimes it extends to as many months. In the other domestic animals the period of incubation varies from two weeks to ten or even fifteen or sixteen months.

As should be well known to every dog-owner, rabies canina presents itself in two forms: as furious, and as still or dumb rabies. It is not my purpose to enter into minute details with reference to this disease, but rather to endeavor to attract attention to the most prominent symptoms in which the disease manifests itself.

Writers have, however, divided the disease into three stages, and, as laymen might suppose that by these was meant three distinctly marked intervals, we will at once say that such do not exist, and that, while the periods may be said to mark different stages of development in the disease, yet these stages extend one into the other so imperceptibly that no intermissions are observable. All this dividing the phenomena of certain diseases into periods is more or less a matter of artificial classification, to suit the conveniences of the clinical teacher.

These three stages have been spoken of as—

1. The melancholic or initiatory.
2. The maniacal or irritative.
3. The paralytic or lame stage.

The first perceptible indication which is manifested by the bitten or infected dog would never lead one to suppose that the most fearful and dangerous disease known to man was in process of development in the favorite of the family.

It consists in little else than a change in the natural deportment of the animal.

This should be emphasized—*every change in the natural deportment of your dog should excite your suspicion,* and render you watchful and uneasy. No time should be lost, not only in confining your dog most carefully and securely, but in seeking the advice of the most skillful veterinary expert at your command. Among the chief initiatory symptoms are surliness, uneasiness, depression, moodiness, a continued desire for change of place, first in one corner, then in another; now *on* the sofa, then under it: if naturally morose, the bitten dog often displays a suddenly developed affectionate disposition; on the other hand, the generally affectionate dog becomes morose and suspicious, snappish and irritable. The most insignificant circumstance will set such a dog in a fit of rage. The eyes frequently give indications of the approaching tempest, the conjunctivæ or linings of the lids being injected or reddened; the eye itself having a peculiar, unnatural expression, which, to be realized, must be seen.

Even in the early part of its development *an abnormal appetite is often apparent, and is to be looked upon as one of the most characteristic symptoms of the malady.* The neat, delicate, and cherished pet of the family turns away from the usual loved tidbits, to fill its stomach with masses of filth, such as its own fæces, straw, rags, and the like.

The sexual functions are frequently abnormally irritated, which, has probably given occasion to the absurd theory with reference to the genesis of the disease previously considered.

Such animals are more or less resistant to attempts at control, and the once true and trustworthy house-dog, or the inseparable lady's companion, suddenly develops a most marked desire to get away from the favorite door-step, or the handsome rug, and to run off over the country.

The muscular movements soon begin to demonstrate a certain want of concord; they become uncertain, wavering, or weaker than usual.

Such dogs frequently lick the place where the wound causing infection has been, even gnawing it, as if it itched; but a far worse enemy than fleas is at the bottom of this trouble, and a more energetic remedy than "Persian Insect Powder," or great "Doctor Go-it-cure-all's Magnetic Enemy to Worms and Insects," is needed to rid the poor beast of its troubles.

Without any signs of intermission, but rather with a gradual increase of these phenomena, is ushered in the so-called maniacal or "mad" period of the disease. Nearly all the previously considered phenomena are presented to us with a tenfold intensity. The whole external appearance of the animal becomes changed. The appetite is wanting; the once docile and affectionate dog is now a fiend incarnate, seeking to bite and tear all within its reach; the cheery bark of welcome, which once greeted the approaching master or mistress, is changed into an indescribable *howl*. The tendency to wander from home, or break away from its fastenings, is unbounded; the parlor pet seeks to get out, and the chained watch-dog bites and tugs at its chain in its endeavor to break away. If confined in cage, they bite and tug at the bars with the fury of a maniac, which they, indeed, fully resemble. If, up to this time, the unfortunate dog has displayed more or less respect for the master's presence and voice, it now begins to know him no more, although some cases are recorded where the ties of affection have even ruled, in a measure, such a canine maniac until life was almost extinct.

Once free, they do not pursue any regular course, as if following some intellectual perception, but roam here and there, often returning home, and behaving like disobedient children, afraid to face the owner's displeasure.

According to the previous nature of the dog is its inclination to bite during this period of the development of the malady, some being more dangerous in this regard than others. The slightest irritation, such as the presence of a stranger, another dog or animal, the presentation of a stick, is sufficient to set such a dog into a paroxysm of rage; these paroxysms decrease in severity as the dog becomes exhausted by disease.

Such animals seem frequently, like the human maniac, to be gifted with supernatural strength and energy. Chains thought to be unbreakable are ruptured as if made of straw; walls or fences thought to be unscalable are easily sprung over; barn-doors or partitions so solid and thick that escape is thought to be impossible are easily gnawed through, and an infuriated fiend becomes loose to prey upon the community and the balance of the animal world. *Hydrophobia, or fear of water, is never seen in the dog,* public opinion to the contrary. During my stay at the Royal Veterinary Institute of Berlin, I had quite a number of opportunities for observing rabid dogs, and have frequently seen them bury their noses in the dish of water in their cages, in their vain attempts to drink, which the paralytic condition of the muscles of deglutition rendered absolutely impossible.

As all severe exertions must have an end, so in this disease these maniacal phenomena gradually pass over into those of the paralytic form; the paroxysms slowly become weaker, and the remissions less and less perceptible.

The suffering and pitiable animal has become greatly emaciated; the once lustrous coat dull and staring; the plump and rounded flanks sunken; the bright and intelligent eye becomes dull and expressionless; the tongue protrudes from the mouth, appearing more like half-dried leather than a normal tongue.

Slowly but surely the weakness extends over the organism. The gait becomes weaker and weaker; the hind-legs waver from side to side, until finally, overcome by weakness and paralysis, the animal sits before you, a picture never to be forgotten.

Some lie as if overcome by sleep, but, if irritated, will rise upon the fore-feet and seek to bite or snap at the irritating object.

The voice becomes hoarser and hoarser, the attempts to breathe are painful in the extreme to look upon, the pupil of the eye is distended, and all natural expression is lost.

Death closes the painful drama in from four to seven days, although in extremely rare cases the battle for life may continue to eight or nine days; never more than that.

The phenomena of dumb rabies are so similar to those of the paralytic form that I will refrain from describing them. The disease ushers itself in, in about the same way, but the initiative phenomena pass almost imperceptibly into those of the paralytic form.

This dumb variety, when once developed, is not so dangerous to mankind, or other animals, as the maniacal form: from the paralysis of the lower jaw, such animals are unable to bite; it is dangerous to mistake this paralysis for a bone in the throat, which is sometimes done; the fluids of the mouth are as sure to cause infection as those from a maniacal dog, if they come in contact with a wounded surface.

Prevention.

1. Reduce the number of dogs in each State to the lowest possible minimum, by means of a high and rigidly exacted dog-tax.

2. A quarterly revision of all the dogs owned in a State should be made by the police authorities, and *all dogs*, of whatever age, sex, or character, found without a license number and tag upon their collar for the time in question, and not an old tag, should be peremptorily killed at a time fixed by law, unless a license is at once procured.

3. All dogs found running loose without an appropriate collar and tag should be peremptorily killed.

(*a*.) The police should have power to kill, and not authorized "dog-killers," who, as experience has taught us, are more apt to be "dog-*stealers*" than faithful public servants.

4. In every city, town, or village, there should be, not a pound, but an animal quarantine, where animals in which contagious or infectious diseases were suspected could be quarantined, for a time fixed by law, and remain under the daily supervision of a competently qualified State veterinary official, no empiric.

To this quarantine should be sent every dog in which an abnormal inclination to bite has been observed, and especially and peremptorily every dog which had bitten a human being without justifiable cause. Here it should be caged and confined for a period of not less than five weeks, and at the expense of the owner. If the owner of such a dog will not pay the expense, then at the expense of the city, town, or village, in which said dog is quarantined; the dog or dogs in question, if found healthy at the expiration of such a quarantine, to be sold at public auction on account of said town, city, or village, or killed.

(*b*.) Too much stress can not be placed upon the value of this last clause to the community. No greater mistake can be made than at once killing a suspected animal which has bitten a person. The plan proposed, by ascertaining the real condition of the dog, will do more than any one thing to free the mind of a person bitten by a dog from the danger of hysteric rabies, and also free the minds of the community from an unnecessary and protracted anxiety.

5. These regulations should apply to all dog-owners, whether breeders or not, and no exception to them should be made, on promises of owners to see to them at home.

(*c.*) It is the safety and peace of mind of the community which are to be considered, and not the pleasure of individual dog-owners.

The technical supervision of competent State veterinary officials (in no case of empirics) is the only course which can guarantee any success and protection to the community.

THE HORSE.

Hippophagy, or the Consumption of Horse-Meat as Food.

Horse-meat steaks! Roast horse-meat!

It is really singular what feelings of aversion one finds immediately following upon the suggestion of such articles of food in this country. "Have we not beef, mutton, pork, and other articles of food in such an abundance that you need not bring up such a disgusting idea?" is the next remark.

The "disgust" in all these questions is simply based upon custom. That which is disgusting to the people of one country may be most commonplace or a luxury to those of another. So it is with periods; the tastes of different generations vary in other things than fashions.

Thus we see that hippophagy, or the consumption of horse-meat for food, was at one time an almost universal custom among the pagan people of Northern Europe and Britain. Being a pagan custom, it was but natural that, with the extension of Christianity among these nations, its missionaries should insist that not only religious rites, but other customs of these people, which they looked upon as relics of heathenism, should be given up. We find these efforts of the missionaries supported by edicts from the popes, so that the practice gradually became extinct, to be again taken up in the early part of our century, and to gradually extend, though the custom has never been without its adherents among the nations of the world.

We can think of no justifiable reasons for such aversion to horse-meat among our people. In fact, this aversion is based entirely upon ignorance, and its twin sister, prejudice.

That we have a sufficiency or even a superabundance of animal food in our country is of itself no justifiable reason for heedlessly sacrificing to the knacker a large amount of valuable food each year.

One sees upon our streets, at any time, a large number of horses much better suited for the shambles than for work. Poor men are often compelled, by a tyrannical law, the result of a sickly and gushing sentiment, to sacrifice to the knacker, who pays them nothing, horses that a few weeks' suitable feeding and rest would make worth forty to sixty dollars for meat. Hundreds of so-called weeds are yearly born and raised by farmers and breeders, to be at maturity simply objects of torture from their unfitness for work, that at four to six months old would pay a reasonable profit to the owner as horse-veal, for the expense of raising and breeding. While, so far as we know, no horse-meat is offered for sale in the markets or provision-stores of this country and Britain, it is fast becoming universalized among the cities of Northern Europe, as may be seen from the following:

For the first six months of the year 1877 the horse-butchers of Paris slaughtered 5,283 horses, donkeys, and mules; the same furnished 959,730 kilos (1,919,460 pounds) of flesh; while, for the same part of the year 1876, the number of animals of the same species which were used was 4,422, and the net amount of flesh sold, 803,500 kilos (1,607,000 pounds). In 1878 the number of horses and mules thus slaughtered was 11,319, while in 1877 there were 10,619, showing an increase of 700 head in one year.

Decroix,* a most enthusiastic hippophagist of France, says that "for some years hygienists and pathologists have been directing their attention to the progressive invasions made by tape-worms in the human species, and they have applied themselves to discover the cause of these invasions, and the means by which they may be opposed. Notwithstanding several very interesting works, some points are still controverted; but it has been demonstrated that we are attacked by the armed tape-worm, *tænia solium*, as well as the unarmed, *tænia mediocanellata*, or better, *tænia inermis*; that the germs of these entozoa are introduced into the intestinal canal of man by the flesh he eats; and, finally, that the armed tape-worm is derived from the pig, and the unarmed from the flesh of cattle and sheep. The former, says Dr. Cobbold, are found chiefly to infest people of the poorer classes, while the latter are more frequently found among the wealthy. It is well known that the larvæ of this parasite (*tænia inermes*) are derived from imperfectly-cooked veal and beef. M. Regnault has made the interesting remark that the number of armed tape-worms has not notably increased, while the unarmed worm has become more and more frequent. The certain cause of this frequency has been considered to be the therapeutic

* "Veterinary Journal," iii, p. 47.

employment of raw meat, nowadays very common; also the custom of eating it raw. The latter cause has not been sufficiently impressed upon the public.

"Beef and mutton, then, frequently contain, in addition to their nutritive principles, morbific germs, the existence of which is not apparent to the meat inspectors or consumers. In the first place, the custom of eating raw flesh must be abandoned; roasted flesh is generally well cooked, even burned externally, while in the interiors it is in many instances still raw. In the second place, when physicians have to prescribe raw meat, *the flesh of the horse* should be chosen in preference, *as it is more healthy and nutritive* than that of the ox, sheep, or pig. The horse, in fact, is not liable to those verminous affections which produce the germs of the different kinds of tape-worms of which the human body is the receptacle. Horse-flesh is *more digestible* than that of the other animals, which are prematurely and excessively fattened. It suits more especially weakly, anæmic, or chlorotic people, and those who undergo severe muscular exercise. During the first quarter of the year 1875, 1,821 horses were slaughtered in Paris for food; while, for the same period in 1876, 2,370 were used, an increase of 549."

Dr. Hugo Hertwig, the first assistant of the market-inspection bureau at Berlin, gives a very interesting account of the different equine-slaughtering establishments in that city and the regulations to which they are subjected. He says: "More than a thousand years have passed since our forefathers ceased to use this valuable article of food, which is principally due to the influence of Christian priests, and their desire to wean the people away from all relics of the heathenism in which they were supposed to have lived up to their time. Boniface III played an important part in this matter. Dr. Spinola, and a singer at the Royal Opera-House, Blume, played an important *rôle* in bringing it again into use. Notwithstanding much opposition, the consumption of horse-meat has gone on steadily increasing among the people, not only of Berlin, but other German cities. A most favorable influence was exerted by the order issued by the police president of Berlin, whereby a most exact control of the horse-meat market was ordained, and the quality of the meat offered for sale guaranteed to the people. The regulation of March 24, 1854, ordered: "That no horse could be slaughtered, under a penalty of a fine of five thalers ($3.75), before it had been subjected to veterinary inspection, and pronounced suitable for food." For this purpose, a legal certificate was given, which must be kept by the butcher, for a period of four weeks, and shown to the police officials at any time during that period. An improvement in this regard has been since introduced, by which all certificates of this nature are written in a book having prescribed printed forms, which are kept by each butcher, and are open to the police at all times.

"All places where horse-meat is sold must be made known to the public by an appropriate sign, and no other kind of meat can be sold from them. . . .

"The slaughtering of a horse, ass, or mule for human food can only take place at the slaughter-houses appointed for the purpose, and regulated by the Government."

The plan of the book for each butcher of horse-flesh to keep for reference is as follows:

1. Number of horse, mule, or ass killed.	2. Description of same, giving age, size, color, or other special points.	3. Date of inspection.	4. Name of butcher, with number of license.	5. Attest of veterinary inspector, with reference to hygienic condition of animal slaughtered.	6. Day of killing, or other disposal of animal.

It was of great benefit to the public when the numerous horse slaughter-houses were done away with, and a general one instituted for the city of Berlin, known as the Central Horse Slaughter-House.

The increase of the consumption of horse-flesh in Berlin is shown by the following figures:

1847..11	butchers	slaughtered	3,000	horses.
1853.. 5	"	"	686	"
1854.. 4	"	"	400	"
1855.. 4	"	"	700	"
1856.. 4	"	"	759	"
1857.. 2	"	"	367	"
1858.. 2	"	"	450	"
1859.. 4	"	"	443	"
1860.. 4	"	"	618	"
1861.. 3	"	"	519	"
1862.. 7	"	"	1,042	"
1863.. 7	"	"	1,307	"
1864.. 8	"	"	1,742	"
1865.. 8	"	"	2,142	"
1866..12	"	"	3,115	"
1867..17	"	"	2,911	"
1868..18	"	"	4,026	"
Total..............			25,226	"

"In Berlin, during the years 1877–'78, 4,739 horses were slaughtered for human food. Of these, 74 were condemned as unsuitable before slaughtering, and 89 after; of the latter, 20 were found infected with glanders. . . .

"In 1877 at Altona 1,442 horses were slaughtered, of which ten were given over to the knacker; of these, three were condemned on account of glanders, three suffered from pulmonary gangrene, and four from entero-peritonitis. The greatest number of horses are slaughtered in the winter months, their flesh being made into sausages." *

The central horse-slaughtering establishment of Berlin is a completely inclosed locality covering about an acre of ground, upon which is situated a two-storied building answering for the residence of the inspectors, and a bureau for the police officials; further, two stables for the horses destined to be slaughtered, and two large slaughtering-places with all necessary conveniences; and two smaller rooms, one for the hides of the slaughtered animals, and the other, to which only officials have entrance, for the reception of slaughtered but condemned meat, i. e., such as was proved to be unsuitable for consumption after the animal had been killed and dressed, but not such as came from animals having a contagious or infectious disease; further, for the examination of animals, a room having almost entirely glass sides, so as to give the greatest possible amount of light to the inspectors.

For such horses as on inspection demand the attention of the veterinary police, there is a special quarantine station, which is completely disinfected and cleansed every time it is used. The greatest cleanliness is observed in all parts of this establishment, special places being designated for the blood and other offal, and after each day's slaughtering each part is cleansed and disinfected under the supervision of the inspectors.

The following plan is carried out in the inspection of the animals:

Each morning, from nine to ten, the horses to be slaughtered are mustered for inspection, their breed and nationality, and all other results of an external examination, entered in the appropriate book. To this end notice is first taken of the external appearance of the animal, and then its temperature is carefully noted, to ascertain that the animal is absolutely without fever. On completion of this examination, the character of the respiratory phenomena, the visible mucosæ, the lymphatics and glands, the cough, etc.; only

* "Mittheil. aus der Praxis, 1877–'78," p. 97.

when all this is completed is the official permission to slaughter given. It is self-evident that only horses suitable for slaughter are brought forward for inspection, and not such as are hastily brought in. If, in a given animal, any suspicious phenomena are observed, which under other circumstances would scarcely be taken into consideration, a definite opinion as to its suitableness for food is withheld until the animal is slaughtered and dressed, which is done under the supervision of the inspector.

If a horse is found suitable for the purpose, it is at once slaughtered, otherwise its slaughter is peremptorily forbidden. The latter takes place in all infectious or feverish diseases, in emaciation, in all cachectic conditions, and in all animals having suppurating wounds. Animals not suffering from infectious diseases are allowed to be killed for knackers' purposes, a special certificate being filled out for this purpose. Horses, in which symptoms are observed suspicious of glanders, are either consigned to the quarantine station until a telegram is sent to the knacker, or are given back to the seller (of the horses), when due notice, by telegraph, is at once given to the proper veterinary police authorities.

To the honor of the horse-butchers, it should be mentioned that this seldom occurs; on the contrary, good horses are generally bought for this purpose, the butchers often making journeys of one hundred to one hundred and fifty miles to procure them, often buying from breeders young horses which from deformities or other reasons are not considered suitable for rearing. They often pay thirty or forty dollars for such horses, which makes evident the value of the business of horse-slaughtering to the community; for not only is a cheaper article of food, of good quality, offered to the people, but in case of a broken leg, or other misfortune, rendering a horse unsuitable for the work required of it, the owner frequently receives money enough to supply him with an animal suitable to his purposes; at least he does not suffer a dead loss, as is at present the case in this country, and frequently lame animals are thus relieved from torture, to the material benefit of the owner. In Vienna, similar conditions to those in Germany prevail, and the inspection and regulation of the traffic are carried on with the greatest circumspection.

The inspection which is exacted at the horse-slaughtering establishments should be extended to those where other animals are slaughtered.

Aside from the great benefit which the poorer classes of the community derive from having a cheaper meat than beef for food, is the great saving of material. Many horses are each year killed and sent to the knackers which, were hippophagy a custom in this country, would bring to the owners money enough to buy animals suitable for certain work. Horses condemned to death on account of broken limbs would not then become a dead loss to owners, but would bring from forty to sixty dollars for food-purposes. Also, from a humanitarian point of view, the question is deserving of consideration. Many a person has an old horse which years have rendered unsuitable for working purposes, yet the owner's circumstances will not permit the killing of the animal. Were it the custom to consume horse-meat, such animals could be very easily brought to a fairly fat condition, and at small expense, thus bringing far more money to the owner, from the shambles, than could possibly be their worth from a working point of view.

GLANDERS.

French, Morve; German, Rotz.

HISTORY.—Williams says glanders was described by Aristotle, which is an error; in Aubert's and Wimmer's German translation of his "Natural History" with the original text, it says: "The ass —but not the horse—suffers especially from one disease, which is known as 'malis.' It at first attacks the head, a viscid yellow slime running from the nostrils; when the disease extends to the lungs it is deadly, but when limited to the head it is not so."

It is impossible to see how any one can affirm the above to be a description of glanders, for it is equally applicable to strangles, especially when complicated with malarial pneumonia, commonly called influenza, the proper name of which should be pneumo-pleuro-enteritis equinæ infectiosum.

The first writer of antiquity to describe anything like glanders was undoubtedly Apsyrtus, who lived in the fourth century A. D. He united under the name of "μαλίς" several dangerous diseases, while he describes farcy as elephantiasis. Vegetius followed in the same direction in the next century.

Long before the disease was known to be transmissible to man, it derived a certain pathological interest from the assumption that it was a cause of syphilis in man, due to improper cohabitation with mares. This idea seems to have sprung from the coeval outbreak of glanders among the horses, and syphilis among the soldiers, at the famous siege of Naples in the sixteenth century. Syphilis is not inoculable in animals.

Rufus (thirteenth century) gave a very fair description of the symptoms of the disease; he declared for its contagiousness, but considered it to occur in all manner of ways.

Ruini (fifteenth century) held the same opinion. Winter von Adlers Flugel, a quaint German author of the sixteenth century, had many odd ideas of the nature of the disease. He describes it as occurring in two forms: the one known as "white" or stone-glanders, which is curable in the early stages; and the other called "yellow," and which gives forth an offensive odor, and is incurable. According to him, the symptoms of glanders are:

1. The horse appears as if suffering for breath when ridden hard and stopped suddenly, a point which has some practical diagnostic value.
2. The material which flows from the nose sinks to the bottom of a vessel when filled with water. This idea is even asserted to have diagnostic value by modern writers. Ditmar's report on glanders, in the report of the United States Agricultural Department, 1878, says "it has some value."
3. The flow is constant.
4. If the discharge is white and odorless, it is "stone-glanders."
5. If yellow, reddish, or mixed with blood, the case is incurable.
6. Such horses often have a "rotten moisture" coming from the mouth.
7. When given water, a profuse discharge is to be seen issuing from the mouth and nostrils.
8. The ears and head droop.
9. Difficult respiration.
10. Cough, and have tucked-up flanks.
11. The nostrils are cold.
12. Appetite is poor.
13. Emaciated and lazy.
14. The mane falls out.
15. Such horses have an offensive odor.

The disease occurs in three ways:

1. The discharge comes from the brain.
2. The animal has chronic disease of the throat.
3. One horse can infect others.

When the discharge comes from the brain, it is due to a superfluous amount of fluid in that organ, which causes corruption.

Chronic pharyngitis often causes the disease.

From the latter part of the last century there has always been an active controversy as to the genesis of glanders: two schools have existed, the one affirming it to be of a purely contagious character; the other admitting its contagiousness, but affirming its genesis from all sorts of circumstances. These two opinions still oppose one another, though at present those affirming the abiogenetic or spontaneous generation of glanders are becoming less and less. In France, even to this day, there may be found many advocates for the spontaneous generation of glanders, while in times past many asserted the non-contagiosity of the disease. This was essentially due to the teaching of Bourgelat and the Alfort school; while the Lyons school obstinately defended the contagiousness of the disease.

One of the most important French authors of the last century, and the first of this, and one who has exerted no mean influence upon veterinary literature, was Lafosse the younger, and it is both interesting and instructive to read what he has to say upon so important a subject, particularly as he represents the most advanced veterinary thought of his period.

In his "Cours d'Hippiatrique," Paris, 1772, Part II, p. 263, he says: "The ancient authors knew nothing more of the seat of glanders than they did of its treatment. Some of them looked upon it as seated in the head, others in the lungs, others in the kidneys, others in the stomach, and confounded the different kinds of discharge; to all of which they have given the name of glanders."

"To assume that glanders was seated in the lungs was pardonable—1. Because they have a communication with the nose. 2. Because a discharge from the lungs by means of the nose does take place (as in pneumonia). 3. Because the discharge from the lungs bears some resemblance to that from the pituitary membrane (the lining of nasal cavities). 4. Because glanders is often complicated with pneumonia, or, which is the same thing, the discharge from the pituitary membrane is often mixed with that from the lungs. The ancient veterinarians were less scrupulous in their researches than in naming maladies—they were deceived by appearances. They were in a good way, but erred in distinction. To assert that glanders is situated in the kidneys, spleen, liver, or in the brain, is contrary to the best teachings of 'hippotomie.' They utterly ignored the fact that there was no connection between these parts and the nose."

It is evident that even this great luminary of our art knew very little himself about glanders, and that his knowledge of the seats of the peculiar products of glanders was equally as fallacious as that of the ancients whom he condemns. But we will let him speak for himself:

"I distinguish glanders according to its nature; as glanders properly speaking, and glanders improperly so called."

"True glanders is the discharge which comes alone from the pituitary membrane. It is not proper to speak of any other form of glanders than this."

"Every other disease than this is not glanders."

1. "True glanders may be distinguished as simple and complex."
2. As primitive and secondary.
3. As initiative, as confirmed, and as inveterate glanders.

Simple glanders is that which comes from the pituitary membrane.

Complex glanders is that which comes from the same, and the trachea or the lungs at the same time.

Primitive glanders comes independent of all other complications.

Secondary glanders is that which follows on other diseases.

As to its cause, Lafosse takes a most sensible position when he says: "The primary causes of glanders are not known. Some persons think that it is due to some acrid and acid material."

The *ens* of the disease is to be sought in an inflammation of the glands of the pituitary membrane which produces the discharge.

He considered glanders curable in its early stages, which should be treated after the manner of all inflammations. When the disease had become chronic it was incurable.

So much for the ancient authors.

Of modern English authors, Fleming and Williams are the best known.

In his "Veterinary Police," Fleming speaks of glanders "as a special diathesis peculiar to the equine species."

Glanders is not a "diathesis." Diathesis is from the Greek *τιθημι—to dispose;* and the word means a peculiar condition of an organism, predisposing it to certain diseases; as scrofula disposes to tuberculosis. We may speak of a glanders dyscrasia. It can not logically be applied to that peculiarity of the different animal species by which certain diseases originate in them primarily, or only in them. We can not speak of a measles diathesis, or a rinderpest diathesis, any more than a glanders diathesis.

A diathesis is something inherited or produced. It is a weakness causing a tendency to secondary complications.

Fleming says again, "It has been grouped with that class of diseases termed 'granulomes,' and defined as a malady having a tendency to the formation of granular cells and destructive processes."

Here we see another error, which, had our author been personally acquainted with the pathological processes of glanders, he could not have fallen into.

Glanders is not characterized by destructive processes, as we understand them in pathology.

In general, the processes of glanders have more of a formative than destructive character. The tubercles of glanders seldom form secondary tubercles in the immediate vicinity, but are generally isolated neoplastic growths. Even in the mucous membrane of the nose, the destructive processes are far exceeded by the formative, and the permanent cicatrization of the ulcers of glanders is no rare occurrence.

"Acute glanders has been occasionally supposed to be merely the expression of purulent infection in the equine species, from the frequency with which it has been observed to follow severe operations, purulent fevers, or inflamed blood-vessels."

Glanders is in no sense of the word a purulent infection, and when it appears under any of the above circumstances it was either present in a latent form anticipatory to their occurrence, and they acted as the *causa sufficiens* to the visible outbreak of the disease, or the animal acquired it after either of the above conditions were produced.

"The highest Continental authorities, and those who have most attentively studied the etiology of the affection, *are absolutely unanimous in their opinion* as to its being at times directly developed and without contagion having anything to do with it."

It is surprising that a man of Mr. Fleming's erudition could write such as the above, for, in 1868, long before his book appeared, Gerlach, no second-rate authority, had come out absolutely for the strictly contagious nature of glanders; and his opinion had been adopted by the most eminent Germans at the time of Mr. Fleming's publication.

An equally fallacious opinion is, that "it appears among horses when unduly exposed, poorly fed or watered, etc., as in the army at times, or where hygienic measures are neglected, and the laws of health ignored; or in large towns, or in large establishments, if the horses are suddenly called upon to undergo severe exertion during bad weather and upon an insufficient allowance of food or forage of an unsuitable character."

Were this so, then nearly, if not more than, half of the work-horses among the poorer class of horse-owners would have the disease. Neither faulty ventilation nor the most arrogantly absurd non-hygienic condition can ever produce of itself, or themselves, glanders.

Within the last year Mr. Fleming has given up all the above views, and joined with emphasis the contagionistic party.

Williams says: "The remote causes of glanders, though not yet clearly understood, are often found to arise from many debilitating influences, such as old age, bad food, overwork, exhausting diseases and general bad management; from specific miasmatic or animal poisons, such as those generated in localities where large numbers of horses are congregated together, even where the stables are well ventilated, lighted, drained, and the animal well attended to in every way, but more particularly where the contrary is the case."

Nearly all veterinary authors seem still to adhere to this opinion, but Roell has come out a specific contagionist in the last edition of his "Special Pathology."

Fleming quotes, in proof of the theory of spontaneous generation of glanders (spontaneous means the development of something out of nothing), the well-known extension of glanders among horses of armies during campaigns, as illustrated by the late Franco-German War, and other such experiences.

It would seem as if the whole veterinary profession had never had eyes or brains, or else this manner of extension would never require the theory of spontaneous generation to support it. One would think that pulmonary and constitutional glanders was as much a myth to the veterinarians of the day as it was to Lafosse at the end of the last century, who ridiculed any form of true glanders other than nasal.

Lesering* gives a case illustrating the ease with which glanders can occur among army-horses, and still the cause be unsuspected. I will give it as nearly as possible in his own words:

"When glanders occurs more frequently in times of war or mobilization of the army, the explanation is to be easily found in the fact that great numbers of horses are centered upon a small extent of territory, and the opportunity to infection greatly increased thereby."

"This assertion is amply illustrated by a personal experience of my own. In Prussia, where there is no want of mobilizing the forces, statistics have proved that after such occasions glanders acquires a shocking extension among the horses. The open nature of these manœuvres, as well as the known care and careful revision to which in the Prussian army horses are subjected, make it absolutely impossible that undue labor, bad feed, etc., should have any influence

* "Bericht a. d. Vet. Wesen im Sachsen," 1862.

on these eruptions. In such manœuvres, I once had occasion to review some one hundred horses that were turned loose into a riding-place for the night, and ran about among each other 'pell-mell.' Of the one hundred, seven were found having glanders. How many of the balance, the further life of which I could not follow, could also become infected? How different would be the ideas of another veterinarian who should examine the balance of these animals after the manœuvres were over! What cause could he surmise for their infection other than the vicissitudes of the exercises, unless he were a contagionist?"

But the utter ridiculousness of the spontaneous-generation theory—the bad air, bad hygiene, and composite evil theories—finds an easy explanation when we come to study the peculiarly insidious nature of pulmonary glanders, which often leads to years of support of a contagious center, without even exciting the suspicion of any one, especially in a country like ours, where the average animal practitioners—I will not call them veterinarians—know less than nothing of the principles or practice of veterinary science.

The very insidious nature of pulmonary glanders, when the specific processes of the disease are so deeply seated as to be beyond our positive recognition, is very nicely illustrated by the following cases, which could be easily enough augmented by reference to veterinary literature:

Case I.—*Chronic Glanders in the Horse.*—"A ten-year-old mare was brought to the Munich school by its owner on the 10th of April, 1876, which had been suffering for several weeks with a nasal discharge, accompanied by some general disturbance.

Status præsens.—Examination on seeing the animal: No fever; the left intermaxillary gland swollen, with a node in it as large as a hazel-nut; the right less swollen; not sensitive to touch; the overlying cutis not attached; a profuse muco-purulent discharge from left nostril; the mucosa, so far as visible, diffusely hyperæmic, swollen; some serous secretion from the right nostril; the mucosa less red than that of the left side; an occasional dry cough." *

Such a condition as the above, while it lacks all positive symptoms of glanders, justifies the strongest suspicion that such *is* the case; said suspicion, and a consequential police supervision of the horse, must exist, either until the symptoms entirely disappear, or the diagnosis is confirmed in some other way.

The owner of this horse, and the veterinarian who attended to

* "Deutsche Zeitschrift für Thiermedicin," Erstes Supplement, 1878.

his stable, both declared this and all the horses in the stable free from any suspicion of glanders.

Three inoculative experiments were made with the nasal discharge, by saturating threads in the same, and drawing the latter through the cutis of a live rabbit's ear. All three gave negative results.

Haubner (of Dresden) introduced the (at times valuable) idea of trepanning the sinuses of the head in case glanders is suspected, which will frequently lead to the discovery of the disease.

It was done in this case this; "the sinus Highmori contained a moderate amount of muco-purulent secretion, the mucosa of both divisions was somewhat thickened, hyperæmic, and had a tense but *perfectly smooth feeling. Not a single sign of unevenness could be distinguished.* All this seemed to justify the conjecture that in this case we had only to do with a case of chronic catarrh of the sinuses of the head."

The cavity was treated by injection of a two-per-cent carbolic-acid solution twice a day; the same flowing out of the left nostril indicated that the opening was still free.

On the day following the operation a rise in temperature took place, 39·1° C.; pulse 56, which again disappeared in time.

"From the seventh to the tenth day after trepanning the head the intermaxillary glands became very much swollen, but neither abscess formation nor resolution in any degree took place."

"On the 14th of May the temperature again increased and continued augmented until the animal was killed. In the mean time the trepan-wound healed completely, and was entirely closed on the 22d of May."

Autopsy by Bollinger, May 28th:

"Extensive nasal and pulmonary glanders. In the left sinus Highmori (a cavity of the head) a considerable quantity of yellowish, thick, viscid, purulent material; the mucosa having a swollen, uneven nature, clouded with occasional hard neoplasmata (nodes) projecting above its surface; the infiltration common to glanders to be seen at places. The mucosa of the sinus Highmori dextra (right cavity of skull) presented nothing abnormal, aside from a slight catarrhal swelling."

In the above, we see that all diagnostic assistance failed to discover the disease. Even the trepan-wound healed normally, and not with long-continued ulceration, as is frequently the case in glanders, and yet the disease *was present.*

We have seen that three inoculative experiments with the discharge from the left nostril gave negative results. Three others made in the same manner with thread saturated with material directly from the ulcerated surface of the supernasal parts, gave positive results.

This shows that even inoculative experiments are not always to be depended upon.

Case II.—*Chronic Glanders.*—This case is still more interesting and has much more practical value, as it illustrates perfectly how one horse can be the means of infecting others, and yet not excite attention to itself for a long time. This horse had been in the possession of its owner for over two years anterior to the time it was brought to the Munich clinic; *two years before this time* glanders had appeared in the man's stables, and *one* horse was killed on that account, the others being quarantined. These quarantined animals —among them was a somewhat wind-broken but otherwise apparently healthy work-horse—were declared to be free from the disease at the expiration of the time fixed by law. No other horse was bought in the mean time to take the place of the one killed.

In February, 1878, the mate of the above-mentioned wind-broken horse died from pneumonia, but at the autopsy it was found to be diseased with chronic glanders.

"Upon this an active veterinary inspection of the animals in the stable again took place. The wind-broken horse—which had a very insignificant swelling of the left intermaxillary gland, and a slight pellucid, viscid nasal discharge—was isolated from the others. As, however, after six weeks' careful quarantine, no further symptoms appeared among the other horses, they were declared free, the above-mentioned horse still being quarantined." *

Friedberger, who makes the report, had this horse a long time under observation; he says as follows: "*Status præsens.* The highly wind-broken horse was in a comparatively good condition, feverless, good appetite and spirit; but the hair did not have the same luster as that of the other horses in the stable. The left intermaxillary glands were somewhat swollen, attached but slightly to surrounding tissues, and evinced no tenderness on pressure. From both nostrils flowed a clear, viscid fluid, the discharge not being at all constant in quantity, but in general more profuse from the left than right. Nothing suspicious could be seen in the nose by the ordinary method of examination."

"The first diagnostic aid to which I resorted was the endeavor

* Ibid., Zweites Supplement, 1879.

to produce self-infection, by eroding the nasal mucosa so that the discharge would necessarily flow over the wounded surface. A completely negative result followed.

"The nasal discharge was very variable, being on some days scarcely visible, and on others very profuse; at times it assumed a thick, muco-purulent character."

"On the 7th of May (1878), I succeeded (by means of Gunther's nasal speculum) in discovering a radiating cicatrix on the septum in the superior parts of left nostril, which occasioned me to request the owner to give it over to the school for further observation and eventual slaughter."

"Numerous attempts at self-inoculation were made, but were entirely unsuccessful, but the constant presence of the cicatricial formations in the nasal membranes permitted an unquestionable diagnosis, so that the animal was killed on the 23d of May, 1878."

Autopsy (*Bollinger*).—"Chronic glanders of the nasal cavities, the superior part of the sinus sinistra marred with large stellate cicatrices; perforation of the septum, cicatrices and ulcers of the mucosa, and miliary tubercles in the moderately swóllen glands."

"Glanders of the larynx, trachea, bronchial tubes, bronchiectasis; glanders of both lungs, cicatricial atrophy of left lung."

"The nature of the pathological conditions makes it evident that they had been present for a very long time, the exact period not being ascertainable, but, as is shown, for over two years, during which time this non-suspected animal had been the means of causing the disease in others."

Having very cursorily looked over the views of some of the representative authors of veterinary medicine as to the nature of glanders, it becomes us to endeavor to define our own ideas.

Glanders is, then, a peculiar infectio-contagious disease, which occurs protópathically only in the horse; the original cause of which is unknown and lost in history, but which, in our day, owes its genesis entirely to contagion.

Spontaneous generation of glanders is for us an absurdity; even so is the so-called metamorphosis or degeneration of other diseases, such as strangles, influenza, diabetes, or marasmus—a condition—into it; equally absurd are the assertions of authors, that bad hygienic influences, of whatever kind or nature, overwork, etc., can directly cause the development of the disease.

Were this so, we should have glanders constantly raging in certain districts, as an en- or epi-zoötic disease, which is not ever the case.

Transmission to other Species of Animal Life.

Glanders also occurs in the ass and mule, but I am inclined to the opinion that it is originally an equine disease, and that when it attacks these other solipeds, it is due to infection from, or by means of, a diseased horse.

It is also transmissible to man and all the domestic animals, *except to cattle.*

Sheep are especially susceptible to infection. Goats have been known to acquire the disease when kept in the same stable with diseased horses. The disease has been observed, or intentionally produced, in dogs, cats, prairie-dogs, white bears, lions, mice, Guinea-pigs, rabbits, and, according to Gerlach and Spinola, the hog also, although no generalization of the disease appeared to take place in them.

Geographical Distribution.

Glanders is fast becoming a regular cosmopolite. With the extension of civilization, diseases of man and animals follow a similar course. If the march of empire makes its way westward, disease accompanies it. While nearly all the contagious diseases of man and animals are lost in history—that is, come to us with the earliest historical records—still, during this period, we can follow their westward movement along with the tide of Aryan civilization.

In civilized lands the extension of all contagious diseases bears direct relation to the intelligence of the government in taking means to suppress them, and the frequency and ease of travel and intercourse.

This is naturally limited, in one way or another, by the peculiar characteristics of the inficiens (cause) in each disease.

Glanders has followed the same course. At one time it was said not to prevail in hot climates, but we now know that it has acquired an alarming extension, and frequently breaks out at the different cavalry stations of the British forces in India and other tropical countries.

Where there is little or no intercourse with other parts, there is little or no glanders, as in Iceland and other northern countries.

This led to the assumption that it did not thrive in such a climate, and that it steadily increased as we proceeded from the north to the south, until we arrived at tropical limits.

This is all wrong; the occasions to infection—with lack of sanitary police—being given, glanders will appear as frequently in one climate as another.

We have said that intercourse had much to do with the increased extension which glanders may acquire—this is well illustrated by the experiences of different wars. In our own country, glanders has acquired much more prominence since the war. In consequence of the late Franco-German War, the percentage of glanders among the horses of Prussia increased (reported cases) from 959 cases for 1869-'70 and 996 for 1870-'71 to 1,729 for 1871-'72 and 2,058 for 1873-'74.

In France, during the anti-contagionistic influence of the Alfort school, especially of Dupuy and Bouley, the one looking upon the disease as tuberculosis, the other as a form of pyæmia, and defending these absurdities with all partisan bitterness, the disease acquired a perfectly frightful extension, so that in a mortality of 75 per thousand among the army-horses, an average of 35 was due to glanders.

As the contagionistic idea began to gain ground, to the honor of the Lyons school it always adopted this side of the question; the yearly average slowly but steadily diminished: the deaths falling from 75 to 44·5 per thousand, and the cases of glanders from 35 to 20·5 per thousand horses. While in 1846 the French army lost 4·7 per cent of its horses from glanders, the mortality in 1864 was only 0·9 per cent from the same cause.

A most remarkable and extensive eruption of glanders occurred at the royal stud of Mezöhögyrs, Hungary, between the years 1809 and 1816, nearly 20,000 horses perishing. In 1812 alone 12,000 perished. This was all due to the disease not being looked upon as contagious, but a simple dyscrasia, in accordance with the humeropathological tendency of the veterinary medicine of the time.

In London, and the large English cities, glanders is reported to be steadily on the increase.

It is so also in this country, without ANY effective measures being taken to prevent it.

In Massachusetts we have a useless institution, which bears the name of "Cattle Commission," and is supposed to look after glanders, but in *all truth* it looks after nothing, and investigates *nothing*, except what it finds by the merest accident, or is reported to it by others.

Mr. Charles P. Lyman, formerly veterinary surgeon at Springfield, Massachusetts, writes me as follows:

"Your letter is received, and, although I fear that I can not give you the data as minutely as you wish, yet I will do my best to give the outlines of the outbreak of glanders which we had here during the past year. The first horse that can properly be said to belong to the outbreak was owned by an express company here, and, with the others of the company, was kept in a livery-stable. This horse was taken by a quack to treat, upon the 'no cure no pay' principle; the man promising to be able to bring about the result in a few days. It so happened that I was called into the same stable to see another horse, and while there one of the grooms, who had recognized the disease, called my attention to this horse. I examined the horse, and told the owner of the stable that he should have him removed. My advice was not heeded, however, and the animal was allowed to linger along until it died in its box. After this had taken place, the stable was subjected to disinfection, but it was too late, for four other horses, which had stood near the stall of that first named, were killed on account of glanders. It is perhaps worthy of mention, for it shows the absolute ignorance of Dr. Quack No. 1, that upon the morning that the horse of the express company died, when Dr. Q. came to make his usual morning call—the horse had already been drawn away to the knackers, the doctor (?) not knowing that he was dead—a hostler remarked to him that 'they had taken the horse out for a little'; to which the doctor (?) answered, 'I do not think it will hurt him any. I was going to tell them that they might put him to work to-day.' On the 8th of March I was called to look at a horse belonging to Messrs. ——, whose store was next to the office of the express company, but whose horse was kept at a different stable. This horse, on the night when I first saw him, seemed to have an attack of acute pleuro-pneumonia—remember, I had myself as yet had no case of glanders—however, glanders unmistakably developed itself in the next thirty-six hours, and the horse was killed. Following this was a roan horse in the same stable in which I diagnosed farcy, and ordered isolation. The owner would not believe the fact, at least he said he did not, and called in the services of another Dr. Quack, who said, 'The horse must have fallen through some hole in the floor and made his leg sore.' This horse was then sold to a Frenchman for twenty-five dollars, Quack No. 2 treating him for a while, and I lost sight of him, to follow him up about two months later, when I was called in by a woman to see a horse in a different part of the city, and found the same horse, in a moribund condition from glanders. It was immediately killed and taken away. The husband of the woman had bought this horse of the above-mentioned Frenchman for thirty-five dollars some four weeks previously, with the assurance that he had fallen through a floor, and that that was all the trouble with him. At my instigation suit was threatened, and the money recovered without the case coming into court. In the mean time four or five other horses that had been in the same stable with the second horse were condemned and killed, among them a fine mare worth some five hundred dollars. In these cases, all the horses had stood upon the same side of the stable with horse No. 2. After this experience the other horses were all removed from the stable, which was most carefully cleansed and disinfected, and allowed to stand empty three or four weeks. Since then no new cases have occurred at this stable. During this time the disease had become well dispersed around the city, and isolated cases were a frequent occurrence, the days being rare in which we were not compelled to condemn one or more of these animals. There was no great amount of trouble in getting most of the owners to consent to the destruction of the diseased horses, but a few would not consent, and would quietly sell the horses, so that I generally lost sight of them, as they were taken over into Connecticut, and there disposed of. The first one for which I was compelled to call in the services of the State Commissioners was owned in Chicopee, Massachusetts, and after being condemned and the board of selectmen notified by me, the horse was turned loose in the streets, it being summer, to wander about at will; this fact coming to my knowledge, I decided to call in the commissioners. The horse was killed, but not before four or five others had contracted the disease from him, which were also killed. Another center of infection had in the mean time come into existence at the southern part of Springfield, due either to the carelessness or ignorance of the previously mentioned Quack No. 1, who had been called upon to see a sick horse at a brick-yard; this person treated the horse, and he finally died in a small stable containing nine other horses. A few days subsequent to the death of this horse, a second animal sickened, and my services were requested; the horse appeared as if it had some foreign substance in his windpipe, owing to a drench which had been given it, and, while I was debating what to do with him, the owner said there was another sick horse in the stable, that I might look at before departure, remarking, '*Dr. Quack* says it has strained its leg.' I found it to be another good case of farcy, which let in light upon the sickness of the other horse. I ordered the horses removed from the stable, and to be separated, the stable at the same time to be thoroughly cleansed and disinfected. Five of these horses died of glanders. In all, from March 8, 1878, to March 19, 1879, fifty-six horses have been killed on account of glanders, which is a large number for a small city like ours. It is but natural to assume that many cases escaped my observation, *and you can well realize the difficulties which a person without the proper authority meets with.* Although after June 1, 1879, I had every assistance which the mayor, Mr. Powers, and the city solicitor could give me, the State law seemed *so vague to him*, that he did not feel like doing what he would have liked to do, or what seemed necessary in the matter. It is to be hoped that we shall soon have some better legislation with reference to these matters. Foremost, it should be *some one's* business to look up and attend to these matters exclusively. A competent veterinarian should at least have an active connection with every Board of Health in the State, and one also with the State Board. These matters are too intimately connected with the public health to have them governed by separate boards. We have not yet been able to completely eradicate the disease."

The following letter was kindly furnished me by Mr. Firth, Secretary of the Massachusetts Society for the Prevention of Cruelty to Animals:

DEAR SIR: In response to your request to be furnished with a report of the number of farcied and glandered horses coming to the notice of the society the past two years, I herewith transmit the same, as follows, viz.:

Farcied horses	2
Glandered	27

of which number twenty-four were killed at once, three were isolated by the health authorities (and, as we were informed, subsequently destroyed), while the final disposition of the remainder was never known to us. And in this connection permit me to say that the earliest operations of the society (in the year 1868) developed the frequent presence, in public places, of infected animals, and also the not unfrequent complaints at our office of men who had been duped into their purchase; and not only were the diseased animals destroyed, but in some instances others to whom they had communicated the disease.

The growing necessity for such legislation as would make it the especial duty of local boards of health to take cognizance of such cases, led the society and the Board of Health of this city to present to the Legislature of 1878 the draft of a bill that, it was felt, would effectually aid in stamping out the disease. The result was the passage of chapter 24 of the acts of that year (amended in chapters 160 and 178 of the acts of 1879).

It is well known to all competent authority, and it was in evidence before the legislative committee, to whom the matter of a statute was referred, that the most *dangerous* are the *most obscure* cases, and, inasmuch as the *general* condition of an animal under those circumstances is not such as to render him unfit for labor, it is not reached by the particular statute (chapter 344, acts of 1869) our society seeks to enforce; yet, on the other hand, the presence of such an animal in a public place is dangerous, and in such cases we make it our duty to *at once* bring the matter to the attention of the health boards.

We feel the subject to be all-important, and trust we have been instrumental in securing a measure of protection both to animals and their owners.

Very respectfully yours,

CHARLES A. CURRIER,

Special Agent of the Massachusetts Society for the Prevention of Cruelty to Animals.

I have made exertions to get reliable information from other quarters, but only received the two following letters in reply, for which I desire to publicly thank the authors.

My friend and colleague, Dr. Liautard, of the American Veterinary College in New York city, writes:

"You ask me for a letter with regard to the extension of glanders in New York city and State. With reference to the latter, I have but little to say, as my experience is entirely limited to the city of New York.

"From my connection with the city Board of Health, and the American Veterinary College, I have been enabled to observe, to no inconsiderable degree, the extent to which this disease prevails in our metropolis. Although it has found a powerful enemy in the Society for the Prevention of Cruelty to Animals, I am well satisfied that it exists in our private and public stables, and can be seen traveling upon our streets every day in the year.

"In connection with my duties at the college, I have had occasion to condemn quite a number of horses brought to our free clinics. In 1876 I condemned 40 horses; in 1877, 49; in 1878, 62; and from January 1 to March 1, 1879, 49. This does not include animals found by me in my private practice.

"But the most important of all my observations with regard to glanders, the one which has no equal in all my experience, is that of the summer of 1877. I was at that time requested by the Board of Health to inspect the different large public stables of the city in relation to glanders, as the disease had become so prevalent as to cause numerous complaints to be made. At the same time I was requested by the president of one of our large horse-railroad companies to call on him. Upon visiting him, I examined and condemned in one day thirty-six horses, and, after impressing upon him the dangers to which the entire stock of the company were exposed, I was authorized to extirpate the disease from their stables. I inspected the entire stock (over twelve hundred horses) weekly, then semi-monthly, then every three months, until, after over nine months of hard work, I finished my task, not having found any more glandered horses in my last three visits. *The company lost by this procedure some three hundred horses.*

"On retiring from duty, I warned the president of the danger that existed of the disease again appearing, and endeavored to impress upon him the necessity of professional inspection of the entire stock weekly, or at least semi-monthly, as is done in the large Continental companies. Whether my advice was regarded or not, is shown by the fact that glanders again appeared, and is still existing in the same stables to quite a large extent.

"Another company also requested my services. It had about nine hundred horses, and in about the same length of time, and after similar work, I condemned to death about *one hundred* horses. I also gave the same advice on this occasion which I had given to the first-named company, and it was followed to such an extent that I am not aware that there is a single case of glanders among the horses of this company to-day.

"In another stable, which I visited by request of the Board of Health, where there were over two hundred horses, twenty-five of them were condemned at two visits. These animals were kept in the hospital of the stable, and were under the care of the so-called 'doctor' (!). I had no authority to subject the entire stock to revision, but if I had, I am sure that the results would have been fully equal to those of the other examinations. I am perfectly sure that I could find numerous cases of glanders among the horses of this company to-day.

"Is it not indeed surprising that such a condition of things should be allowed to exist; and how can one comprehend that the president of a company could so overlook the interests of the stockholders as to allow so many diseased horses to remain among those of the company, without continually being on the watch to prevent such disasters? Let us take, for example, the first case: 300 horses, valued at the lowest estimate at $125, amounts to $37,500. The same amount to replace those destroyed makes $75,000. Add to this the loss by food, labor, the danger of infection to other horses, the costs of cleansing and disinfection, and $100,000 would not cover the loss to the company. In spite of all this, these companies still continue to employ as veterinary advisers men entirely ignorant of the phenomena of this disease, or, if they know them, men who are false to their duties to the public, by persisting in treating animals they refuse to condemn even with the most manifest symptoms of glanders.

"Still at times an animal is recognized by one of these practitioners, but the symptoms are of a mild type, the animal is in good health and condition, it represents a certain sum of money: he allows it to be sold to some low dealer (if he does not recommend it), or perhaps to some countryman. In the first case the horse goes to some horse-market, and is sold again to some poor but licensed vender, cartman, or cheap livery-stable keeper, unless it happens to be seized by an agent of the Society for the Prevention of Cruelty to Animals, who has it destroyed upon my certificate. In the second case the animal is taken across the river to Long Island or New Jersey, spreading the seeds of this loathsome disease wherever it goes. In the face of such evidence as this is it not high time that either our State authorities, or those in Washington, paid more attention to the contagious diseases of animals, and enacted laws for the protection of our animal property, as well as human beings, from infection? Is it not high time that American veterinarians used their influence toward the establishment of a general sanitary veterinary system for the country, with its appropriate head in connection with the National Board of Health at Washington, looking toward the suppression and prevention of these damaging animal pests?"

Dr. Gadsden writes from Philadelphia thus:

"Dear Sir: In answer to your inquiry respecting the prevalence of glanders in this city and State, I am glad to inform you that disease is seldom met with now in this city. I can not answer for the State, but no doubt there are many cases that do not come under my notice.

"I need not tell you that I have them destroyed as soon as possible after examination. During the twelve years I have been in practice in this city, I think it is safe for me to say I have condemned two hundred (200) horses with this loathsome disease and had them destroyed, so you will see I have not been idle. About six years ago I was called to one of our best horse-car stables, to examine some 'sick' horses that a quack was 'treating' by contract (so much per year). I found several of them suffering from glanders in its worst form. I told the president of the company the consequences if he kept them longer in the stable; he ordered me to pick out the diseased ones at once, and if I remember right we destroyed between forty and fifty of them in about two weeks. I have had that same unpleasant duty to perform at four other horse-car companies in this city; the quacks used to treat them for 'distemper.' We have no special law on the subject. If I find any trouble about having the diseased horse destroyed, I call at the office of the Society for the Prevention of Cruelty to Animals, and ask them to send an officer to look after the horse, and see that it is not worked (as that would be cruel), also to see that it is not kept near other horses (as that would be cruel to them); so you see it very soon answers the owner's purpose (pocket) to have it destroyed.

"I have known of three men that died with this terrible disease in this city from inoculation (through sores on their hands), while attending glandered horses and mules; all of them suffered very much. I hope you will do what you can to teach the public the danger of this disease, as it is worse than this (so-called) pleuro-pneumonia in cattle, and that is bad enough."

It is just the same in every State, and our national Government is as incompetent and culpably negligent as those of the States.

Cattle commissions are unnecessary, and one-sided affairs. What we must have are boards of animal hygiene in each State.

A great noise has been made about pleuro-pneumonia among our cattle. The Government and the cattle interest most emphatically denied that we had any, as they do now about porcine trichiniasis; but finally had to admit that we have a little of the former. We should never have heard of either of them, unless some one had felt his pockets *touched*. Then, like cowards, we sneaked behind a false assertion, and said, "We have not such things." But Europeans did not believe our assertion, and finally we retracted, and admitted that we have just a few cases of pleuro-pneumonia along our Atlantic seaboard.

How is it with glanders?

Glanders has much in common with pleuro-pneumonia; it is even more stealthy in its progress. Should we, unfortunately (or fortunately, I should say), ship a few lots of horses with this disease to some European country, we should probably again have the

12

stereotyped denial on the part of the Government and the horse interests; yet I venture to assert that there are to the thousand fifty per cent more glandered horses in this country than cattle having the contagious lung-plague, and that the former disease is extending with more rapidity among our equine than the latter among our bovine population.

The government gives the people no means of knowing the facts from trustworthy statistics. The United States Agricultural Department of Statistics, with regard to animal diseases, is a disgraceful farce.

Etiology.

In our remarks upon the views of different authors with regard to the nature of glanders, we have unavoidably touched upon their ideas as to its cause, which renders necessary some repetition in this place.

We have not time to discuss all these views in detail; but we, as those before us, are all children of the period, and can not well separate ourselves from the opinions prevailing at the time; yet we must, *in all things*, ever entertain a certain degree of skepticism: to doubt is the beginning of self-education. A person who has never doubted is an ignorant believer, and has no self-knowledge —a mere puppet, unfit to be a member of any profession.

So in glanders, one party has looked upon it from the iatro-chemical stand-point, looking upon an abnormal degree of oxidation, or an undue degree of acidity of the blood as the cause; others, of the humoral-pathological school, saw its origin in all sorts of dyscrasies—not diatheses, as Fleming has written—and even from our stand-point we can speak of glanders dyscrasia, but not in the way of humoral pathology, whereby the dyscrasia was the cause of glanders, but from the natural scientific sense, the dyscrasia being a part of the disease, the same as the neoplastic processes; that is, the result of the action of *the* inficiens. Others saw in it a form of equine scrofulosis; and still others looked upon it from the neuro-pathological stand-point; while others saw in it a form of tuberculosis, and with the eruption of the pyæmia theory, we find it classed with that kind of diseases. Nearly all these different views led to the more or less strong opposition of the contagious nature of the disease, and, as we have seen, to great losses on the part of the people.

Is glanders pyæmia?

The whole theory of the autochtone development of glanders is more dependent upon a few experiments with pyæmic material than anything else.

Renault and Bouley injected pus into the jugular vein of a horse, supposed to be healthy. On the sixth day pustules were observed to develop in the nose, and soon afterward ulcers. Death resulted in eight days. The autopsy gave numerous tubercles in the lungs, and ulcers of the nasal mucosa. A positive result followed the re-inoculation of another horse, with nasal discharge from this one. Laisné reports a similar result. Others report the same, but Vines exceeds all in absurdity, when he asserts that he produced glanders by means of injections of vitriol into the trachea, and other such procedures.

These experiments are openly opposed by others in the same direction, and are not conformable to the results of pathological experiments in our day. In fact, it should be well known that the introduction of pus into a jugular vein *will* lead to processes in the *lungs* which, taken by themselves, might lead one to suspect glanders.

Furthermore, in old horses, nodulated bodies are frequently met with which the inexperienced might take for tubercles—such is the condition known as bronchitis nodosa.

Whether genuine tuberculosis occurs in the horse is an open question!

Lauret, Billroth, Guenther, Spinola, Gamgee, Lee, and others, have made numerous injection and other experiments, with both laudable and ichorous pus, but have in *no case* produced glanders.

It will be observed that *only* in *one* case was glanders proved to exist by second inoculation, in Renault and Bouley's experiments. In *all* the others no case of proof, or secondary inoculation, is given.

Were glanders *ever* due to pyæmia, we should have far more proof of it than at present exists.

That it could ever have been assumed to be generated in this way, must be sought in the hitherto all too much neglected fact of the long latency which the pulmonary form may have, extending over years without even a single detectable symptom of the real disease. A wound, a cold, undue exposure, or any of the causes hitherto looked upon as protopathic, may cause the acute eruption of the disease.

The theory of the spontaneous generation of glanders again finds full contradiction in the observations of practical experience, made on islands distant from the mainland, and out of general communication with it.

Krabbe * reports that, on the Island of Bornholm, with over

* "Deutsche Zeitschrift," i, p. 286, 1878.

7,000 horses, the disease is unknown, and the same is true of Iceland, with about 35,000 horses.

No one would, I think, be bold enough to assert that these animals are not as much subjected to the evil influences of exposure, poor feed, pneumonia, etc., as the horses of more favored climates.

While we can not help expressing our surprise that authors of undoubted practical experience should still hold to the spontaneous generation of glanders, and give it up for nearly all other similar diseases, it is still more surprising that any person of sense can hold to the utterly illogical, metachemical, or degeneration theory by which one disease transforms itself into another, without the aid of cause.

Such a thing is opposed to both common sense and experience. What, then, must we consider the cause of glanders? In our day, contagion, and nothing else!

A specific but unknown inficiens enters the organism and produces results, in general, only observed in this disease.

In accordance with the best results of modern pathologists, we must assume this inficiens to be of an organic, formative nature; that is, belonging to the bacterial world. Chauveau has looked upon peculiar cells as the etiological moment, but this is not in accordance with our present views, though in one sense, but not in his, the bacteria are cells. Frank has looked upon some chemical material as the inficiens, and has demonstrated that the nasal discharge and blood of glandered horses possessed catalytic action, and could transform peroxide of hydrogen into O and H_2O.

Hallier, Mueller, Semmer, Zurn, and others, have all described bacteria found in the blood and secretions. Schutz claims to have discovered, cultivated, and produced the disease by inoculating them. These germs must either act of themselves, which, from the nature of the disease, is scarcely probable, or, which is more likely to be true, by means of some irritants which they themselves produce by certain unknown metachemical processes.

Such an irritant is absolutely necessary to explain the slowly-developing processes of chronic glanders—the (as we shall see) gradual complication of the stroma, or interstitial tissues of many of the most important organs.

It is not in conformity with our knowledge of germ-life that they can directly act in this manner. Zurn * describes the bacteria of glanders as follows: "In the blood of horses diseased with glanders I have found micrococci, and strings of the same—streptococci—

* "Pflanzlichen Parasiten," p. 375.

consisting of from four to eight single cells. The micrococci did not have a uniform size, yet they were always round, and had an average diameter of 0·0002 millimetres. I observed that they multiplied by fission. I saw these objects in warm blood taken directly from the horse; they were principally to be seen in and around the white blood-cells. The red cells also seemed to be invaded by them, but to a less degree. The smallest capillaries were often obstructed by colonies of micrococci."

"In the diseased lymph-glands I also found great numbers of the same, and also staff-like bacteria—bacilli. They were either isolated or in joints of two or three members. Such objects were also present in the mucous lining of the cavities of the head."

Whether these objects seen by Zurn have really any etiological connection with glanders is still an open question. Pure cultivation, extended experiments, etc., can only finally discover the immediate inficiens.

One must be careful not to attribute too much importance to micrococci or bacteria, found in any part of the nasal cavity or pharynx, or bodily cavities which connect with the open air; for they are not to be considered of any diagnostic value, and their isolation is too difficult a task for our present means.

The germs must be seen and collected elsewhere than here, or from open wounds, on account of these foreign admixtures—even though such material be highly infectious at the same time.

The inficiens of glanders is both *transportable*—by that I mean suspendible in the expired air to a limited degree—and *fixed;* that is, attachable to any foreign vehicle as a purveyor and supporter of infection.

With relation to the inficiens being based upon the perspiration and expired atmosphere, we have the very illustrative experiments of Gerlach and Viborg.

In these, horses having glanders were driven in cold weather, so as to get into an active perspiration; the steam arising from them, as well as the expired air, was caught in glass receivers prepared for the purpose, and allowed to condense.

Healthy horses were then inoculated with this material, and the phenomena of glanders observed to develop. The expired air was found to be far more active than the transpiration from the cutis.

These experiments go to prove two things:

1. That the inficiens is transportable to a minor degree.
2. That the inficiens must be of a *formative nature.*

No other conclusion is possible; for, in our studies on bacteria, we have already learned that neither gases nor chemicals have the power of multiplication within themselves; yet even in this case, multiplication of the inficiens must have taken place to have produced infection, for Gerlach says that "only some twenty drops of the condensed fluid was used for the inoculations." Viborg, who lived early in the century, could not well have discovered form-elements in these fluids, and it is doubtful if the microscope which Gerlach used in 1868 was equal to it. At least, he reports that none were to be seen, and concludes that the infectious elements exert a chemical action, which was also Virchow's opinion at that time. Negative experiments (which, however, have always but little value in the face of positive, as the individual immunity peculiar to all species must always be taken into consideration) have been made by Hertwig, Regnault, and others, with reference to the expired air causing infection by means of the lungs. Diseased horses were caused to breathe into a canvas bag at one end, while healthy ones breathed from the other, yet in these cases no infection took place. These experiments are, however, only too abundantly contradicted by daily experiences.

THE BLOOD.—Numerous experiments made with the blood of glandered horses have shown it to be infectious.

Schimming* gives the following *résumé* upon the results of his and other experiments:

1. "Venous blood from a glandered horse injected into the veins of a healthy one causes glanders.

2. "The quantity of infected blood injected appears to exert an influence upon the duration of incubatory stadium; the stage of the disease in the animal from which the blood was taken may not be without influence also.

3. "Three months may elapse after the transfusion of such blood before we can recognize any pathognomonic symptoms. This will probably serve to explain the negative results which followed some of the experiments of Viborg, Gerlach, and Hening; that is, the period under which the animals were kept in observation was too short to allow the disease to develop.

4. "The blood from glandered animals appears to have a less intensive action upon healthy animals than the nasal discharge, and secretions from wounded surfaces."

5. "Transfusions with such blood in dogs, cats, and swine, gave negative results."

6. "The subcutaneous injection of six grammes of defibrinated

* "Ansteckungsfähigkeit d. Rotzblutes," Dorpat, 1875.

blood, taken from a glandered horse, in dogs, produced the disease, which would seem to indicate that in this way the blood was more actively infectious than by intravenous injection."

Chauveau looks upon the active principle of infection in the blood as being based on certain suspended particles, leucocytes, or other form-elements, and not upon the serum.

Time failed me to make any search over the literature as to the existence of the infectious principle in the secretions of the parotid and other glands, or the urine, although Gerlach casually mentions that the latter is infectious, without giving any experimental proofs.

Both practical and experimental experience sufficiently prove the fixedness of the infectious principle of glanders.

We know that it is contained in the discharges from the nasal cavities, in the secretions of the cutaneous ulcers, and that whatever becomes polluted with such material, be it the harness, cribs, bedding, or any other accidental vehicles, may retain its dangerous properties for a long time.

A valuable experiment could be made as to infectiousness of the fæces from horses diseased with glanders.

Tenacity of the Contagium.

The infectious principle of glanders retains its activity for a long time, and under varying influences. When a vehicle—nasal discharge—is spread out, and quickly dried, on any hard substance, it soon loses its activity, but in stables where it pollutes the crib, etc., it retains it many months. It loses its activity on exposure to a temperature of 45° R.; by exposure to scalding water, or by the action of chemical agents—disinfectants—such as chlorine, carbolic acid, etc.—but only when brought into actual contact with the same.

Decomposition does not appear to thoroughly destroy it (Gerlach). It seems to lose its virulence when introduced into the intestines (as flesh) of man, the dog, swine, and hens, but while not so active, is still capable of causing infection in the horse.

The dispersion of the infectious principle over the organism is by means of the blood and lymphatic systems.

The Entrance of the Infectious Principle into the Organism—that is, Natural Infection.

Experience goes largely to prove that while the infectious elements of glanders have a fixed character, that is, are not capable of being taken up by the atmospheric current, and carried to any great distance from the point of original generation, or lodgment, still that, in by far the greater number of cases, *infection must take place by means of this principle* when suspended in the atmosphere; that is, by means of the expired air from glandered horses. Were this not so, cutaneous glanders (farcy) would be far more common than it is; in fact, it should, under this circumstance, be the primary form.

Again, were the infection not generally due to a suspended principle, we should have far more cases of ulceration in the lower or exposed parts of the nasal passages, which is rare, while deeper seated ulcerations are more common.

Again, that a suspended principle is commonly the cause of infection, is proved by the numerous cases of pulmonary glanders which occur with little or no nasal complications; in the numerous cases of pulmonary glanders, accompanied by cicatrices in the mucosa of the bronchial tubes, trachea, and pharynx, all indicating the long continuance of the disease, but, with RECENT complications in the super-nasal parts, with no evidence of older complications.

Disposition.—Immunity.

As in every other contagious disease, not every horse exposed to infection has glanders. Of 138 healthy horses which Lamirault caused to stand among diseased ones, and to be cleaned, etc., with the same utensils, and to work with the same harnesses, only 29 became diseased—28 with glanders, 1 with farcy.

According to Lydtin, 40 to 50 per cent of the horses exposed to natural infection became diseased.

By inoculation of 23 horses, only 8 became infected.

The almost invariably fatal character of the disease does not allow us to judge whether an acquired immunity is possible or not, by animals that have once had it.

With the present French mania for all kinds of vaccinations with cultivated virus, we shall probably hear of a modified form of glanders being able to give an acquired immunity to natural or further infection, at least for a time.

I always stand skeptical to all such assertions—ready to believe, but doubting until the evidence is overwhelmingly *pro* or *con.*

At present I do not believe in the generalization to which the few Pasteur vaccine experiments have led.

Inoculation for glanders is no new thing, but has as yet always signally failed. Furnival,* an enthusiastic Briton, claims "to have cured seven bad cases of farcy by inoculation," and was anxious to

* "Fleming's Veterinary Journal," vol. x, p. 51.

continue this method of equine salvation, but, as we have heard nothing more from him in this direction, we may conclude that there are backsliders in his equine salvation army.

Phenomenology.

According to duration, glanders may be spoken of as acute or chronic; according to seat, as nasal, pulmonary, or cutaneous glanders (farcy).

Pulmonary glanders can occur without either the nasal or cutaneous forms being present, but it is very questionable if either of the latter can occur without evidences of pulmonary complications.

Chronic glanders is the common, acute the rare course which the disease assumes.

Incubation.—Duration.

In inoculations the incubatory period is generally from three to five days, but in natural infection it is very hard to say, the authorities varying from five to six days to as many weeks. In that form which is known as chronic glanders, a period of apparent latency may exist for months, yet even here there must be a period of incubation.

Acute glanders may terminate in from ten to fifteen days, while the chronic variety may continue for months or even years, how many is an open question.

Chronic glanders terminates invariably with the acute form, but when the acute variety follows known infection, it never assumes a chronic character.

Acute Nasal Glanders.

Under this name we usually find both the acute processes in the mucous membranes of the head and those of the cutis treated.

It is generally the conclusion of chronic glanders, where the disease occurs by natural infection. It also may follow directly on infection.

Although, according to Fleming, Reynal denies that acute glanders generally terminates the chronic form, the evidences to the contrary are so strong as to leave no doubt of its correctness.

The acute form is ushered in by more or less fever, by hyperæmia of the mucosa of the nasal cavities, with tumefaction of the same, and sometimes with slight epistaxis (bleeding from the nose). In a few days the nodes begin to develop in the mucosa, or diffuse yellowish infiltrations of the same take place; a discharge from the nose follows the first stage of congestion: the same is at first thin, viscid, and contains but few cellular elements, but it soon becomes thicker, more viscid, of a queer yellowish-green color, and adheres more or less to the nostrils.

These nodes and infiltrations soon begin to show evidences of breaking down, the edges become swollen and ragged, resembling rodent ulcers; they extend by the formation of new nodes, or proliferations in the circumference, and the sequential breaking down of the same; frequently such ulcers coalesce, giving rise to extensive ulcerated surfaces. When these conditions last a long while, perforation of the septum sometimes takes place.

It has been noticed that the discharge is often limited to one nostril, and particularly to the left, for which we have no explanation, but, whichever side it is, there is the locality of the most serious disturbances.

The submaxillary and retro-pharyngeal lymph-glands soon become complicated, the infectious elements gaining access to them by means of the lymphatics of nasal cavities. The lymphatics may often be seen as swollen cords, and, if not seen, felt. The processes in the glands are essentially of an indurative character. The breathing is frequently labored, from the complication of the larynx, so much so that death may sometimes result from œdema glottidis. The fever increases, the animals become more and more depressed, lose their appetite, etc. If this condition appears as a conclusion of chronic glanders, we have mucous râles in the bronchi, sometimes pneumonic infiltration, with the usual respiratory symptoms.

Soon follow œdematous swelling of the legs, sheath, the sub-abdominal region, with the characteristic farcy-buds over different parts of the body, especially the posterior, the swollen lymphatics, the complications, induration of the sub-cutis, etc. With the progress of the disease, and breaking down of the tissues, the discharge from the nose and cutaneous ulcers becomes more profuse, diarrhœa frequently sets in, albuminuria is present, and, if not killed, the animals die a miserable death in from eight to fourteen days.

In a case of chronic glanders, inflammatory conditions may be ushered in by a variety of circumstances, viz.: an infected horse may, in the same manner as a healthy one, be attacked by any acute feverish disease, let it be from any mechanical injury, from the influences of cold, or miasmata, or any such thing. Catarrhal disturbances of the respiratory tract are especially favorable to the transformation of chronic to acute glanders. Bad weather, cold and dry east winds, in fact, any influences which tend to irritate the mucosæ, exert a similar influence. The same is true of severe surgical operations, wounds, fever, etc.

Bollinger has shown by numerous experiments that the nasal mucosa is a favorite place for the local disturbances of glanders without regard to the point whence infection took place.

Pulmonary Glanders.

In general, this form of glanders may be looked upon as the same thing as chronic glanders. The true importance of this form of the disease has scarcely had due appreciation even from the profession.

It can exist for months, or even years, without the appearance of any outward signwhich could be at once considered as pathognomonic.

Gerlach and Bollinger both give numerous cases where glanders has been suspected, but in which characteristic symptoms entirely failed, yet on the autopsy the pathognomonic phenomena in the lungs were found abundantly represented. Gerlach says:

"On November 2, 1863, three horses belonging to a coal-dealer were brought to the school clinic at Hanover. No. 1 was killed on account of farcy; Nos. 2 and 3 were kept for four weeks under observation. They were both emaciated, and had an ill-looking coat. No. 3 had no other suspicious symptoms. No. 2 had, at first, a slight tumefaction of the intermaxillary glands, which gradually diminished, and a somewhat retarded respiration. After four weeks' observation, both horses were returned to the owner, the police being notified that they were still to be looked upon as suspicious. On the 10th of February, 1864, horse No. 2 was again brought to the school on account of epistaxis. It was much emaciated, and asthmatic to a high degree; the respiration was much retarded, and the animal had a short, dry cough; the intermaxillary glands were not diseased, and the nasal mucosa presented nothing abnormal. Fever and symptoms of disease were entirely wanting. On account of the antecedent circumstances, pulmonary glanders was suspected, and the horse killed.

Autopsy.—The mucous membranes of the head and the intermaxillary glands healthy, the lungs filled with glanders neoplasmata, etc.

On account of this result, the third horse was killed. It was *broken-winded*, otherwise not a single sign of glanders could be perceived.

Autopsy.—Not an indication of glanders in the nasal cavities or cavities of the head. Intermaxillary glands healthy. In the lungs tubercles, and the characteristic growths of glanders, phenomena which may be looked upon as justifying the strongest suspicion of the presence of chronic glanders, especially pulmonary.

Gerlach says: "It can be almost axiomatically asserted that a continuous hard nodulated condition of the intermaxillary glands in a horse is sufficient to excite the suspicion of the existence of glanders, even when no suspicious phenomena are to be seen in the nose. I have never seen a tumefied condition of these glands which had any deceptive resemblance to the bubo of glanders, in any simple inflammatory or catarrhal complications of the mucous membranes of the head.

Further, a horse must be looked upon with suspicion—

1. "When it has a dry, dull, wheezing cough, with retarded respiration; when the general condition of the animal is poor, the hair staring, the body emaciated."

2. "When horses in this condition have stood or worked beside, or otherwise been in relation with others known to have had glanders.

3. "When the dyspnœtic phenomena have been anticipated by suspicious glandular or catarrhal phenomena.

4. "When a horse that has been much in contact with such a broken-winded horse acquires the disease, the latter should be suspected.

5. "When, in the course of the above condition, any suspicious glandular or catarrhal complications make their appearance."

Veterinarians have made a mistake all along in judging glanders too much from the clinical stand-point, that is, *from visible* symptoms, and have neglected to appreciate the true value or teachings of the processes in the larynx, trachea, lungs, and other organs, which are only revealed by a necroscopical examination.

At the Berlin school, where very exact records are kept of the results of each autopsy, it was found that in 216 cases of glanders, upon which examinations were made between the years 1871 and 1874, the location of the disease in the lungs failed in but ten of them, while they were wanting in thirty-three cases in the nasal cavities and those of the head.

Pulmonary glanders, it must be repeated, is as frequently the primary lesion of the disease as that of the head or cutis. Of the above 216 cases, the lesions of the lungs were found to antedate those in the nose, or cutis, in more than half the cases.

Bollinger says, from much experience, that the conclusion of Virchow and others is erroneous, that the nasal mucosæ are as frequently the atrium of the infectious principle of glanders as the genitals in syphilis, and that the pulmonary complications complete the disease.

In proof of which he gives the following cases from the records of the Munich school:

1. A horse was brought in with a tumefied condition of the right hind-leg. The animal had a slight mucous flow from the nose, occasionally coughed, and had some fever. The leg continued to swell, the fever augmented, and the animal was killed, being considered incurable.

Autopsy.—Subacute glanders of the larynx, the trachea, and lungs. Nasal cavities completely normal.

2. A nine-year-old horse, in a fair condition, was taken into the clinic with the appearance of severe dyspnœa. Nasal outflow from both sides, considerable fever, accelerated pulse and respiration, a weak, painful cough. The diagnosis was acute œdema glottidis, or muscle paresis in larynx. Tracheotomy. After eight days the horse was killed.

Autopsy.—Chronic and subacute glanders of the larynx; acute glanders of the nose, the trachea, and lungs.

Upon the septum of the right nostril was to be seen a fresh ulcer, and in its neighborhood, as well as higher up, several smaller ones. Retropharyngeal and laryngeal glands acutely swollen. Extreme œdema glottidis. The inner surface of the larynx showed a diffuse ulceration, partly covered with fresh granulations. Isolated nodes in the lungs.

3. *Autopsy.*—Chronic glanders of the larynx and lungs, with acute nasal glanders, and swelling of the glands.

Pathological Anatomy.

Glanders is essentially characterized by neoplasmatic processes, which are represented by tubercles, nodes, the diffuse infiltrations known as glanders-growths, and by pneumonic conditions, which in general come under the head of dry *catarrhal*, also by complications of the stroma of the large glandular organs, and in very chronic cases by thrombosis of the pulmonary veins, and the formation of gelatinous infiltrations of varied extent in the lungs.

The unknown inficiens of glanders undoubtedly has a specific tendency to act upon, irritate, or excite into a state of proliferating activity the interstitial tissues, which compose the stroma or framework of the organs.

The works on veterinary pathology absolutely fail, either in noticing this fact, or calling sufficient attention to it.

I can not at this moment recall a single paper upon the "shrunken kidney" of chronic glanders, which is a very common occurrence, and many of our text-books make no reference to the clinical phenomena by which it is indicated; but when present we can almost, if not always, find casts and *détritus* in the urine, as well as albumen.

It is also worth recording that this shrinking of the equine kidney in chronic glanders—I have never seen it in any other disease, but my own experience is very limited—which is due to proliferation of the elements of the stroma, and thus anticipated by a swollen condition of these organs, does not give rise to that granulous or hob-nailed appearance, which occurs in man under like processes, and produce the condition falsely called *cirrhosis renalis* —*κιρρος*, *yellow*—a name given to the yellow appearance of the cut surface of the liver—rum-drinker's liver—due to stocking of the gall, under similar processes, upon the hepatic stroma. The framework of the liver of the horse is complicated in a like manner, giving rise to brown atrophy.

As the disease assumes an acute character, we find the organic parenchyma also affected, which makes itself anatomically apparent in the clouded swollen condition of the cells, the fatty metamorphosis of their plasma, and finds its expression in the weak movements of the organs, muscles, and the gradually approaching marasmus.

The very frequent occurrence of *ante-mortem* coagula in the heart, and formation of extended and bleached-out thrombi in the pulmonary veins, is to be attributed to the weakness of the heart, due to parenchymatous carditis.

In the report of Ditmars (to the Agricultural Department, previously alluded to) on glanders, may be read quite a dissertation upon glanders-cells as something specific. This idea is borrowed from Gerlach, and is simply a product of the period when Gerlach studied the disease, and the minds and endeavors of pathologists were all bent toward the discovery and description of specific cells.

Singular to say, Gerlach, who was in general not only a skeptical but most logical man, fell into this error.

Gerlach says: "The neoplasmatic processes of glanders consist of round cells, spindle-cells, the last in part derivatives from the former, and the proliferation of the connective tissue, which, by-the-way, is only a secondary phenomenon in glanders, and has nothing specific. These round cells have nothing singular in their form, they are like granulation and pus cells; *nevertheless, they are specific* and the true basis of the disease—they are therefore glanders-cells."

In the above we have two serious errors:

1. There are no such things as specific cells.

2. The complications of the connective-tissue, stroma, of the organs, in which proliferation takes place, is essentially *peculiar* to glanders—that is, in the general manner in which it occurs, though the process itself has nothing specific in it, and may and does occur under other conditions. The irritans, the infectious principle of glanders, is the specific element; and also, we can say, the general manner in which the interstitial tissues of the equine organism are complicated, is also something peculiar to the disease. Gerlach contradicts himself when he calls these round and spindle cells "glanders-cells," especially the former, and says they constitute the "*specific and true basis of the disease.*" In another place he tells us, "they originate from the cells of the connective tissue and epithelial elements."

Were they specific to glanders, they should be peculiar to it, and not occur in anything else.

This is not so: *they are the simple products of inflammation.* Just such cells may be found in simple but severe ulcerations of the nasal mucosæ, from wounds, chemical irritants, or such like. We can produce them at pleasure.

Specific cells are a physiological impossibility, so far as abnormality is concerned.

They may be heterotopic, that is, produced at a place where they do not belong; as an epithelial production in the brain, or in the uterus, or a bone; then we call it cancer.

Or the singular phenomenon of an embryonal tooth in the parotid region, which is sometimes met with in the horse.

Neither the cells nor the teeth having anything peculiar in themselves, they are normal elements in a wrong place.

Cells may be heterochronic—that is, normal cells may be produced at an abnormal time.

In Fig. 2 of Gerlach's illustration of glanders-cell, he give as first-class picture of the gelatinous connective tissue of the embryonal umbilical cord; a specimen, by-the-way, which offers the very best opportunity of studying the appearance and connections of spindle-cells.

Glanders-cells, cancer-cells, tubercle-cells, are all without any specificity. It is not the *cell* alone which makes the *cancer;* it is the seat, and the peculiar anatomical arrangements, with its physiological characteristics, which constitute the specificity of that malignant neoplasm.

The genesis of these cells in the nasal discharge was pretty correctly given by Gerlach, but since his day we have been taught that the greater portion of them are migrated leucocytes; this is true for pus-formation, but in *inflammations* it is certain that proliferation also takes place—hence some of our round cells may be *proliferated*, epithelial, or connective-tissue elements. This question of the origin of spindle-cells by formative processes or inflammations is still an open one, to my mind, notwithstanding the authority of Cohnheim. I, for one, do not believe a white blood-cell can transform or develop into a spindle-cell. We can not tell the difference between a white blood-cell and the intermediate or round cell condition of the developing spindle-cell.

Like begets like, and in inflammations, where *formation* takes place, it is my opinion that the migrated cells perish by fatty degeneration, and the formation is due, as long ago asserted by Virchow, to the permanent elements.

In glanders we have more or less circumscribed forms of neoplastic formations. The first of these are the tubercles, which vary in size from submiliary to that of a cherry or acorn; 2. The glanders-growths, varying from the above to the size of an apple, but of irregular form; 3. The glanders-infiltrations, which are less circumscribed in their *outlines*, and extended along the surface; these are particularly to be found in the nasal mucosa and sub-cutis.

The Glanders-Tubercle.—There has been and still exists much discussion and difference of opinion as to what should be considered a true tubercle.

While this discussion is valuable, from an anatomical and practical sense, it has still led to much unnecessary mystification among students.

It has always been the old hunt after specific cells, or specific characteristics, by which to decide between two (macroscopically) apparently similar objects. In the energy of this hunt the true specific has been lost sight of to a much too great degree.

The cause, irritans, is the specific element; the product may or may not have specific characteristics. We find tubercles occurring under a great variety of circumstances and among many different species of animals. Different causes lead to their production in one and the same species.

In the horse, tubercles occur in glanders; an idiopathic miliary tuberculosis has been reported, however.

I can not at present tell whether there are any marked structural differences in these tubercles in the horse.

Again, a peculiar *chronic production* in old horses, with more or less bronchial catarrh, is known as "bronchitis nodosa"; this has been mistaken for glanders and for true tuberculosis. The nodes are mostly composed of connective tissue, with round cells between the fibers, and consist of a circumscribed proliferation of the walls of the finest bronchioli, as they lose themselves in the infundibula. At times one can make a differential diagnosis, macroscopically, with ease, a transverse section of the object revealing the lumen of the air-tube. Carefully executed microscopic section will *always* reveal the true nature of these nodes.

Hereditary influences do not appear to play any part in the production of tuberculosis in the horse.

The *glanders-tubercle, in the lungs*, is of a permanent character; it does not extend, as in human tuberculosis, by infection of the neighboring tissues, forming large masses of degenerating material, which break down and lead to the formation of cavities—one form of phthisis pulmonum. They do not occur in any such quantity as in the human lung. They are inclined to calcify, although fatty degeneration of their centers is by no means uncommon.

They are due to a specific cause, the irritans of glanders.

I have no doubt that miliary tuberculosis can be produced in the horse, by the entrance of foreign substances into the lungs, as the aspiration of a spray containing in it the sputa from human phthisical subjects, as has been done in dogs.

We know nothing of the cause of the very rare miliary tuberculosis in the horse.

In men and cattle we have an hereditary predisposition to *tuberculosis.*

Here comes the ridiculous part of the assertion of many authors.

The diseases are *identical.* Why? Because in both cases giant-cells are found in the tubercles. The tubercles of glanders are not *true* tubercles.

1. Because they have no giant-cells.

2. Because they have a central vessel, which these others do not.

Both forms have a vascular circle, or rété, embracing them.

Giant-cells are not specific to tubercles. They are not present in all stages of the development of the neoplasm. According to Kölliker, their presence is always indicative of retrogressive or destructive processes; they are the *rodents* of cellular pathology, or physiology.

They occur in the medulla of the bones, in sarcomatous tumors, and, according to Kölliker, are one of the *active* causes of the normal indentations of the bones—at least, they are found under the periosteum. Tuberculosis also comes to pass in swine, rabbits, Guinea-pigs, monkeys, and other animals. Does the same cause work here as in man, the horse, or cow?

Again, etiologically speaking, we have several varieties of tuberculosis in man: First, hereditary causes; second, *idiopathic infection*, from antecedent conditions, *scrophulosis*, *cheesy* conditions of glands due to other causes; third, infection from persons having phthisis, by means of the aspiration of some specific irritans with which they pollute the air; and, fourth, the questionable infection due to milk from tuberculous nurses, or cows.

In *cattle*, we may briefly assume an almost similar line of causes.

This will do for our present purpose.

The tubercular neoplasm of glanders is, and always will be, a *tubercle*, having its peculiar cause, anatomical construction, and course.

Undoubtedly, in some unknown way, the physiological and anatomical characteristics of the different species, as well as the variations in the cause, exert some influence upon the structure and course of life of the tubercle. With regard to the structure and nature of the tubercles in glanders, Virchow says that "they are formed chiefly by cellular proliferation. In the youngest neoplasm I found large numbers of small, delicate cells, as well as numerous nuclei; in older tubercles, the cells are longer and contain nuclei; these cells are very abundant, composing the greater part of the node. These cells undoubtedly proceed from the pre-existing elements, and especially in the mucosæ from the connective-tissue cells of the mucosa and sub-mucosa. The greater the number of cells, so much more dense and yellow is the node; retrogressive processes soon take place in the older nodes; the cells undergo fatty metamorphosis, and break up and shrink.

Leisering, who has made very extensive studies upon the neoplasmata of glanders, says: "In whatever form the neoplasms of glanders may appear, the cells constitute their prevailing element. They are generally found varying in size; the majority bearing the strongest resemblance to pus-cells; others are from four to six times larger. Aside from these, numerous free nuclei go to make up the largest part of the node, as well as the cells of proliferating connective tissue. The neoplasms have a varying character, according to the predominance of the cellular, or stromatous, intercellular tissue over one another. The more rapid the development of the neoplasm, the more prominent the cellular elements; on the contrary, in slow development, the connective tissue prevails. The dissolution is hastened or retarded by the same. In slow development, the vascularization is less marked than in rapid. Wherever the processes of glanders are present, there may be found the tubercles, although the lungs are the favorite seat. They are sometimes present in great numbers, and at others it is very hard to find even solitary examples.

Why the tubercles in the lungs have so little tendency to break down, and those in the nasal mucosa are so prone thereto, must be sought in two circumstances:

1. Their development is far slower in the lungs.
2. The matrix is different.

Those in the lungs are absolutely from a connective-tissue matrix, while those in any mucosa are from a far less consistent matrix.

At any rate, they occur in the nasal mucosa much more as they develop in the human lung, that is, *en masse*, which, on account of their transient character, accounts for the tendency to breaking down, and here they seem also to have the infectious character of the human tubercle, new ones springing up in immediate proximity to antecedent ones, which gives to the ulcerated surfaces thus caused their rodent or extending characters.

The development of tubercles in the sinuses of the head does not occur to any such degree as in the mucosa proper to the nasal cavities; the nodes, or neoplasmatic productions which we find here, have a different character, to which we shall again refer.

In farcy, the tubercles lie chiefly in the cutis, although they also develop in the subcutaneous cellular tissue, and frequently attain considerable size.

"Histologically, the tubercles of glanders are exactly alike, whether we find them in the lungs, nose, or cutis. In a fresh condition they are more or less soft, transparent, and of a pearl-gray color. In this condition they each have an individual central vessel, as may be seen by injected lung specimens."

Do those of the other localities have this central vessel?

"In the examination of these nodes, we may often find at the center a hæmorrhagic point, which probably proceeds from this vessel.

"They may continue for a long time in the above condition. When newly developed, they are immediately limited by healthy lung-tissue; later they become a special limiting membrane of connective tissue. They are frequently surrounded by a circle of congested vessels, outside of which we frequently find more or less desquamative pneumonia.

"They undergo different metamorphoses; sometimes fatty degeneration or calcification.

"These calcified centers can often be removed as small calculi from the connective-tissue capsule, or limiting membrane. The development of ulcers most frequently occurs in the mucosa of the respiratory tract and in the cutis; neoplastic and degenerative processes following successively on each other."

Infiltrated Neoplastic Processes.

"By this is meant diffuse, not sharply circumscribed, neoplastic growths, composed of a gelatinous, pellucid, yellowish, reddish, or grayish mass.

"This condition is most frequently met with in the mucosa of the nose, the sinuses of the head, the larynx, and trachea; they extend but little above the surface of the mucosa proper.

"They undergo, generally, two forms of metamorphosis:

"*a.* Desquamation of the epithelium takes place upon the diseased localities, leaving an ulcerated surface. The cellular elements prevail to even a greater extent than in the nodes. They vary much in size. They undergo dissolution very rapidly, and give the most pregnant examples of glanders ulceration.

"*b.* The fibrous character may predominate, and it is in this form that cicatrization takes place."

Virchow differs from Leisering, in that he thinks the cicatrices proceed from the *ulcers*, rather than from the infiltrated form glanders. Bollinger looks upon the cicatrices as processes of natural healing of ulcerated surfaces, whether the same come from ulcerative or infiltrated disturbances.

In nasal glanders we frequently find intensive thrombosis of the veins of the septum and turbinated bones, as well as of the lymphatics.

The mucosa of the sinuses of the head is very delicate in a normal condition; in many cases of glanders we find it the subject of neoplastic processes, mostly of the diffuse form, interrupted by numerous circumscribed places of a more fibrous character, which project above the general surface. The mucosa and periosteum of these cavities form one membrane, and it is self-evident that one can not be complicated without the disturbance extending to the others, which leads to the developmont of osteophytes and hyperostoses, which remain after the mucosa has been removed by maceration.

Haubner, of Dresden, has endeavored, and often successfully, to make use of these complications of the sinuses of the head as aids to diagnosis in doubtful cases of glanders. By trepanning, the diseased nature of the mucosa and bones may frequently be seen, and in many cases the true nature of the disease may be determined by the ulcerative character which the healing wound of the operation assumes, although this can not be said to be an invariable rule.

We also find these diffuse neoplastic processes in the lungs of varying size and quantity. Sometimes they are on the edges, and at others in the body of the lung. In their substance tubercles may be often found; the adjoining tissue is generally more or less hyperæmic.

At first, these places consist of a yellow, gelatinous mass; later, the cellular or fibroid character may prevail. In the first case, they present some characteristics of *gray hepatization;* in the *last*, the cut surface is dry, and the resistance to the knife greater in making a transverse section.

These infiltrations undergo the same metamorphoses which we have learned in the tubercles, and complicate the pulmonary tissue in their dissolution. In general, caseification and calcification take place. They are frequently circumscribed by a sort of connective-tissue capsule.

The processes in the cutis and limiting muscles have the same characteristics as those in the lungs and nasal cavities, except that the lymphatics are more considerably complicated. They frequently terminate in extensive sclerosis of the subcutaneous cellular tissues or the development of ulcers, farcy-buds, or abscesses. Erysipelatous and phlegmonous complications of the cutis and subcutis are by no means uncommon, especially in the extremities.

As secondary complications of glanders, we often find bronchitis and broncho-pneumonia in the lungs, especially in the anterior and deeper portions.

Another peculiar pulmonary complication, though not specific to glanders alone, as it comes also in aged and worn-out horses, is known as gelatinous infiltrations.

This condition being so common, and so little noticed in works on veterinary pathology, I feel justified in touching upon it here.

Schutz, the able pathologist of the Veterinary School at Berlin, says, "This condition occurs quite frequently in the lungs of horses complicated with glanders, and I must admit that I have had no little difficulty in following its genesis." *

* "Lungenkrankheiten des Pferdes."

Gelatinous, infiltrated portions of the lungs are more or less transparent, densely filled with fluid, and extended to a moderate degree. The fluid in such parts is viscid. The changes in these parts become more marked as the fluid in the alveoli augments. When we make a transverse section of such parts, this fluid does not flow over the cut surface, which is smooth and lustrous, unless we exert pressure upon the lung. The contents of the alveoli strongly resemble mucus, but, as there is no mucous membrane in the alveoli, it terminates with the bronchiolus; if this fluid contains mucin, it must then be aspirated with the air. It does not, however, contain mucin. This fluid is very viscid and much like the white of eggs; it also contains cells, most of which strongly resemble the white blood-cells; some of them are larger, and are undoubtedly desquamated and swollen endothelial cells.

Accordingly, the disease product in the lungs consists of a viscid fluid and cellular elements; this mass seems to be of a movable nature, and it is quite interesting to know why it is not expectorated.

At first, however, I will remark that I can not accept the terminology, "inveterate œdema," which Rindfleisch has given to this condition, especially as he attributes it to the extravasation of the serous elements of the blood in consequence of mechanical hinderance to the circulation. On the contrary, we have here to do with an inflammatory process, as is indicated by the presence of so many round cells in the fluid. Laennec was the first to give the name of "gelatinous infiltrations" to these conditions, and Brückmüller has also treated it as an inflammatory process. In it the extravasation of fluid far exceeds that of the cellular elements of the blood, which, with the desquamated epithelium of the alveoli, make up the mass. When this occurs alone we have a desquamative pneumonia, which is similar to the desquamation which occurs from the cutis, except that the loosened cells are here inclosed in a cavity; the presence of the fluid in this case causes them to swell, and become more or less transparent, the same as when we put the desquamated cells of the cutis-epithelium in water. As in most pneumonias, there is also an exudation of fluid from the vessels into the alveoli; the name of catarrhal pneumonia is better than Buhl's terminology, "desquamative pneumonia." Horses have, in general, this form of pneumonia, although not every catarrhal pneumonia is complicated with gelatinous infiltration.

The conditions to the development of gelatinous infiltration are:

1. "*Atelectasis of the complicated pulmonary tissue*—i. e., the

complicated portion of the lungs must first be *airless* before the inflammatory processes take place. The atelectatic parts have a more or less homogeneous character, and, when they become filled with this fluid substance, they have the above-mentioned gelatinous, pellucid character. The atelectatic parts are rendered œdematous by the inflammation; fluid and cells distend the alveoli instead of air; such parts are tense, yet elastic to the touch. We have, then, atelectasis—airlessness—plus inflammatory œdema."

"It may be remarked that we have two forms of œdema: the one mechanical, due to some interference with the circulation, by which the vessels become so distended that the serous elements of blood exude through the vessels; this is exemplified by the *collateral œdema*, which often takes place in the non-complicated parts of the lungs in pneumonia, that causes death by a sort of internal self-drowning. The other is due to inflammation, which you should know all about."

2. "A second condition proper to gelatinous infiltration is anæmia; or, in other words, bloodless atelectasis is a *sine qua non* to gelatinous infiltration. This anæmia is the reason that such parts have a yellowish or yellowish-gray color. According to Rindfleisch, a hyperæmic condition develops in every atelectatic part. This hyperæmia is the cause of the exudation of the blood-serum in the alveoli, and causes a condition which he names splenization. His 'inveterate œdema' is only to be distinguished from splenization by the absence of hyperæmia, and the anæmia by the pressure caused by the continued transudation of fluid into the alveoli."

According to Schutz, neither splenization nor gelatinous infiltration are due to mere serous transudation. Both owe their genesis in atelectatic tissues to inflammation, except in splenization the atelectasic tissues are in a hyperæmic, while in gelatinous infiltration they are in an anæmic condition. The splenized and gelatinous infiltrated tissues contain not only serous fluid, but the products of inflammation, i. e., water, which is rich in albumen and cellular elements. Gelatinous infiltration is, therefore, not the second stage of splenization, as Rindfleisch asserts, but either can occur *sui generis*, and we have therefore to consider why at one time we have gelatinous infiltration and at another splenization of the lung.

"I have only seen gelatinous infiltration in emaciated and weak horses, which were anæmic. It makes no difference whether this latter condition was produced by poor dietetic conditions or chronic disease. In such horses all parts are pale, also the atelectatic portions of the lungs; and slight catarrhal processes in such parts easily produce gelatinous infiltration. The grade of the anæmia present decides the grade of the paleness, and the latter is not the secondary but the primary condition of the lungs, into which the transudation of fluid, etc., takes place. When, however, the atelectatic parts are at the same time hyperæmic, as in vital hypostasis, and, in such hypostatic-atelectatic parts, inflammation takes place, then we have splenization.

"Gelatinous infiltration, therefore, consists of atelectasis, *anæmia*, transudation of fluid, and a moderate filling of the alveoli with cells; splenization, of atelectasis, hypostasia, *hyperæmia*, transudation of fluid, and a moderate filling of the alveoli with cells."

The conditions to atelectasis and anæmia are always present in emaciated horses. In such, the respiratory movements are weak, and they frequently suffer from bronchial catarrh. Atelectasis is naturally to be found in those portions of the lungs where the conditions to the free circulation of the air are the least favorable; that is, the middle and anterior portions of each lung. The extent of the atelectasis is dependent upon the extension of the bronchial catarrh, and the degree of weakness of the respiratory functions. As such horses are also anæmic, the atelectatic portion of the lung must be in a like condition. Atelectasis and anæmia are both quite common in horses suffering from chronic glanders; their respiratory functions are also weak, and they often suffer from bronchial catarrh. Therefore, in such horses, the lungs are already prepared for gelatinous infiltration, and we see it occurs the moment they acquire a catarrhal pneumonia. Gelatinous infiltration is, however, a secondary complication, and has no idiopathic connection with glanders. Each can occur without the other, though the former is a frequent complication of the latter. We frequently find the pathological processes of glanders in small and circumscribed portions of the lungs, while the gelatinous infiltrations complicate extensive portions of the same. When the latter are very extensive, we often see striking clinical phenomena, caused by local catarrhal pneumonia, which has come in as a secondary complication to glanders. Clinicians have then said that the glanders has become acute, though in truth it has only become complicated by an acute catarrhal pneumonia.

"If they die in this condition, glanders has not been the cause, but the accessory complication. If such horses have laid upon one side for some time *ante-mortem*, we shall find hypostatic hyperæmia in the diseased portions of the lungs, and then, instead of gelatinous infiltration, we shall find a splenized condition in the deeper-seated portions of the lungs. Such parts derive their name from their resemblance to the spleen.

"Gelatinous infiltration and splenization occur under peculiar circumstances; both of them represent the beginning of an inflammatory process, or a cellular infiltration of the alveoli—red hepatization. Frequently, however, the alveoli become filled with cells, when we have the condition of full cellular alveolic infiltration—gray hepatization. These places are situated in the vicinity of the bronchioli, and bespeak a high degree of irritation of the pulmonic tissues. The causes of catarrhal pneumonia find their atrium by means of the bronchi, so it is natural that these conditions should develop in their vicinity. Broncho-pneumonia has always a local character; it is circumscribed, not diffuse; centers of pneumonia, therefore, develop in the gelatinous, infiltrated, or splenized parts. In the first, the centers are of a whitish, in the latter of a grayish-red, color. Persons who look upon all circumscribed inflammatory centers as indications of glanders, could easily mistake these for the same. They have nothing whatever to do with glanders, however, and can occur in any horse under the above conditions."

We have already spoken of the general complication of the interstitial tissue, or stroma, of the large glands of the organism in glanders, which does not find mention in the books, and have only to mention that circumscribed neoplasmata also develop in these organs, and sometimes within the bones. In the liver they possess a great inclination to calcify. Clouded swelling and granular degeneration of parenchyma of these organs also take place. Leucocytosis, or an unnatural number of white blood-cells, is also common in chronic glanders; the increase of these cells is sometimes so great as to produce a veritable leucæmia; ten white to twenty red cells have frequently been counted. The cause of this condition is to be sought in the constant irritation which the lymph-glands undergo in this disease.

Diagnosis.

The diagnosis of glanders is often extremely difficult; especially is this the case in the chronic form, where all external pathognomonic symptoms are wanting; but the fact of infection of other horses, the prevalence of the previously detailed dyspnœtic, debilitated, and other suspicious phenomena are generally sufficient to warrant a questionable diagnosis, and the exact quarantining or slaughtering of the animal by the authorities.

Prognosis.

Always unfavorable; treatment is never justifiable, on account of the danger of the extension of the disease to man and other animals.

Prevention.

No one but accredited veterinarians should ever be permitted to examine either glandered or suspected horses by the civil authorities. If the disease is confirmed, or if there is a justified suspicion of its existence, the veterinarian should at once inaugurate careful inquiries as to the period during which the suspicious symptoms have been present; the number of horses stabled with such diseased or suspected ones; whether they have worked with them; which have stood beside them, and for how long; have any been sold, or otherwise removed from the stable, and carefully examine each horse in detail. The results of such an examination should be reported in due form to the civil authorities. The examining veterinarian should at once isolate the diseased or suspected horses in a place distant from the healthy ones, or better, the healthy ones should, if possible, be removed from the infected stable. The owner and attendants must be notified of their duties in this regard, and of the danger to themselves from carelessness.

Special persons should be detailed to take care of the suspected animals.

The veterinarian should make an accurate and detailed description of each horse upon the place, or in the stable, a copy of which, with owner's name, should be given to the civil authorities.

If glanders be diagnosed in a horse, it should be at once killed, and in a way to guarantee, as far as possible, no further extension of the disease.

When the suspicion of glanders exists, the animals should be killed—

1. When it can be proved that the suspected animal has been in intimate relations with one known to have had the disease.

2. When there exists a suspicious nasal discharge; tumefaction and nodulated conditions of the intermaxillary and other accessible lymph-glands; when suspicious cutaneous conditions are present, especially when in unison with these conditions we have more or less marked difficulty in respiration, and want of condition in the animal.

3. When, after the lapse of three months, a suspected horse can not be declared free from suspicion by a majority of three qualified veterinarians.

4. When the owner can not supply suitable conveniences for quarantining such a horse, or where reasons exist which render such a procedure necessary to the public good.

5. If the owner refuses to comply with the veterinary police regulations.

When necessary, suspected horses should be branded in a manner to be fixed by law.

A horse must be looked upon as "suspected" when it has stood in the same stable with one known to have or have had the disease; or when it is known that it has been exposed to infection from such a horse.

Suspected horses or stables must be subjected to periodical examinations by an accredited veterinarian; these revisions should occur at least once in eight days.

Such horses may be allowed to be used within certain limits and according to certain regulations of the civil authorities.

Such horses should be kept under veterinary control for a period of not less than three months. If the restrictive regulations of the civil authorities are not rigidly adhered to, suspected horses must be subjected to stable quarantine, where veterinary revision should also take place at least twice a month.

The animal should be peremptorily killed, should the owner attempt to evade these rules, and the evasion punished by law.

Should the disease extend from an infected locality, a careful examination of the horses in the vicinity should be made.

The cadavers of horses killed on account of glanders should either be chemically destroyed or securely buried, after the hide had been destroyed by slashing and the carcass rendered uupalatable by saturation with kerosene. Three feet of earth should cover such cadavers, and the burial-place be either fenced in or paved.

Public watering-troughs are to be condemned, and faucets put in their place. Hackmen, teamsters, etc., should be obliged by law to carry buckets to water their horses.

The disease may be declared as ended—

When all diseased or suspected horses have been killed, or when the latter have been declared free from suspicion.

When the infected stables, utensils, harnesses, etc., have been thoroughly cleansed and disinfected.

Glanders in Human Beings.

As I said of anthrax, it seems to me indispensable that the veterinarian should also know the essential points of glanders in man. In detailing these I shall give the facts directly from Bollinger's description.

Etiology.

It must be self-evident that equine glanders is *the* source whence human beings derive the disease. In most cases it is possible to trace the disease to the cause, although in some we are unable to; this latter variety has been looked upon in times past as of spontaneous origin.

The inficiens gains access to the human organs by means of wounded or abraded surfaces, either in the care of diseased animals, or by persons examining them, or by persons in knackers' establishments, and occasionally through accident or sheer carelessness. In some cases the nose, mouth, or eyes may serve as the atrium, when horses snort and blow such material into these cavities. A few cases have been reported where the bite of a glandered horse has caused infection.

It is undoubtedly a fact that the flesh of glandered horses is infectious, as is proved by the disease occurring in lions and other animals that have fed upon it.

Decroix, the noted hippophagist of France, had the temerity to eat it in both a cooked and uncooked condition, and saw no evil results therefrom. Röll and others report cases of infection of grooms and others by drinking from the stable water-pails, or by wiping a wound with a rubbing-cloth, or among veterinarians by using one's handkerchief to wipe the horse's discharge from off the clothes, and then using it about the person.

When the disease occurs without any known *locus infectionis*, we must assume that it is through the aspired air, especially where a constitutional complication antedates any local disturbances.

This has been observed to occur in grooms, etc., especially where they sleep in the stables, or by the accidental sleeping upon the straw which had been used to bed a glandered horse.

In this regard the following two cases are interesting:

1. A groom had the habit of taking the warm blanket off the horse and replacing it with another. He would roll himself up in it perfectly nude, and cover himself with others, and thus sleep in the stable. The man acquired glanders, though no one had suspected its existence in the horse, nor were there any ul-

cerations, nasal discharge, or tumefied glands, to indicate its presence.

The autopsy developed the presence of pulmonary and constitutional glanders.*

2. This is a most remarkable and instructive case. A family lived *over* a stable, with steps leading down from the tenement by the stable-door. The mother had an infant at the breast, and one day, when taking it down to give it fresh air, a horse which was being led out snorted and blew some discharge from its nostrils into the child's face. The child was taken ill, and glanders diagnosed. An elder sister, who was in condition to act as wet-nurse, one day took the child to nurse; she had excoriated nipples, and some of the discharge from the child's nose probably came in contact with them. Both child and sister died from glanders.†

3. A young man purchased a glandered horse at Detroit, Michigan, not knowing what it was. He contracted the disease and died.

The Massachusetts State Board of Health have recorded thirteen cases of glanders, between the years 1859 and 1875, in that State.

Cases of the transmission of glanders from man to man have been reported; one where a family of man, wife, and four children all became diseased from sleeping in the same bed with the father.

Predisposition.—It can, in general, be said to be very small, when we consider the frequent occasions offered to infection to those whose business brings them among such horses.

In general, glanders among human beings may be said to be a "calling" disease; that is, occurring among the above-named classes.

Of the 106 cases collected by Bollinger—

41 were grooms.
11 coachmen, teamsters, and riders.
14 horse-owners and farmers.
10 veterinarians and veterinary students.
6 knackers.
6 horse-butchers.
5 soldiers.
4 doctors.
3 gardeners.
2 horse-dealers.
1 each in a policeman, shepherd, smith, and an anatomy servant at a veterinary school.

* "Mittheilung an d. Praxis im Preussischen Staate," 1879–'80.

† "Veterinary Journal," vol. ix, p. 144.

Incubation.—The incubatory period is from three to five days; sometimes extending to fourteen days or three weeks.

Course.—The disease assumes either an acute, subacute, or chronic form.

ACUTE GLANDERS.

Of twenty-eight cases, of which but one ended fatally, the average duration, aside from the period of incubation, was 16·5 days. Cases of seven to eight days' duration are rare; in general, it lasts two to three weeks, sometimes four.

The introductory phenomena are frequently a general feeling of disturbance, weakness, headache, shivering, often combined with uncertain pains in the extremities, especially in the muscles and joints.

If a trauma (wounds) formed the atrium of the inficiens, we may remark on the *locus infectionis* hyperæmia and inflammation of the parts; swelling and inflammation of the lymphatics. In rare cases the disease begins with shivering. When the pains are intense and intermittent or continued, fever is present. The ulcers increase, the edges and base acquire an evil appearance, the ulcer frequently a chancrous, rodent character. When the wound is upon a finger, the whole arm may be the seat of an erysipėlatous or phlegmonous inflammation, which is often complicated with pustular or ulcerous eruptions. The constitutional disturbances increase at the same time: the patient loses appetite; the evacuations are retarded; the weakness increases; the pains in the muscles and joints become more intense, and the fever augments.

When the anamnesis is wanting, and when the infection has taken place from a volatile inficiens, or when all signs of outward infection fail, the disease might often be mistaken for typhus. As the disease progresses, reddish spots appear on the cutis, which transform into pustules resembling those of variola or pemphigus. These pustules often appear in great numbers, and are of varying dimensions. They frequently coalesce and form ulcers, giving off an offensive odor. Large ulcers often develop on the extremities, which extend to the sinews and bones. These cutaneous affections are frequently so extensive as to leave scarcely any part of the body uncomplicated. Sometimes the joints become tumefied with fluctuating swellings. At others these eruptions appear within twenty-four or forty-eight hours; again, only within two, three, or four weeks, after the appearance of nasal catarrh, tumefaction of the muscles, pain, etc.

The mucosæ, particularly of the nose, are frequently the seat of inflammatory and ulcerative processes. When the nose is complicated, we observe in the beginning a secretion of a thin, viscid, whitish discharge; swelling, hyperæmia, and pains in the nose and surroundings, gradually develop. The nasal discharge is frequently unilateral, and later becomes thicker, muco-purulent, and offensive. In a few cases nodules may be diagnosed. In many cases we can diagnose, *intra vitam*, the development of pustules and ulcers in the nasal mucosa, which in malignant cases lead to erosions of the perichondrium and perforation of septum. The uni- or bilateral nasal discharge appears often only after two or three weeks, coeval with diffuse redness of the nose, which may extend over the face and forehead. In few cases the nasal discharge fails, although nodular eruptions take place.

As in the horse, so in man, we frequently observe that the nasal affection appears to be the closing complication of the disease.

Later, or coeval with the cutaneous eruptions, there develop catarrh and inflammatory ulcerative processes in the other mucosæ, which stand in more or less intimate connection with that of the nose, as in the conjunctiva, the mouth, œsophagus, and trachea. In some cases abscesses develop in the joints, particularly those of the hands. The submaxillary and lingual glands, which often contain abscesses, become swollen and painful. The respiratory tract is frequently the seat of serious complications, such as bronchial catarrh, with accompanying symptoms. The pulse is small and frequent; the temperature increases to over 40° C.

The participation of the nervous system is made evident by vertigo, headache, ringing in the ears, want of sleep, uneasiness, somnolence, delirium, etc. Albumen is sometimes present in the urine. In pregnant females, abortion often takes place.

Chronic Glanders

Assumes the above characteristics in varying form and less rapid development. The medium duration—recovery is quite frequent, slow, and incomplete—extends over four months.

Pathological Anatomy.—In this regard the phenomena in man bear a strong resemblance to those of pyæmia.

The chief difference between those of man and horses is the greater prevalence of tubercular eruptions in the former; otherwise we have almost similar conditions, except the greater tendency to abscesses in man.

Diagnosis.—This, when the cause is known, is easy, otherwise often very difficult, especially on account of the resemblance of the processes to those of pyæmia.

Prognosis.—This is far more favorable than in the horse, although in the acute form it is generally fatal.

Of 38 cases of acute glanders, healing by	1
Of 7 cases of subacute glanders, healing by	2
Of 34 cases of chronic glanders, healing by	17

Therapeutics.—This belongs to medical men.

Prevention.—Keep down equine glanders, and see to the proper instruction of those about horses, that they exercise great care about those having glanders, or in which it is suspected.

PART II.

THE HISTORY OF VETERINARY MEDICINE.

In the foregoing pages I have endeavored to place before the public some of the principal dangers to which mankind is liable from animal diseases themselves, or from parasites which, while infecting the so-called lower animal organism, do not in some instances cause any very serious disturbances; still, when introduced into the human organism, may cause disturbances of a very serious if not of an absolutely mortal character.

The only known means by which prevention of these disturbauces, or maladies, may be hoped for, is by the enactment of laws and regulations by the different State governments—which should, however, be uniform in all States. These laws and regulations should be rigidly executed. Their execution, however, does not come within the province of human medicine *per se.* It belongs to another branch of medical science, which has been, up to the present time, utterly neglected by the people of this country, whether represented by the respective State governments or by the General Government at Washington. Coming under the same head, and therefore to be considered with it, are the suppression and prevention of those ravaging animal pests which in past ages have almost depopulated the older Continental nations of their animal wealth, and which can any day be landed upon our shores; in fact, as I have already shown, some of them are already "domesticated" with us, and the sole reason that their real nature and their ravages among our animals are not more immediately felt by the American people is the utter failure of reliable statistics upon the subject to bring it *home* to every American statesman and citizen as well.

The Commissioner of Agriculture, at Washington, gave out, for the year 1879, a pamphlet entitled "Investigations of Diseases of Swine, and Infectious and Contagious Diseases incident to other

Classes of Domestic Animals." The title is high-sounding enough, but while Messrs. Law and Detmers, veterinarians, give us some valuable knowledge with reference to *one* contagio-infectious disease of swine, the so-called "hog-cholera," the "report" is absolutely wanting in any reliable statistics with reference to the same. Numerous medical men have also given contributions with reference to this swine-disease, many of which are most absurd: for instance, calling it "typhus," and comparing it with the specific infectious disease of man known by that name. Veterinary-Surgeon Detmers also gives a compilation with reference to the glanders of the horse. Aside from the pleuro-pneumonia of cattle, *no other* contagious disease of our animals is mentioned in the report. This is not to be wondered at. In a country where there are very few well-educated veterinary surgeons, where there is no appreciation of the true value of veterinary science; in a country where quacks and empirics of every form are nourished and appreciated before the well-educated practitioners, in only too many instances; in a country where there is no official examination of the products from food-producing animals, and where there are neither laws nor regulations for the suppression of contagious animal diseases; in a country boasting, as it does, of its civilization and the extent of education among its people, where there is no well-organized veterinary school, or a medical school devoted exclusively to the scientific study and development of science, and regulated by the State—it is not surprising that it is impossible for the Government to gather reliable, or any, statistics with reference to the devastations caused by pests among its animals.

The prevention of the already described human *diseases due to causes originating in our domestic animals, the suppression and prevention of devastating animal pests, can* ONLY *be attained by the development of veterinary science, and at the hands of scientifically educated veterinarians.*

This can only be attained by having a completely organized and State-regulated veterinary institute, and for reasons which I shall presently give. One national institute is far more in the interests of the people of this country than State institutes.

Before, however, entering upon the discussion of that subject, it is not inappropriate to cursorily trace the history of veterinary medicine from its beginning to our time. The history of veterinary medicine *per se* can be logically divided into two periods: the ante-school, or crude, empirical period, extending from the earliest antiquity to the year 1762; and the scholastic or educational period, extending from that date to our own day. Both of these periods are capable of subdivision. The pre-scholastic period may be subdivided into the ante-Greek, the Græco-Roman, and the period of the "Stahlmeisters," "mareschal," or master of the horse, while the scholastic period may be divided into the educational-empiric and the scientific-educational, which saw its birth about thirty years ago.

"Westward the march of empire takes its way!" So true as this is, it is no less true that with the "westward" movement of humanity and civilization, the contagious and ravaging pests which have preyed and still continue to prey upon a suffering human and animal world have kept up a uniform extension. So it is of science. So it is with the endeavor of medical science—prevention. So it will be with that branch of medical science which I am endeavoring, however unsuccessfully, faithfully to represent—veterinary medicine.

Philologists have taught us that the civilized races of the day took their rise from the Aryans, a pastoral people who conquered the nomad tribes living on the high plateaus of the Caucasus Mountains in the north of India. These Aryans attained a wonderful degree of civilization, which is detailed to us in records of an age some 1000 years B. C. With their civilization was mixed an immense amount of superstition, a great awe and reverence for all the startling phenomena of nature, as well as all natural creations. These records are ingrafted in the beautiful poems of the "Artharva," "Rig" and "Ayur Veda," the last meaning the "Science of Life," and the great war-poem, the "Mahabharata."

The reverence which these people bore to their Brahmans, as the ministers of their gods, and their worship of the sacred cow, and tender care of all animal life, are well known to the student of these ancient writings. With suffering comes naturally an immediate search for relief. Behold, then, the birth of empiricism! The results of these experiences were handed down from mouth to mouth; these sayings being frequently collected and recited for the benefit of the people by the priests and wise men. The wealth of these early people, and also of many of their immediate descendants of our day, was in their immense herds of grazing animals. Fleming, "Animal Plagues," says: "The immense steppes of Central Asia still furnish us with examples of this condition of the unsettled races who wander over them with their countless herds." A recent traveler* in that region of the world pleasantly describes some of

* Atkinson, "Oriental and Western Siberia."

the scenes he witnessed among them: "Just as the day dawned I turned out to examine our position, when I discovered the snowy peaks of the Sian-Shan. They appeared cold and ghost-like against the deep-blue sky; presently they were tipped with the sun's rays, and shone forth like rubies. I sat on the ground, watching the changes with much interest, till the whole landscape was lighted up. Immediately near me was a busy scene; on one side the men were milking the mares, to the number of more than one hundred, and carrying leathern pails of milk to the 'koumiss' bag in the 'yourt,' the young foals being secured in two long lines to pegs driven in the ground. In front, and on the opposite side, the women were milking cows, sheep, and goats, and a little distance beyond these the camels were suckling their young. Around the camp the steppe was filled with animal life. The sultan told me that there were more than two thousand horses, half the number of cows and oxen, two hundred and eighty camels, and more than six thousand sheep and goats. The screams of the camels, the bellowing of the bulls, the neighing of the horses, and bleating of the sheep and goats, formed a pastoral chorus such as I had never heard in Europe." On another occasion he writes: "All were out with the dawn, and then appeared a scene highly interesting to me. The whole of the herds are brought to the 'aoul' at night, where they are most carefully guarded by watchmen and dogs placed in every direction, rendering it almost impossible to enter any 'aoul' without detection. The noise at first was almost intolerable; there was the sharp cry of the camels, the neighing of the horses, the bellowing of the bulls, and the barking of the dogs, and shouting of the men. I counted one hundred and six camels, including their young; there were more than two thousand horses, one thousand oxen and cows, and six thousand sheep and goats. Even these, large as the number may appear, were far short of the total number belonging to the patriarch chief. It was, indeed, a wonderful sight, when they were marched off in different directions, spreading themselves out in living streams as they moved slowly along the steppe."

Disease then, as now, especially the ravaging pests, robbed these early agriculturists, not only of their means of sustenance, but of their wealth. As in our day, when such visitations endanger the animal property of the people of a country, so in those by-gone days did our Aryan fathers appeal to the gods for protection, and make choice offerings from the fairest and best of their flocks for their amelioration. They knew nothing of *prevention*, in a modern sense. The gods were manifesting their anger, and wreaking their wrath on the children of men. Appeasement was their only source; and, at the cessation of the ravages, choice offerings of thankfulness betokened the gratitude of suffering man.

"Charaka" and "Susruta" are the names which have come to us of the two earliest medical authors in the Sanskrit tongue.

The earliest source from which our knowledge of Indian medicine is derived is taken from the hymns of the "Rig-Veda," about 1500 B. C.* In the "Artharva-Veda" diseases are looked upon as evil spirits which overcome human beings, or as the results of the displeasure of the gods, or as the influences of the sorceries of wicked men. The most wonderful healing attributes were accorded to the soma-plant. The Aswin, a twin god, were looked upon as Hygeia by the Greeks, i. e., as the gods of health: they made the lap of woman fruitful; they knew the plants which were endowed with health-giving properties; they kept the altar-fires burning. At a later period they are described as the physicians of the gods. Besides them, the god Agni, the god of fire, was looked upon as the new awakening of spring; Rudra, of the air, the winds, and the earth.

These early authors also ascribed healing qualities to the action of cold water:

"Two winds move slowly here and there, from ocean, and from distant lands;
Power move thee, move thy suffering forth;
Wind, move healing this one to, and move, wind, his suffering forth.
The gods have thee hither sent with all the means of healing overspent."

"Full of healing power is the watery wave; the water cools the fever's heat:
Full of healing power against all pests, health bring to thee the water's flood."

"The good magi are under the protection of gods, in order that they may combat evil spirits."

The essence of life is embodied in the air (the respiration). Vital Power, Vital Spirit, are often spoken of. The doctor *per se* is only mentioned in the more recent sections of the "Rig-Veda." "The wishes of men vary: the wagoner seeks for wood, the doctor for patients, and the priest for libations."

In the Brahmanical period of the Aryan people, the priests appear to have also busied themselves with the practice of healing. At this period the doctor seems to have taken a much-respected place among these people. A completely educated doctor must

* This information with regard to ancient medical history is taken from Haeser, "Geschichte der Medicin."

command all the principles and practice of medicine. Susruta says that "the practitioner who does not perfectly unite in himself a knowledge of both surgical and inner diseases is as a bird with but one wing."

The studies of the medical student began with the twelfth and ended with the sixteenth or seventeenth year. At no one time should a teacher instruct more than four or at the most six students. Charaka gives the rules for instruction in detail, and the requirements necessary to both teacher and student, in a manner not unworthy of imitation, in many respects, by the same classes in our own day and country.

He says: "The student must, above all, pay great attention to selection of the most suitable text-books from the great number which are presented to him; he must select a teacher who is familiar with all the scientific, technical, and moral qualifications of his profession. He must devote himself unceasingly to the study of the text-books of his profession. The teacher must not be less circumspect in the selection of students of honorable birth, morality, physique, and intellectual and manual ability. The students must begin their studies in winter, and at a time when the moon is becoming full; on a day known in the calendar as favorable, and at a time when a favorable constellation is in the ascendency; they must be introduced into their profession in the presence of the holy Brahmans and the doctors, and with the offering of milk, butter, prayers, and sayings of wise men, and presents to his teachers. The celebration should end with an address to the students by the teachers, in which they should be cautioned to be chaste, modest, and reticent, to wear a beard, to speak the truth only, to eat no meat; above all things should they be obedient to their teacher, and endeavor to gain favor in his eyes. The practitioner who wishes to have a successful practice and to acquire an honorable name, must look to the health of the living; above all, that of the holy Brahmans *and the sacred cow*, and pray daily at the time of his uprising and retiring. He must seek, with all the strength of his soul, to restore the sick to health; though his own life be called in sacrifice thereby, he dare not on any account neglect the sick; he must never seek to ingratiate himself with women. In dress and all external things he must be simple, no drinker, and must always remain distant from bad company. In speech the practitioner must be gentle, clear, and pleasant, speaking only to the point, and with moderation; he must weigh seriously the appropriate time and locality; must be diligent in reflection, and seek in every way to increase in knowledge. He must never offer help to persons that have made themselves disagreeable to the king, or to the people; or offer assistance to deformed people, deteriorated, unruly, or wild persons, or even to women, when their husband is absent. The student must never accept a present from a wife, except with the permission of the husband. When he enters a residence, it must be in the company of an authorized person; he must be well clad, and enter with bowed head, reflecting, and with full dignity take due cognizance of all the surroundings. Once in the sick-chamber, his whole attention must be given to the treatment of the patient. The things going on in the house of the patient must never be advertised abroad; he must never inform a patient that a fatal termination to his illness is approaching. The most learned man must never seek to impress upon others the idea of his own importance. Many persons withdraw themselves from such men, however capable they may be. The science of medicine is, in all truth, not so easy of acquisition. He must ever be willing to learn from the experience and knowledge of others. To the earnest man the whole world is full of teaching; only to the ignorant is she an enemy. With this in remembrance, even the words of an enemy may be conducive to the good of many. He must religiously observe every duty to the gods, the fire, the holy Brahmans, the Guru, the aged, and the holy teacher. When this is done, then shalt thou be favored by the fire, the fluids, and the gods. When not, thy life shall be unsuccessful. When this has all been said, the teacher shall respond, 'So shall it be.'"

Susruta gave similar advice to that already given by Charaka, to the students of medicine. He says: "They must utterly abstain from love and hate, from anger and laziness, and from greed for gain. They must pay consideration to external appearances, and have care that their clothing is appropriate and cleanly. They must be servants of the truth. They must show the same respect as to their parents, to the Brahmans, to their teacher in medicine, to their friends, and to all those who turn to them for help. The doctor must wear his hair short; his nails must be clean and closely cut; he must never leave his house except with his cane or sun-shade; above all, must he avoid all undue intimacy with women. He must be handsome, well built, amiable, earnest, but without self-conceit, friendly, and full of spirit; his speech must be soft yet encouraging, as that of a friend; his heart must be pure and honorable; he must be a pattern of cleverness and sagacity, and must love his patients better than relations, friends, or his parents. One may have fear of a brother, a mother, or a friend, but never of his doctor.

The teacher shall read from the holy books step by step, and verse by verse; he must speak distinctly, but without undue exertion, neither too rapidly nor too slowly, neither through the nose, nor with any indications of impatience."

The theoretical education of the student took place in the open air, frequently in groves. The practical instruction consisted in the visiting of patients, the practice of surgical operations upon models made of wood covered with wax, also on soft fruits, and the puncture of leather sacks; the extraction of teeth was practiced on the dead body and upon animals. The students also accompanied the teacher on journeys in search of medicines, and to study the diseases of other regions. In order to practice his profession, it was necessary that the student had the consent of the rajah (ruler), who watched over the execution of the regulations for the practice of medicine.

We see here that these Aryans were further advanced in some things even than the enlightened citizens of this boasted country, for they did not allow even the graduated student to practice medicine without the consent of the recognized authority; and, further, the practice of medicine was regulated by the authorities. Quacks and empirics probably, then as now, were vampires of civilization, sucking the life-blood of the people; but, nevertheless, the people had means of distinguishing the accredited man from the swindler, and the title of "doctor" was worth something more than the paper it was written on, which is not at present the case in the United States of America.

"*Not seldom, however, through the carelessness of the rajah, unsuitable doctors were admitted to practice. Such men flatter the friends of the sick, are very attentive, take less pay, are bold-faced, and never attribute the poor results of their practice to their own ignorance. The educated practitioner must flee the company of such men as a thicket full of ravenous animals.* The reward of the practitioner must be ordered according to the means of the patients. It is dishonorable to demand pay of Brahmans, relations, friends, and the unfortunate. The doctor shall take no other pay from women than refreshment. The kings have especial doctors, who take part in the wars; others must be present in the kitchen to prevent poisoning."

In the "Laws of Manu" it is written that "the doctor who mishandles *animals* shall receive the *lowest*, while he who mistreats *human beings* shall receive the highest punishment."

The Indian doctors possessed but little real knowledge of anatomy. They, however, made studies upon the human body, but in a singular and unfruitful manner. The body must be that of a healthy man, not too old, not deformed, and from a person that had not died from poisoning or the devastations of a long and wearing disease. The body must lie for seven days and nights in the waters of a brook, and then the outer parts must be removed by brushing with twigs. Instead of a description of the different parts of the body, we find numerous calculations, measurements, and classifications of the parts. According to Susruta, the human body consists of seven elements, and seven skins or membranes, three hundred bones, twenty-four nerves, three fluids, one hundred and seven joints, nine hundred ligaments, ninety sinews (the nails were looked upon as the endings of the same), forty principal vessels, seven hundred branches, and five hundred muscles. The navel was looked upon as the central point of the nerves and vessels. The cardinal elements, air, gall, and mucus, find frequent mention. The air is situated below the navel, the gall between the navel and heart, and the mucus above the heart. To the elements making up the human organism was also added ether, out of which sprang light, out of light generated water, and out of them both earth. The seven organic products of these cardinal elements were the chyle, blood, flesh, cellular tissue, bones, the medullary substance, and the semen. The blood generated from the chyle. The chyle is an aqueous fluid; it becomes red in the spleen and liver. Milk formed the exclusive article of food to the end of the first year; to the third year, milk and rice; and to the fifteenth, rice alone, when a mixed diet was allowed. The best means for the preservation of health are the weekly offering of an emetic, monthly a purgative, and twice yearly (at the change of seasons) blood-letting. Diseases were classed as natural and supernatural. Diseases were frequently caused by sin. The most important diseases were due to a want of or surplus of action of the cardinal elements upon the physiological elements—the chyle, blood, etc. The predominance of one cardinal element over the others gave rise to the different temperaments. The soul seeks to equalize the disharmony, dyscrasies of the cardinal elements, by which disease is produced. Disease is, therefore, a disturbance of the activity of the soul occasioned by abnormalities of the cardinal elements. The air contained in the body is the cause of eighty different diseases. To these belong the diseases of the nerves—tetanus, trismus, chorea, also leprosy. Among the diseases of the urinary organs one is surprised to find that a sweet and albuminous urine is mentioned. Diabetes was considered incurable.

A knowledge of poisons and their action is an indispensable part of the education of the doctor, as the food is often poisoned by the enemies of the ruler, wicked women, and unthankful servants. These ancient Indian doctors seem to have been well acquainted with hydrophobia, as the action of the bite of the rabid dog, fox, jackal, wolf, bear, and tiger. The treatment consisted in appropriate local applications to the wound, and the inward offering of antidotes.

In this regard Wise * says:

"*The Bites of Mad Dogs.*—When dogs, jackals, foxes, wolves, bears, or tigers, become mad, they foam at the mouth, which remains open, their tails hang down, they do not hear or see well, and saliva flows from their mouths. In such a state they snap at and bite one another. The part that is bitten becomes senseless, blood flows from the wound, which becomes black, and other appearances are observed, as after a wound with a poisoned arrow. *The person bitten makes the same kind of noise and movements as that of the animal which has bitten him. When such a person sees the shape of the animal which has bitten him, either in water or in a glass, it is an unfavorable symptom. It is also unfavorable when the person is afraid of water, and dreads either seeing or hearing it. This is called hydrophobia, the fear of water.* When the person dreams of the rabid animal, it is unfavorable. Toward the termination of the disease the person is convulsed, becomes insensible and powerless, and dies."

"*In all such cases the first part of treatment should be to scarify the part and squeeze out the blood, after which the part is to be washed and burned by means of hot 'ghee.'* Then apply to the wounded part a mixture of certain antidotes, and give old 'ghee' internally. Errhines are also to be given with the milk of the arka-plant, *Calatropis gigantea.* Susruta recommends the following, which is to be used both internally and externally: Take of 'Shirisha,' 'Kustha,' 'Haridra,' 'Shita,' 'Sharshapa,' of each forty ratas, mix in a pint of water, and boil until reduced one fourth. During the treatment the patient should be kept in a cool situation, without any water. When the symptoms disappear, the person should then bathe, and on the third and fifth days the above is to be administered in half the dose given at first. He is then to take rice and milk. It is recommended in these cases to act powerfully upon the system by strong medicines before the poison has produced its constitutional effects. After the infliction of the wound, and before it has

* "History of Medicine in India," vol. i, p. 280.

produced any general effects, the free use of water in bathing is recommended, and the bowels are to be afterward opened by purgatives and emetics, followed by errhines to clear the passages."

The perfection to which the Aryan doctors developed the practice of surgery is surprising indeed. They made many useful instruments, catheterized the bladder, removed stones, punctured the abdomen, originated plastic operations upon the nose, ear, and lips, set fractured bones, performed "laparotomy," and made skillful operations upon the eye. The Cæsarean operation was performed on the death of the mother to save the infant.

The beginners of veterinary medicine, or, rather, those who first practiced the healing art upon animals, were undoubtedly the shepherds and herdsmen, who were intrusted with their care. This employment was frequently followed in families, and the results of experience thus gained were doubtless transmitted from father to son for generations. These early veterinary empirics must frequently have come in friendly intercourse, and thus the results of mutual experiences were interchanged and criticised; so the fund of empirical knowledge gradually increased, until the sum of these experiences was finally gathered on parchment, and then, with the birth of printing, into books. While many of these men were undoubtedly keen observers of nature, there is no doubt that they were also great admirers of the marvelous, and equally superstitious, so that many most absurd superstitions as to the causes of disease crept into their sayings and writings.

Charaka is said to have written a work upon the diseases of animals, but I have vainly searched for any quotations from it. That the Jews and Egyptians were acquainted with many forms of animal disease must be known to every reader of the Bible, for the plagues with which Jehovah punished the Egyptians, and through which they were robbed of their cattle, are most graphically described by Moses. The oldest Egyptian monuments bear upon them carvings illustrating the treatment of animals.

The Greeks possessed, at a very early date, a more or less extended literature with reference to the treatment of the diseases of animals. With the blooming of Greek culture, medical art took an active move forward. Hippocrates, 460–377 B. C., the honored father of medicine and the compiler of all the knowledge which existed up to his time, was quite well acquainted with the coarser anatomy of some of the lower animals, and we find several notices in his writings which warrant us in assuming that he was not unacquainted with some of their diseases. In speaking of hydrothorax, or water in the chest, he says, "It is a disease which is also frequently met with among oxen, sheep, and swine." * He had probably met with it in these animals much more frequently than others, because of their frequent use in the sacrifices at the altars of the gods at the Hellenic temples. In another place he says: "In cattle, the thighs are apt to become dislocated at the hip-joint, when they are particularly lean, which occurs at the end of winter, at which time they are particularly subject to dislocations. Homer has well remarked that of all beasts oxen suffer the most at that season, and especially those employed at the plow. In them, therefore, dislocations happen most frequently." † The influence which Hippocrates exerted upon medical science for a thousand years after his death is scarcely appreciated by the public, and by far not sufficiently esteemed by his successors of the present day, many of whom have not read his works, notwithstanding their accessibility to English readers, by the above-mentioned excellent and critical edition, for which we are indebted to the Sydenham Society for publication. The young practitioner of to-day seems to be carried away by the desire for new things, and all sorts of *new remedies* are eagerly sought after and experimented with, much to the neglect of the study of the fathers of medicine. The present generation is emphatically one of research, but it is a great and harmful error to think that the microscope and crucible can reveal *all* that is to be known of disease. The works of the fathers of medicine often excelled those of the present day in clinical observation, in the exact description of the intra-vital phenomena of disease, and in detailing the results of experiences gained at the sick-bed from the use of medicines. At present a healthy reaction is beginning in this direction, and the microscope furor is being toned down within the limits of practical possibility, notwithstanding a New York enthusiast purposes to tell us whether two given persons are compatible for marriage, so far as the production of healthy offspring is concerned, by the microscopic appearance of the granulations in the protoplasma of the white or colorless blood-corpuscles. That such an assertion is but the utterance of a visionary and untrustworthy observer scarcely needs to be mentioned.

Hippocrates,‡ also called the great, is said to have come from a family of doctors, descending from Æsculapius and Herucles. Little is known of his life, many relations concerning the same being mixed up with myths and impossible extravagances. He was, how-

* Haeser, *loc. cit.*, p. 173. † Works, Sydenham edition, vol. ii, p. 575.

‡ Wunderlich, "History of Medicine."

ever, greatly honored, and both practiced and taught medicine among his countrymen. He was the author of many books, but few of those which have come down to us are looked upon as genuine; many others attributed to him contain much of his teaching, however. It is a mistake to designate him as the founder of a new system of medicine: he was simply a harvester in the fields of medicine, but also a keen observer of the phenomena of disease. He himself says that "he who scorns or throws away the past, and seeks to make a new way and new theories, or thinks that he has found such, is either a deceiver or is himself deceived"—words which should not be without due appreciation by the Æsculapians of the present day and generation. The followers are many, the discoverers of new truths but isolated phenomena in the march of human progress.

He was a grand observer of nature. He made no new system, but was bitterly opposed to hypotheses. He looked upon the living organism in the Epidoclesian sense, as composed of four cardinal elements, which he named blood, mucus, black gall, and yellow gall. His pathology was simple in the extreme. When these cardinal elements bore a proper relation to each other in the living organism, a crasis or normality existed; any disturbance of this normal condition, any preponderance of one of these elements, either as a whole or locally, produced abnormality, dyscrasis. He laid but little value upon theoretic discussions: "When any one can give a better explanation, it suits me equally well; such ability is but the result of a glib tongue." His anatomical knowledge was quite limited, and he seems never to have made studies upon the human body. He laid great stress upon the value of knowledge with regard to *all* the external phenomena presented by the diseased organism. The conditions, in disease, of many internal organs, did not, however, escape his attention—such as the swelling of the spleen, and its subsequent retraction, in various forms of infectious disease. "The practitioner should be able to recognize the conditions presented to him, without the necessity of referring to the relations of the patient; . . . if perspiration occurs in a fevered patient, without remission of the fever, the disease will be lengthened; the fever increases when the teeth have a viscid coating; . . . a disease in which sleep has a deleterious influence is deadly; when the patient is, however, improved by sleep, it is to be looked upon as a favorable symptom; . . . sleep and sleeplessness, when present to an abnormal degree, are evil symptoms; . . . when a convalescent person has a good appetite, but does not improve thereby, it is a bad symptom; . . . he who would correctly prognosticate as to who will die or who will recover, whether the disease will be of long or short duration, must know well all the phenomena, and be well versed as to their respective value."

His manner of treatment was well considered, and he generally avoided heroic means. He placed great stress upon the value of dietetics, which should be adapted to the individuality of the patient, his constitution and habits. He was, according to his idea of the cardinal elements, much addicted to the employment of local means, by which the supposed centralization of a given element was to be equalized or the surplus removed; therefore, we find in his writings many directions for local bleeding and applications. He invented quite a number of surgical instruments; performed trepanning of the cranium, set bones, and reduced luxations. He highly prized cauterization, and his last aphorism reads: "What medicine will not cure, the iron will; what the iron will not cure, fire will; what fire can not cure, must be considered as incurable."

But, above all Greek writers of antiquity celebrated in the field of medicine, none equaled, in a knowledge of the anatomy of animals, that mighty intellect which has been the wonder of humanity for generations, and which had not its equal in the arena of natural science until long after the middle ages—Aristotle.

"Aristotle was born at Stagyra in Macedonia, in the year 384, and died 326 B. C. He was undoubtedly the greatest thinker of his time, and united in himself all the knowledge which then existed. His father, Nichomachus, was body-surgeon to Amyntas III, of Macedon, the father of Philip. At seventeen years of age, Aristotle went to Athens to study under the immortal Plato, who recognized his great genius, and called him the brightest spirit of his school. Aristotle soon separated himself from his teacher, and began to oppose the doctrines which he taught; he went to Macedon, and became the tutor of Alexander the Great. When the latter went upon his conquests into Asia, Aristotle returned to Athens, where he appeared in the character of teacher, Alexander supporting him, and for his studies giving him the immense advantages offered by the collections of curiosities made in his foreign conquests. The results of his investigations are collected in his writings and speak for themselves. On Alexander's death the enemies of Aristotle became powerful enough to cause his banishment from Athens; he was declared a heretic, a disbeliever in the gods, and so deadly was the pursuit of his enemies that he finally killed himself in his sixty-third year. His body was brought to the place of his nativity, his countrymen erecting a monument to his memory. Aristotle may be justly styled the founder of zoötomy, the anatomy of animals. His writings, subsequent to his death, suffered a rather changeable destiny: they fell at first into the hands of his heirs; then they were buried and barely escaped destruction from decay and worms; afterward they were conveyed to Athens, and finally to Rome by the Romans on the capture of Athens, and from there they have been dispersed over the world, but not without many falsifications and changes." *

His anatomical descriptions,† so far as they had reference to man, were limited to topographical descriptions of the external parts; the formation of the internal was, as he himself says, little known, but they were described according to analogy, from the examinations of similar organs in the lower animals. He describes the brain and its membranous surroundings, as well as its ventricles, cavities; also the optic nerves in their passage from the brain to the eye; on the other hand, he denied any connection between the brain and the ear; he describes also the larynx, uvula, epiglottis, the trachea and its bifurcations in the lungs, also the Eustachian tubes, but had an incorrect idea with reference to the connection between the heart and lungs; he described the œsophagus, and its passage into the stomach, as well as the extension of the latter to the intestines; also the epiploön and mesenterium. Notwithstanding much study, it was impossible for him to come to any definite conclusions with reference to the vascular system; he looked upon the heart as the center of the vessels, but described only three cavities in that organ, missing the septum between the auricles; he notices the aorta and vena cava, as well as the main arteries and veins of the head and neck; also the diaphragm, liver, gall-bladder, kidneys, and their pelvis, the ureters and veins of the kidneys, the urinary bladder and urethra, the testicles and their vessels, as well as the same organs in the female, and the uterus. It is doubtful, however, if he knew of the relation of the secretion of the kidneys to the bladder, or of the organ at present considered as the rudimentary male uterus.

Aristotle had very imperfect ideas of the circulation: the blood was generated in the heart and from there dispersed over the organism; it sprang, coagulated, out of the vessels, and was of variable color. The respiration served as a *cooler* to the organism—its organs are the lungs and gills; his incorrect idea of the connection

* Schraeder-Hering, "Bibliograph. Lexicon f. Thierärzte," p. 16.

† Aubert and Wimmer, "Aristotle's Thierkunde," Leipsic, 1868.

between the lungs and heart gave him the conception that the air came into the heart; he compared the lungs to an air-sac, and does not seem to have had any conception of the changes which take place in the blood by their means. His views with reference to digestion, and the changes which the elements of the organism undergo, were very crude indeed. His description of the senses, seeing, hearing, smell, and taste, is surprisingly clear and explicit. He looked upon the muscles as the organs of sensitiveness, and not of movement; the sinews as motor organs, and the heart as the center of movement. He made an astonishing number of clever observations with regard to the generation and development of animals, and studied the same in the hen's egg; the formation of the heart, brain, and eye, allantois, and chorion; the duration of gestation in many different species. His observations with reference to the instincts of animals are often surprisingly correct, as well as with regard to the variations in their habits of life. Aristotle also described quite a number of diseases among animals, and, as the subject is not without instructive interest, I take the liberty of giving a very free translation of them here.*

"As to the diseases of quadrupeds, swine have three different diseases. One is known as 'bronchos,' and consists in an inflammation of the air-tubes and the masticating organs; it, however, frequently complicates other parts of the porcine organism; sometimes the feet become diseased, and at others the ears. The disease develops rapidly, the swine soon losing their appetite. The herdsmen know of no other treatment than to cut out the diseased part at once. Aside from this, two other diseases occur in swine, both being known by the name of 'kraura.' In one of them we may perceive pain and depression of the head, and in the other diarrhœa is the most frequent phenomenon. This last is reputed to be incurable; the first is, however, cured by rubbing the snout with wine, as well as washing the interior of the same with that material. In this disease, also, but few recover, as it generally ends fatally in from three to four days. Swine suffer most from 'bronchos' when the summer is very fruitful and the swine very fat. Mulberries and plenty of warm baths are said to have a beneficial effect; scarification of the tongue is said also to be resorted to. The swine are measly when the flesh of the limbs, neck, and shoulders is soft; in these places the measles must be sought for. The flesh has a sweet taste when it harbors measles, at the same time it is soft and watery. One can easily tell when

* A. and W., chapters xx, xxii, p. 181.

the swine have measles, for they are to be found under the tongue. Measly swine can not keep their hind-feet quiet; they lose the measles after having fed upon 'tipha,' which also helps their condition. The best food to nourish swine is peas and figs, but one must not give them one kind of food, as mixed diet is best for them. It is said that acorns are greedily devoured by swine, but that they make them have soft and watery flesh. When in a pregnant condition too many acorns cause them to abort, as they also do sheep. So far as we know, swine are the only animals that harbor measles.

"Dogs also suffer from three diseases, known as 'rabies,' 'kynanche,' and 'podagra.' Rabies puts them into fits of rage, during which they bite furiously, and all animals bitten by them when in this condition also become mad, *with the exception of man.* This disease kills the dogs, as well as all animals bitten by them, *with the exception of man.* 'Kynanche' is also deadly to dogs, and from 'podagra' but few recover. Camels are also subject to rabies. Of all other animals, the elephant alone is exempted from this disease, but it is subject to tympanitis."

"Cattle *living in herds* are subject to two diseases, known as 'podagra' and 'krauros.' In the first, the feet become swollen, but they do not die from it, nor do they lose their hoofs; they become better when one covers their horns with hot pitch. In 'krauros,' their breath is hot and respiration accelerated; this is called fever in men, but 'krauros' in cattle. The signs of this disease are drooping ears and loss of appetite; they die rapidly, and the lungs are gangrenous upon examination.

"Horses which live upon *pastures* are subject to *no other* disease than 'podagra.' When afflicted with this disease they sometimes lose their hoofs; but, when this is the case, new ones soon develop, for, as the new hoof grows down, the old one is shed. Among the signs of this disease is swelling of the right testicle, or a corrugated condition of the skin between the nostrils. They are also subject to a disease which is called 'cilos,' which is characterized by the animals placing the four feet together under the body. When horses go for some days without eating, and then become crazy, one has to resort to bleeding and castration. They are also subject to 'tetanus,' a disease by which all the vessels, as well as the head and neck, become stiffened, and the animals move stiff-legged. They soon become purulent. Another disease to which they are subject is called 'krithian,' indicated by a soft palate and hot breath. These diseases are incurable, when they do not cease of themselves, which is also the case in the disease called 'nymphian,' in which the horse becomes stiff when one blows up its nose, or depresses the head; when any one tries to ride them they go in circles until stopped. They always depress the head when rabid. Other signs of the same are that they depress the ears upon the mane, and again elevate them; that they become weak and snort much. Conditions connected with pain of the heart are also incurable: in this the animals have tucked-up flanks, or the bladder becomes displaced, which is easily recognized from the inability of the horse to micturate, and that they draw their legs up and stamp with their feet. According to those who should know, horses and sheep suffer from all the diseases common to man. A poison known as 'sandarac' kills not only the horse but all draught-animals. It is given in water. A pregnant horse aborts when it smells the smoke from a blown-out candle; the same effect is also occasionally observed in women when in the same condition. Horses love meadows and swamps. They drink gladly of dirty water, and when the water is clear they stir up the bottom with their feet, and then bathe in it, for these animals generally bathe gladly and love water. Cattle, on the contrary, do not drink freely of water which is unclean and warm.

"The ass suffers especially from one disease, which is known as 'melis.' It at first attacks the head, a viscid, yellow slime running from the nostrils; when the disease extends to the lungs it is deadly, but when limited to the head it is not so. Of all animals of its kind, the ass can bear cold the least, and thrives, therefore, in warm climates.

"The elephant is subject to tympanitis, and when thus afflicted can neither micturate nor pass fæces. When it eats earth (?) at intervals, it becomes weak; but when it eats it constantly, it does not seem to harm it. Sometimes it swallows stones. It also occasionally suffers from diarrhœa, and is healed by giving it warm water, and hay which has been dipped in honey. When suffering from want of sleep they become weak, but strength returns when the shoulders are rubbed with warm water, salt, and oil. When troubled with pains in the shoulder, they can be helped by placing roasted pork upon the afflicted part. Some elephants will drink oil, others not. When a fragment of iron penetrates their body, it is said that it can be driven out by giving them oil, but those who will not drink it willingly must be given the oil mixed with roots."

The fame of the noted Greek general, Xenophon (349–259 B. C.), is not alone limited to the remarkable retreat of the brave *ten thousand*, for his writings upon the horse and horsemanship have given him a no less lasting reputation. Fleming* says of him: "This celebrated cavalry-officer appears to have carefully studied the character of the horse, and all the precepts which he gives in his treatise on horsemanship are dictated by an amount of wisdom and humanity which has not, perhaps, been excelled since his day. The safety and comfort of that animal and its rider were ever before him; his teachings were principally directed to make the horse peculiarly adapted to service in war. He displays great judgment when specifying the proper form and disposition of the parts which collectively make up the nearest approach to a perfect horse, and markedly shows to what a high degree, in that distant age, this kind of knowledge was cultivated; indeed, from his writings we are led to infer that in *his* time, and perhaps long before, there were accomplished horse-breakers and public riding-masters, as well as men who were excellent judges of the qualities of the horse. In advising as to the good 'points' to be sought for in a horse, he employs the clearest terms to express his meaning. 'A person,' he says, 'may form his opinion of the feet by first examining the hoofs; for *thick* or strong hoofs are much more conducive to firmness than *thin* ones; and it must not escape his notice whether the hoofs are high or low, as well before as behind; for, in high hoofs, what is called the frog is high above the ground, and low ones tread equally on the strongest and weakest parts of the hoof, like in-kneed men, or like cripples among men, who limp on parts which were never intended by nature to support them.' He says, further: 'As attention must be paid to the horse's food and exercise, that his body may be vigorous, so must care be taken of his feet. Damp and smooth stable-floors injure even naturally good hoofs, and to prevent them from being damp they ought to be sloping; to prevent them from being smooth they should have irregular-shaped stones inserted in the ground, close to one another, similar to a horse's hoof in size; for such floors give firmness to the feet of horses that stand upon them. . . . The ground outside the stable may be put into excellent condition, and serve to strengthen the horse's feet, if a person throws down in it four or five measures of round stones, each large enough to fill the two hands, and each about a pound (?) in weight; they should be surrounded with an iron rim, so that they may not be scattered; for, as the horse stands upon them, he will be in much the same condition as if he were to travel part of every day upon a stony road. The feet of horses that have been hardened by exercise will be superior on rough ground to those which are not

* "Horseshoes and Horseshoeing," p. 21.

habituated to it; as persons that are sound in their limbs, to those who are lame.'"

Among later Greek writers upon the domestic animals, we find the name of Absyrtus, and a veterinary, Hippocrates, who lived about the fourth century. The former, born at Brusa, in Bithynia, is by far the most important writer of all the Greeks upon the diseases of domestic animals. It appears that he belonged to a family that was celebrated for its veterinarians; at least, his grandfather, Demitrus, also followed the calling. He was a good observer of the outward phenomena of disease, although not a scientific student of nature; he does not seem to have associated much with the medical men of his time, and thus may have served to give the profession a certain degree of individuality which it had not previously possessed. He especially mentions that the gall-bladder is not present in the horse.

Hippocrates's writings were of but little importance, but were more or less perfectly collected in the Constantinian "Hippiatrica," which we shall find occasion to consider later on. He belonged to that great class of veterinarians who willingly acknowledged the superiority of Absyrtus, and learned from him. Heusinger expresses astonishment that, although Hippocrates lived at the time of Absyrtus, none of the subsequent Greek and Roman veterinarians seem to make any mention of him.

About this time also flourished the noted medical authors Celsus and Galen. Celsus wrote an encyclopædia containing works upon medicine, agriculture, and veterinary medicine; the part treating upon the last two subjects has been, unfortunately, lost to posterity. Of all Roman doctors, however, none has acquired the world-wide celebrity and authority which have been given to Claudius Galenus, 131–200 A. D.* He received a most careful education, studying philosophy and medicine at Pergamos, his native city, also at Smyrna, Corinth, and Alexandria; he was especially diligent in the study of anatomy. At twenty-eight years of age he was appointed medical attendant to the gladiators at Pergamos, and remained there until 164 A. D. He then removed to Rome; but practice seems to have been a secondary consideration with him, and he appears to have been but poorly appreciated by his Roman colleagues. We find him, however, to have been on terms of intimacy with the philosophers, and prominent members of the aristocracy; he held public lectures upon physiology, which for a time enjoyed great popularity, but were subsequently given up on account

* Wunderlich, "Geschichte d. Medicin," p. 33.

of the enmity of the medical profession. He soon after left Rome, traveling over Italy, and returned to Pergamos in 169 A. D., but was again called to Rome by the emperors Marcus Aurelius and Lucius Verus, where he remained until his death, giving public lectures, and busied with his studies and writings. He was the most extensive medical author that has ever lived, and appears to have begun his authorship even as a boy. It has been estimated that he wrote some four hundred books, some of them being quite large. He was, indeed, a polyhistorian, and a man of astonishing learning; many of the views of medical authors antecedent to his time are only known to us through his writings. He possessed great analytical and critical ability; he had seen much himself, and investigated much, and possessed a highly systematic mind, clearing medicine, as it then existed, from much of the superstition and nonsense with which it was burdened. His anatomical knowledge was derived in part from the writings of Herophilus and Erisistratus, and in part from his own dissections, which were made largely upon apes. It had not been possible for a long time to make studies of anatomy upon the human form divine, and this age, which did not pause to sacrifice thousands of human beings at brutal gladiatorial combats, still could not offer *one* for the good of humanity and the advancement of knowledge. Only once, during the German war of Marcus Aurelius, was it allowed the doctors to dissect a human body, but they did not get beyond the situation of the intestines. Nevertheless, the writings of this great doctor remained for a thousand years the source from which a knowledge of human anatomy was drawn, and it was only by earnest endeavors, supported by actual inspection, that his great authority was finally shaken. Galen is accredited with saying that "the education of a doctor was incomplete without a knowledge of the processes of disease among the lower animals."

The writings of the celebrated Roman veterinary authors, Cato, Varo, Columella, and Vegetius, which are mostly compilations from earlier writers, may be found collected in "De Rei Rusticæ," a good edition of which was given out by Gesner in 1735: copies of this work may be found in some of our medical and public libraries. These writings contain descriptions of some diseases, much of which is absurd and ridiculous, in the light of the present day.

"Marcus Portius Cato,* the most ancient of this quartet, was born at Tusculum, or Tivoli, 234, and died 149 B. C. He was of a plebeian family, and served as a soldier under Fabius Maximus, but

* Schraeder-Hering, *loc. cit.*, p. 75.

by his energy of character elevated himself to positions of the highest honor. He became a clever general, jurist, and orator. On account of his steadfast morals, and constant enmity to human frailties, he acquired the surname of 'the Censor.' He was an enthusiastic opponent of Greek doctrines and art, and has the honor of being the first Roman who wrote upon agriculture: in these writings we observe a crude development of veterinary medicine. His writings have been frequently printed and translated into several European languages."

"Lucius Junius Columella* was born at Cadiz, Spain, in the reign of the Roman emperor Claudius, about 42 A. D. He had frequent recourse to the writings of Celsus, and did much for the development of veterinary medicine. His writings upon the diseases of the horse are not inconsiderable, but his descriptions of those of cattle are by far the best which we have received from antiquity."

"Publius Renatus Vegetii † (fourth century A. D.) is noted as the most erudite among the early veterinary authors. He appears to have possessed no inconsiderable degree of knowledge with reference to the diseases of the horse and their treatment, as well as a scholastic acquaintance with the writings of his Greek and Roman predecessors, and some of human medicine, and to have held affectionately to its antiquated theories and methods of practice. I have heretofore said that 'veterinary medicine *has been* but a parasite clinging to human medicine for support.' His writings bear the characteristics peculiar to his time, but are distinguished from those of many of his contemporaries by being written in more scholastic Latin. He used the writings of Absyrtus, but complains of the illiterate style in which they were written. As Vegetius often speaks of the Huns and their horses, and as these people spread over the Volga in 374 A. D., it is evident that he must have lived in the fourth or early in the fifth century, at a time when the Latins also understood Greek. He describes the diseases according to the parts afflicted, and varies but little from his Greek predecessors. It is to his credit that he was the first veterinary author who endeavored to bring some order out of the chaos which had until then existed, and endeavored to formulate some general principles for the diagnosis and treatment of animal diseases. His first two books treat upon the diseases of the horse, the third upon those of cattle, the fourth gives a general description of the bovine and equine form, and the composition of many medicines; among the latter are

* Schraeder-Hering, *loc. cit.*, p. 88.

† Ibid., p. 440.

many which are most ludicrous. While the therapeutic knowledge displayed by Vegetius is frequently good, his knowledge of anatomy was most insignificant, especially of that which was then known in human medicine."

It is in the writings of these authors that we find the words "veterinaria" and "veterinarius" first appearing, indicating the Latin origin of our words "veterinary" and "veterinarian." The art was also called "mulo-medicine," and Vegetius styles himself "Vegetii Renatii sive Mulo-medicinæ." It is at or about this period that we first find intimations of horseshoeing among the Romans, a practice they seem to have borrowed from the Germans and Gauls.*

Veterinarii are also mentioned as attached to the Roman cavalry, and attending to the health of the animals used at the circus at Rome.

During this period numerous pests carried devastation and misery among the Romans and their tributary tribes; the domestic animals likewise suffered from similar scourges. No writer of the period has given to posterity so classical a description of these devastations among animals as the poet Virgil in his "Georgics." I take the liberty of transcribing a few appropriate verses of the same from Mr. Fleming's "Animal Plagues":

"Not whirlwinds from the sea so frequent rush,
Big with storm, as pests 'mid cattle rage.
Nor individuals sole disorders seize,
But, suddenly, whole flocks, with every hope,
At once, and, from the youngest, all the race.

". . . From tainted air arose
A dreadful storm, inflamed by autumn's heat,
And gave to death all cattle, tame and wild,
Corrupting lakes, poisoning the grassy food.

"Hence, midst the springing grass, young cattle die,
And yield their gentle lives at loaded stalls;
Hence, madden fawning dogs, and the sick swine,
With suffocating shake and panting cough, give up their lives.

"Lo! as the bull under the plowshare smokes,
He falls, and vomits mingled foam and gore,
And makes his final groan;

* Any one desiring to read a most interesting archæological study, should not fail to obtain Mr. George Fleming's "Horseshoes and Horseshoeing," which is a work more suitable to general education than for instruction in horseshoeing, though the latter part does not fail in this particular.

The plowman sad disjoins the ox that mourns his brother's fate,
And leaves the rooted plow, his work half done.
Move him not now, nor stream through rocky bed,
That pure as amber freshens all the plain.
His flanks are all relaxed, and his dull eye
A stupor covers, and to earth his neck
Down rushes with the heavy weight it bore.

"What profit, then, their service and their toil?
No change of food affords relief,
And art, implored, destroys."

I have endeavored, briefly, it is true, to sketch the history of veterinary medicine in antiquity, with what success it must be left to the reader to judge. The works which we have already alluded to remained the fountain that supplied nourishment to compiling authors for nearly a thousand years: for it is not until the middle of the thirteenth century that any work of original importance was added to our literature. In the tenth century, the Emperor Constantine Porphyrogenitus, 911–951 A. D., instigated a compilation which included about all the works which had until then appeared.

Schraeder, in his biographical lexicon, says of him that "he was the son and successor of the Greek Emperor Leo. To him we are indebted for about all we know of veterinary medicine up to his time. He favored and nourished science with all his energy, caused public education to be given and schools to be erected, which he made subservient to the uses of the state. He gave his whole attention to the academy at Constantinople, and sought to increase its usefulness with all the resources at his disposal. As author and polyhistorian, he gathered books from all parts of the earth, praised the diligence of compilers, and caused most valuable extracts to be made from innumerable writings upon history, agriculture, and medicine, a task which had never before been undertaken, and even veterinary medicine was not neglected."

Haeser * says of this part of the work, which was entitled the "Hippiatrica," that it consisted mostly of the letters of Absyrtus, Emulus, Hierokles, Pelagonius, Theomnestus, Tiberius, Anatolius, Archedemus, Hippasius, Tetrippus, and Stratonicus. It first appeared in a Latin translation, under the title "Veterinaria Medicinæ," libri II, Joh. Ruello, interp., Paris, 1530. An edition in the original Greek text was published at Basel, 1537, under the title "*Τῶν ιππιατριχῶν βιβλια δυῶ*." Translations of the latter appeared in Italy, 1543; France, 1563; Germany, 1571. It is of general in-

* *Loc. cit.*, p. 546.

terest that Leontius asserts in the Latin edition (the place is wanting in the Greek) *that in the apparent pest-like epizoöties, horses which were healthy were carefully separated from those which were diseased, and their protection was sought by bringing them upon good pastures.* No such regulation is to be found in any work of antiquity against the frequent pest outbreaks of disease among human beings.

We have now, in a very cursory manner, traced the history of veterinary medicine, or better, empiricism, to the tenth century, which may be said to begin the "Stahlmeisters," or master of the horse period. This period continued to the opening of the schools, and in all truth may be said to be still with us; for every one well knows the taste among men occupying such positions to write practical books "on the care and treatment of the horse." While I would not deny more or less practical and empirical ability to men occupying these positions, I must emphatically enter an earnest protest against an American absurdity which leads otherwise intelligent citizens to assume that such persons know anything of disease, and which results in calling in to attend sick animals the first convenient stable-keeper, blacksmith, or cow-herd; that because such men have gained a certain sort of practical knowledge with regard to the care of our domestic animals in health, it is justifiable to assume that they know anything of them in disease. No greater error exists than this, and it has unfortunately extended itself into human practice, much to the cost of a suffering humanity. Experience is indeed valuable, but experience alone has proved a ledge upon which many a man has been wrecked. Times come when your practical man, your man of boasted experience, can do nothing but stand with folded hands and wait. Such times come only too frequently to the man of still greater experience, and that backed up by a most elaborate education and reflective ability. Without education, without that systematic drilling and practice which can only be obtained in well-regulated schools and hospitals, experience is worse than nothing; it results in nothing more than the most absurd guess-work. What idea can a man have of inflammatory processes in the lungs, kidneys, brain, or liver, who scarcely knows the seat of those organs, much less anything of their anatomical construction? In all truth, it is the most abject form of cruelty to give over a suffering dumb animal (alas! it is too often the case with human beings also) to the tortures or futile endeavors of one of these "experienced" quacks. Fortunate would it be for humanity, fortunate for our dumb animals as well, were disease and its treatment the simple thing which such actions on the part of those intrusted with their care would lead us to assume that it was. On the contrary, the study of disease is one of the most difficult tasks which the human intellect has to cope with, and, while many men pass through life with the reputation of successful practitioners, still it is but the limited few who gain entrance to the "holy of holies," and acquire much intimate acquaintance with disease itself. That an occasional quack is rewarded by success is not to be wondered at, when we take into consideration the recuperative powers of Dame Nature herself. Nothing is more amusing, more saddening, than to hear self-important practitioners *boast of their cures.* It is very, very hard, as many distinguished men have admitted, and as every man who has devoted time to experiment in pathological and therapeutical research, but especially the latter, knows, to positively decide whether the improvement which one sees in a given patient is due to the recuperative powers of Nature, to a weakening of the active properties of the cause of the disease, or to the action of drugs which have been offered.

The best and most skillful practitioners are but *handmaids*, servants, to Nature, and he is the best practitioner who most scrupulously holds to the rule, "hands off," and with religious regard aims to support the ever-active recuperative power, efforts, of the physiological functions. It is seldom given to the attendant upon organisms afflicted with inner diseases to *effect radical cures;* this boon is, however, occasionally awarded to the surgeon. Only the quack proclaims to have the radical panacea which *can cure* all and everything. But to return to our subject:

The period which we are now considering in the history of veterinary medicine is marked by the appearance of several works of great historical importance. The first of these was the "Hippiatrica" of Jordanus Rufus, "Marescallus Major" to the court of Frederick II of Sicily. The king is reported to have assisted on the work. Rufus seems to have known but little of the writings of his Greek and Roman predecessors, but, according to Haeser, was not unacquainted with several works of Arabian origin. His mind appears to have been remarkably free from the superstitions of his time. He describes quite a number of diseases, among them laminitis, vulgarly called founder, glanders, tetanus, etc.

Schraeder * says of him: "He was born in Calabria, in the twelfth or thirteenth century, and was from a noble family, and, like many gentlemen of his position, busied himself with training

* *Loc. cit.*, p. 368.

horses, and the treatment of their diseases. That he must have been an important personage, and much esteemed by his patron, is attested by the circumstance that his names appear among the signers of the king's testament: "Ego Jordanus magnus justitia ruis Rufus de Calabria imperialis Marescallus major interfui his et subscribi feci." (Frederick reigned from 1212 to 1250 A. D.) Rufus's work, "De Medicina Equorum," appears to have been written with the advice and consent of the king, but it has been incorrectly asserted that the latter himself wrote it. It appears, from Rufus's own words, that the king had already died at the time of its publication, which accordingly must have taken place subsequent to 1250. It was written in Latin, but at an early date was honored with translations into Italian, and in 1818 Molin, professor in Padua, gave out a Latin edition. None of the ancient Latin works upon this subject afford more pleasure to the reader than this of Ruffus's. From it one can easily perceive that he was a person of considerable experience, far exceeding any of his successors in ability for a period of nearly four hundred years. We do not find in his writings any of the superstitious fables or astrological nonsense which encumbered the works of his predecessors; he was an earnest student of Nature, and gave his conclusions with earnestness and directness. It is certain that he knew little of Vegetius, or of the collected writings of Greek authors; at least, he made but little use of them. Many of his directions are not without value even in our day. Many names which he gave to diseases have been adopted into other languages. Hazard possessed several manuscripts, and especially a French translation of his writings. The contents of one of these manuscripts on vellum, from the fourteenth century, is given as follows: 1. The Creation and Nativity of the Horse. 2. His Capture and Training. 3. The Care and Treatment. 4. The Recognition of the Parts of the Body. 5. The Diseases. 6. The Medicines and Remedies.

The invention of printing gave a great impetus to the publication of works of all kinds—to a degree, in fact, which we of this day and generation can scarcely appreciate. In this regard the publication of medical works kept even pace with those of theology and other branches of learning. In our own field of study there appeared a work of rare value; one, indeed, which marks a turning-point in the development of veterinary medicine. Up to this time there had been no book on the diseases of animals since the days of Aristotle which endeavored to enter at all into the study of their anatomy based on special dissections. This ground was first broken by an Italian work entitled "Dell' Anatomia et dell' Infirmita del

Cavallo," di Carlo Ruini, senator of Bologna, 1598. This work contains numerous illustrations, finely executed, when we take into consideration the period and the condition of equine anatomy. It remained unequaled for nearly two hundred years, when its place was in part taken by the really magnificent "Cours d'Hippiatrique" of Lafosse, *fils*, Paris, 1772.

Carlo Ruini * was born and died in the sixteenth century, at Bologna, Italy, the exact date being unknown. His grandfather was a professor of note at the university of that place, lecturing upon jurisprudence. Ruini also studied the same subject, and, as stated on the title-page of this book, became senator in his native city. But little is known of his life, but in the preface of the book in question it is said that from early youth he displayed a great fondness for horses. The original edition of this work appeared in 1598, and the printing and paper are marvels of perfection. Uffenbach gave out a German translation, and several from French sources soon followed. The book served as a fountain from which subsequent compilers drew much information, using also the illustrations, which, however, frequently lost much credit in the copies made of them. The first part of the book treats of the anatomy of the horse, and the numerous illustrations testify to the diligence of the author in dissections. The second part treats of the diseases of that animal, and is based in no inconsiderable degree upon Ruffus and other authors. As little as the authorship is in general to be questioned, yet it is very doubtful if the "Anatomia del Cavallo" is from Ruini's hand. "I harbored this doubt," says Schraeder, "very early in my study of this book, and the more I have reflected upon it the more have I become confirmed in my doubts. It is my opinion that some young doctor had at his own instigation, or perhaps incited by Ruini, studied the anatomy of the horse, and drew the illustrations, and had them engraved upon copper, which could not be done save at considerable expense, which the wealth of Ruini made possible."

Ercolani, one of the most learned veterinarians of Italy, and celebrated for his researches into historical veterinary literature, questions the above assertion, and gives full credit to Ruini.

I have casually mentioned the brilliant contribution to veterinary literature, the "Cours d'Hippiatrique" of Lafosse *fils*. While Ruini's work was the first illustrated book of any account which had until then appeared, that of Lafosse was the first book with colored plates which appeared upon equine anatomy. The work is divided

* Schraeder-Hering, *loc. cit.*, p. 369.

into three parts, and is embellished with a fine copper print of the author. The first part treats of the anatomy of the horse; the second, of its diseases and their treatment; the third, of horseshoeing. It is impossible to doubt the influence of Ruini, when one thoughtfully compares the plates and the arrangements of both these works. At this period two men, father and son, occupied most prominent positions among the veterinarians of France. I must beg leave to nourish the opinion, heretical as it may seem, that it was an unfortunate thing for France, unfortunate for the development of veterinary science, not art, that the first veterinary schools established at Lyons and Alfort, France, were not established under the direction of the younger Lafosse, rather than under that of his great rival, Bourgelat. Bourgelat was a horseman, *eminently practical*; hence we see horseshoeing and all *practical* routine assuming a place in French veterinary medicine, at the cost of the scientific investigating spirit, which would not have been the case had the more scientific and original but not the less practical Lafosse been the guiding star. I wish to call particular attention to this opinion, for here in America we are in great danger of losing the true union of science and practice, before the great *practical common sense* that our people are so fond of assuming to themselves. We have not yet learned, at least so far as the study and development of medicine is concerned, that experience is a dear task-master. I would not have it inferred that I would neglect the practical—I am too much of an American for that—but *true practice* must ever stand upon the results of scientific research; upon an empiricism based upon something else than the traditions and errors of our forefathers; the things which have been, but which have never at the same time been subjected to the skeptical crucible of the experimental, scientific researcher.

As the two Lafosses, especially the son, exerted such an influence on the development of veterinary medicine, a short notice of their lives can not be out of place here.

"Etienne Guillaume Lafosse,* the father, was born in Paris, and died there January 24, 1765. Little that is authentic is known with reference to his life—he appears to have been lost sight of behind the greater renown of his glorious son. Yet it was to him that the son owed his careful education in the scientific and practical elements of his profession. The father had, however, given us some idea of his ability by his investigations on the seat of glanders, published in 1779, in a treatise entitled "Le véritable siége de la

* Schraeder-Hering, *loc. cit.*, p. 234.

morve (glanders) et les moyens d'y remédier"; in 1750 he gave to the Academy a *brochure* upon lycoperdon as a hæmostatic, anti-bleeding medicine; and in 1754 published a work on horseshoeing. Other writings upon horseshoeing and practice followed, several of which, as also the above, were honored with translations into other languages."

"Phil. Etienne Lafosse, the son, was born at Montaterre, near Paris, and it is said died at Villeneuve, upon the Yonne, June, 1820. He was the eldest son of the former Lafosse, and at thirteen years of age decided to follow the calling which had been so honorably followed by his father and grandfather." (It should be mentioned here that this family has been one of the most noted among those which have given worthy veterinarians to France, and that it is not without honorable representatives at the present day.) "At the conclusion of his school-days, his father required him to serve for a time in his stables, where he acquired proficiency in the handling and care of horses; he then went into the forge for two years, and at the same time devoted himself to the study of human anatomy. He also received instruction in fencing, drawing, and music. Then followed practical experience, gained by accompanying his father upon professional visits, at the same time continuing the study of equine anatomy. By visiting knacker establishments, and making autopsies, he constantly enriched his collection of specimens. At eighteen years of age he received an appointment to lecture upon equine anatomy to the members of the light cavalry stationed at Versailles. He also did the same at the house of his father for the students in the forge. In 1758 we find him stationed as army-veterinarian, and accompanying the army in two campaigns into Germany during the Seven Years' War. On his return he studied medicine at Paris. In 1767 he built an amphitheatre, and gave therein free lectures and demonstrations upon equine anatomy; these lectures enjoyed great and deserved notoriety, but in 1770 he gave them up in order to bring to completion his great work, "Cours d'Hippiatrique"; the same cost Lafosse seventy thousand livres, and gave him an immortal reputation, especially in foreign countries. He did not, however, enjoy the same good fortune among his own people, for, not only in this work, but also in his "Dictionnaire d'Hippiatrique," 1775, he displayed a most active opposition to the schools at Lyons and Alfort, or rather, against their founder, Bourgelat. He nourished a great ambition to become a teacher, or even director, at one of these schools, but his severe polemics seem to have completely shut him off from the desired end. Bourgelat was a far more politic character, and stood in high favor with the ministry, and his scholars gave him such ardent support that the severe critique of his opponent passed him harmlessly by. The disappointment to his ambition, in unison with sufferings caused by a stone in the bladder, made him sell his house in Paris and remove to Russia, where he remained from 1777 to 1781. It is not definitely known what positions he occupied while there. But in no case could he find himself at home in the despotism ruling in Russia, and soon returned to Paris, where he rapidly assumed a position at court as veterinarian, and was also appointed to a similar position in the carabiniers and gendarmes. From his discontent with the government, it is not to be wondered at that we find him taking an active part in the acts of the Revolution, which soon followed: he was present at the storming of the Invalides and Bastile; became a member of the armed commission, division commander, and municipal officer of Paris. But we do not find his revolutionary ideas confined to politics alone; his hatred against the existing veterinary institutions and Bourgelat again found full vent, and he easily saw reasons for the suppression of both, and the removal of the schools to Paris; among other things, he accused the existing powers of supporting a costly and unnecessary menagerie, besides unnecessary instruments, and of accumulating a debt, in the years between 1782 and 1785, of thirty thousand livres. Lafosse was a hippologist *par excellence*, and this exclusive devotion to the horse was used successfully in the arguments against his polemic attacks on the existing institutions. Although the authorities took so little notice of his polemics, yet Lafosse did not fail entirely of public appreciation, for we find him appointed to several important positions as inspector and examiner in connection with the army. In all these he displayed his usual activity. On the 29th of July, 1794, he narrowly escaped death upon the scaffold. He then left Paris, occasionally revisiting it, however, and retired to the country, where he busied himself in scientific studies, occasionally appearing before the public. In 1797 he read a paper before the National Institute, entitled "Mémoire sur une maladie epizoötique vaccinique dans le Canton de Bray, qui a regni pendant l'été de l'an V, jusqu'à la fin de vendémiaire an VI." Other papers followed this of no less importance. In 1796 he was elected associate member of the Institute, but, notwithstanding earnest endeavor on his part and that of his friends, he did not succeed in becoming virtually a member. In 1819 he again vented his hatred against the schools in a writing entitled "Nouvelle Théorie pratique d'equitation." He possessed his great activities until the close of his days, and frequently complained of the unthankfulness of his fatherland —an ingratitude which, notwithstanding his failures, is still discreditable to his countrymen, for if Bourgelat deserves a monument to his memory for what he did for France, Lafosse no less deserves one for his services to the world at large, for none of the literary work of Bourgelat equals that which has given a world-wide reputation to the greater Lafosse.

Other books, which have acquired at least a certain historical importance, but which are of but little practical value, with a few exceptions, at the present day, were the "Parfait Maréchal" of Solleysel, 1664, which was honored with translations into several foreign languages; the writings of Saunier, mostly based upon books which had preceded him; Diaz, in Spain, Von Zind, Newcastle, Winter von Adler's Flugel; Marx Fugger, on Breeding; the "Foure Chiefest Offices of Horsemanship, whereto are added, Diverse Medicines not Heretofore Mentioned," by Thomas Blundeville, of Newton Flotman, in Norfolk, England: London, 1609. (Blundeville is, I believe, the originator of the term "Poll-Evil"); the "Hipponomia, or Vineyard of Horsemanship," Baret, 1661; "Master Peese, Containing all the Knowledge Belonging to the Smith, Farrier, Horse-Leech," etc.; the "Complete Horseman," of William Hope, 1696; "The Farrier's New Guide," by Gibson, 1719; Snape's "Anatomy of the Horse," 1751; and a very remarkable book from Stubbs, on the "Anatomy of the Horse," 1766. During this long period the Continent of Europe and Britain had been frequently overrun with animal plagues. Interesting as a condensed history of these invasions would be, it is not my purpose to enter upon it here, but gladly refer those who care to pursue this subject to the very elaborate work of Mr. George Fleming, entitled "Animal Plagues," where it is treated in detail. Of these plagues, the rinderpest and pleuro-pneumonia of cattle caused the most serious devastations, and I shall presently have occasion to quote largely from the above-mentioned "Animal Plagues," from the writings of three men who played an important part in their suppression, but better still, in instructing the people and governments in the means of combating them; instruction which is as applicable to our day as it was when written, over one hundred years ago.

It is scarcely possible for the people in this country to form any conception of the devastation and misery caused by these plagues in Europe during the eighteenth century; and not only these, but plagues unknown to us, carried death and misery among the people themselves. Wars on wars, with all their accompanying evils, had impoverished both the governments and people. Epidemic on epidemic had almost broken all the binding ties of kindred and affection. Plague on plague had driven people to the last verge of hope for sustenance and wealth, by robbing them of their animals, more especially cattle. "It has been computed that from 1711 to 1714 no fewer than one million five hundred thousand cattle died in Europe from cattle-plague." A competent authority tells us that between 1719 and 1769 "not less than two hundred millions of cattle were destroyed by rinderpest alone." * These figures might easily be augmented to a degree almost beyond human conception. In our own day millions of dollars' worth of valuable animal property is yearly swept away by these ravaging destroyers. Ignorance and superstition prevailed among the people. Where should they look for aid? The doctors were powerless. The veterinary empiricism of the day sank as an imbecile before the furious storm. The Church cried that the Almighty was angry, and punishing the world for its sins. "Come to me—I alone can save you!" said an equally imbecile priesthood. The people went! Instead of help, they found husks. In spite of the invocations of anointed bishops, in spite of the sacred and all-preserving charms which the Church affirmed were possessed by the consecrated oils, or by the burning cross, or heated key of the all-holy saints, Martin and Angelo, in spite of Inquisitional tortures inflicted upon an already suffering animal world by these barbarians of the Church, in spite of all the powers of man, on went the ravaging pests, carrying death and misery in their path.

Empirical curers, then as now, were to be had on all sides, but their medicines were as empty of effect as their brains were of knowledge. The so-called veterinary profession was as powerless as the mighty Church; priestly imbecile and veterinary quack joined hands in producing nothing. Woe, woe was on every side! Hope alone was all that poor humanity had to depend upon. Men felt that they were indeed deserted by God, and that the Father of the heavens was no more mindful of his children. But this was only so in appearance.

We have arrived at the latter part of the eighteenth century, and found—what? That no veterinary science existed; that no veterinarians had added anything of much value, other than a few things of practical import, to human knowledge. But the medical profession had not been idle. While Luther was battling, as a son of Mars, for the freedom of the human intellect from the trammels

* "Animal Plagues."

of an imbecile superstition, and in part demoralized priesthood, Truth was not without her able representatives in many fields of science. Vesalius was following in the path of Luther, and bringing things which had been, until then, hidden in an impenetrable darkness, to the light of the world; the human body was, for the first time, subjected to the analytical power of the human intellect, and the anatomist's scalpel was daily revealing truths before which the superstitions and myths of thousands of years disappeared as the mists before the morning sun. The Church shouted her anathemas, but in vain. In spite of curse, hatred, persecution, and calumny, on went the bark of truth, emphatically testifying to the wisdom of the words of the Eastern sage, "Truth alone is the mightiest of all things, and will live forever." Vesalius was a reformer of the truest type; but to progress, other elements are also necessary. They seek to pull down, not to build up; they serve to tear away the cobwebs, which, as superstitions, prevent the new light from gaining entrance into dark corners. The sun of revolution in medicine found its representative in Paracelsus, a wonderful mixture of superstition and common sense himself, but nevertheless a man who did no small work in preparing the way for the truth to enter men's minds. On went the march of investigation. "More! more!" was the cry of a hungering humanity; and the answer came in the great and immortal Harvey's unlocking the keys to an unknown fountain, and teaching men how the flowing blood was forced through their organisms. England then denied her child, to honor him in future generations as among the "anointed" of the sons of men. The great Hunter laid the foundation of a new science, and made the world a debtor, by laying the foundation of the first museum for pathological anatomy. Boerhaave was teaching a mighty class of scholars, whose fame was to make his great name still more famous. Van Zwieten laid the foundation of the first hospital in Vienna. Glisson started the doctrine of the irritability of the tissues, which found its more complete elucidation at the hands of Haller, immortal physiologist, poet, philosopher, statesman, and naturalist. Harvey and Haller must be looked upon as the fathers of modern physiology. It is not an uninteresting fact that Harvey freed the world of errors which had been held ever since its beginning, in the same year (1620) that our "Pilgrim fathers" broke the ground in favor of human rights on the Western Continent. Haller, Lancisi, Ramazzini, Bates, and others, did the work that an incompetent veterinary profession could not do, by describing the animal plagues, especially pleuro-pneumonia and cattle-plague. Not only did these men describe, they also made most careful observations as to the manner in which these pests extended, and elucidated means of prevention entirely applicable to our day, and which had we, in this country, sense enough to study and follow, would save us untold millions in the future. So true are the descriptions given by these men, so far-seeing the instructions they give for prevention, that I feel myself impelled to give them here.

Speaking of the animal pest which devastated Europe in the eighteenth century, Fleming says: "The cattle-plague—rinderpest—continued its ravages in all the countries named in the preceding year (1712). In Russia, it had enlarged its boundaries. In Germany, it was reported at various places. It was still spreading in Switzerland; but in Holland its violence was excessive; it was said that there alone, between 1713 and 1723, it destroyed two hundred thousand cattle. In Italy it was steadily marching on, and causing havoc on all sides. In Naples, Calabria, and Romagna, its advances were causing the utmost apprehension and fear. The learned doctor and physician of Pope Clement XI, Giovanni Lancisi, was sent to investigate the nature and prescribe measures for the suppression of the pest. To the ability of this man, while obeying his instructions, we are much indebted for an accurate description of the symptoms and *post-mortem* appearances of the malady, as manifested in that part of the Roman dominions. His report is as follows: 'In the middle of the summer of 1713 there was a rumor at Rome that a large number of infected oxen from districts on the Mediterranean were being driven from the market of Frusinoso to us; wherefore it was wisely decreed that no markets should be held, or any cattle be driven into the place. *But merchants introduced oxen into the city secretly by by-ways, because their hopes of selling them publicly had been frustrated; and these, being driven about in all directions, and becoming mixed with our hitherto healthy stock, spread abroad the disease. For, when foreign merchants had doubtful or suspicious cattle, which they could not sell in their own country, they brought them to Rome surreptitiously, and sold them for less than the usual price.*' " *

This philosopher and far-seeing patriot gives us such a high opinion of his wisdom and truthfulness in his work on this plague, that we must quote more largely from his report. He had no doubt whatever as to its being an imported disease. As quickly as possible, when its presence was discovered, all traffic in cattle was to be prohibited, and the law enforced with the utmost rigor in the case of

* Fleming, "History of Animal Plagues," p. 198.

those who moved cattle about. But the disease was still raging; "as a neglected spark at first, it had at length set Italy in a blaze," and was extending everywhere. Lancisi described the disease, dwelt on its terrific character and the hopelessness of medical treatment, and then recommended what he deemed the wisest course. "I advised that every diseased animal should be killed; for, I maintained that, should they be left to a slow death, the cost of medicines, veterinary surgeons, attendants, and other means, would be very great, and not only this, but their very presence would assist in the diffusion of the contagion. The Sacred College, however, ordained that this measure was too severe, and that remedies should be tried; and, in truth, they were greatly influenced in this decision by the number of people who pretended that they had infallible cures for the affection. But the fact is," added Lancisi, "that in the cattle, as in the human plague, not every one who takes the disease dies of it. Some recover, thanks to Nature, rather than to the remedies which are resorted to." The attempts to cure the disease only resulted in failure, and its indefinite extension. Edicts were issued, forbidding the bringing of cattle from the Campagna into the district of Rome, under the penalty of death to a layman, and of the galleys for life to an ecclesiastic. The sale of hides was interdicted, and the flesh, horns, and fat of the animals were ordered to be buried in deep pits and covered with quicklime. Measures were taken to prevent the sale of diseased meats. Inspectors were appointed to visit the markets, and only those pieces of flesh which were stamped with a hot iron by the inspector were allowed to be sold. Skinning the dead carcasses was forbidden, as it might lead to the further extension of the disease. The severity of the edicts was complained of; "but it is a fact," he adds, "that *here*, where the laws were strictly enforced, the plague was arrested much sooner than in other parts of Italy."

The various edicts issued by the Sacred College are given at length by Lancisi. He thinks "they will be of great service to posterity if a similar misfortune should ever again happen—which may Heaven avert!"

Posterity has heedlessly passed them by many and many times, and has consequently paid the penalties of its neglect.

The last chapter of this invaluable work sums up his admirable reflections upon this disease: "The steps which a wise government should instantly take, whenever the pestilence may again appear upon our borders, are these: all roads and by-paths should be carefully guarded, so that no ox or dog be allowed to enter the country. Any animal so entering should be forthwith destroyed and buried.

Should the pestilence, however, gain admission, the separation of the sick from the healthy must be enforced by decree. *Indeed, in my opinion, by far the safest course is instantly to destroy the animal with the pole-axe, so that no infected blood may escape on the ground;* for, in attempting to cure the diseased animal, the veterinary surgeon may convey the disease to healthy animals. The healthy cattle must be removed from their former pastures, which must be regarded as contaminated. The diseased oxen should be kept in stables, to which no one is admitted except the veterinary surgeon or the herdsman. The fountains and vessels used by the animals should be frequently cleaned with quicklime. The clothes of the shepherds should also be fumigated. The dead carcasses, from which not one hair is to be removed, must be buried in deep pits; any saliva or secretions which may drop from them on the way to the pit are to be carefully removed. If any cows are infected, their milk is instantly to be thrown into a hole in the ground; and the severest punishment should be inflicted on those who disobey this order. The passage of all rustics and dogs should be forbidden."

That Lancisi's teachings have not been entirely neglected is shown by the following letter, written to Mr. Fleming while I was a student in Germany: *

MY DEAR SIR: I have just read your very judicious and reasonable letter in the "Times," on the "Cattle-Plague," and being here at Berlin, the headquarters of this outbreak, it may not be uninteresting to you to hear from me as to what I have seen.

The whole state, we will say, is divided into thirty-six departments, and these again are subdivided into districts; over each of these districts is an official veterinarian, known as the "Kreis-Thierarzt," or district veterinary surgeon, and the same arrangement is carried out over the entire Empire of Germany. All these men are selected for their ability, and especially for their knowledge of contagious animal diseases; in the smaller towns the "Kreis-Thierarzt" is one of the men of the town, and has for society those who are considered the leading men of the place. The "Departements-Thierarzt" is a much greater character; he is an unusually well-educated person, who must be thoroughly posted in regard to the laws of the empire relative to his profession and duties, and is responsible to the local state authorities, as well as to the ministry, for the faithful performance of his duties; the "Kreis-Thierärzte" are responsible to those of the departments. These officers all receive salaries from the state, varying from fifty to four hundred

* Published in the "Veterinary Journal," 1879.

pounds per year, and also are permitted to receive fees for their official attendance in addition to their regular fees. They are further favored in their practice by their official positions, it being a guarantee to the public of their competency. Prussia does much to encourage graduated students to continue their studies. This winter some thirty men, from twenty-five to forty years of age, are receiving about forty pounds each from the Government to pay their expenses in Berlin, while they are attending lectures and studying; and at the time I write they are being examined for higher positions. Every year a new set arrives; so you will understand that *our science* is properly encouraged on the Continent, and a man has some incentive to work. In Prussia, to every 4·75 square miles (geographical) there is a veterinary surgeon, and to his care are confided 1,544 horses, 4,592 cattle, 14,221 sheep, 2,192 hogs; and there are (these figures apply to 1875) 1,290 veterinary practitioners. This has no reference to the number of official veterinarians.

These few remarks will serve as an introduction to the remainder of my letter. Early in January there was an unusual excitement to be noticed around our school; messengers were to be seen rapidly passing between the offices of the Minister of Agriculture and the school officials. It soon transpired that "der Teufel's los," as it was expressed to me, or, in other words, the "rinderpest" was in Hamburg. It took but a short time to arrange matters. Professor Müller, whom you know as an anatomist, and a great authority upon this scourge, was dispatched to Hamburg with a high government officer. Another great expert was sent to the Russian frontier; every department veterinary officer was notified by telegraph, and in less than twelve hours an embargo was placed upon every head of horned cattle in Germany. If I mistake not, your Government was officially informed of the sailing of the Castor with infected cattle from Hamburg, in sufficient time to have stopped her before reaching London. She should have been stopped some distance from that port, her hatches battened down, and the vessel and cargo towed somewhere, sunk, and paid for by the Government. If this was in reality the first infected cargo, then England would perhaps have been preserved from a serious loss; the future can alone prove what the loss may be.

To return to the outbreak in Germany. The Berlin and all other markets were most vigilantly watched, and no cattle or other animals were allowed to be removed from them alive for slaughter in the city. (All cattle moved at any time from the markets in Berlin are moved only in large cattle-wagons; the same is true of every other marketable animal, except horses. Glandered horses and suspected horses are invariably moved in wagons, either to the school for inspection, or to the knackers, to be immediately killed.) All cattle that had to be removed were first rigidly inspected, and then conveyed in wagons, and put directly upon the cars; and so it was all over the country. Alluding to your remarks in the "Times," on the futility of inspection when the disease is latent, a fine instance occurred here, which our mutual friend Professor Dieckerhoff unraveled with his customary ability. He was called to Westphalia, it being reported that a cow there was suspiciously diseased. On his arrival the cow in question had been killed, or had died, but her illness was said not to have been rinderpest. It was, however, reported that another cow was sick, and this animal was immediately placed under lock and seal, and the case proved to be one of rinderpest. As the story is interesting, it may be useful to relate it in full: This cow had been bought in Berlin by a butcher, who was a Jew; it was there inspected and passed, put on the cars with others, and taken to the town, the name of which I have forgotten. The other cattle were at once killed; but the butcher having a child suddenly die, the remaining cow was sent to a friend for a day or two, for him to keep, and during the interval the disease had time to develop. Professor Dieckerhoff traced the whole affair from beginning to end; the cow was killed, and rinderpest proved to be present. If this cow had been killed with the others, the disease might have been spread without the real cause ever becoming apparent, or brought to light. I have purposely refrained from saying anything about the action of the authorities in these special cases; in the investigation of some others it was my good fortune to be present. Early one morning about two weeks since, Professor Dieckerhoff sent for me; it was just daylight, and, with him and four other students, we started for a village, about thirteen miles from Berlin, where a cow was reported to be sick. I should state that the Government keeps a very nice "turn-out" and four horses for this purpose, and Professor Dieckerhoff has this clinic (at present he has charge of the school hospitals)—taking four students each time with him, your humble servant going when anything interesting is likely to turn up. We arrived in about two hours, the roads being heavy; we met the local officers and proceeded to the suspected farm-house, but did not enter until we had proved our right to do so; the house being guarded, and not a person allowed to leave or enter the premises, but to speak or pass things in or out through a window. I omitted to state that Professor Dieckerhoff and the renowned Hertwig had been there the previous day, and it had been decided to allow another to pass, in order that the symptoms should become sufficiently developed to prove the existence of the disease, the place being well guarded. During the night a trench had been dug some forty feet long and some fourteen deep in an entirely isolated wood, which we could reach without crossing a public way. We removed the cow, made a necroscopical examination, proved our case; her nine companions were brought after her to the same place, with their chains and stable-utensils: the cows were then shot, after the decision of the proper officers had been given, and they with the utensils were at once buried—a military guard over the place, another about the farm from which they were taken, and also on the streets leading to the village; the inmates of this particular place being confined strictly to their own limits for a time prescribed by law. No cattle or farm animals were allowed in the streets, and only persons permitted there with teams who had received sanction from the authorities. All those who had had to do with the infected cattle were most effectually disinfected; while those that buried them had no cattle themselves, and were not allowed to go near any within the lawful time. I heard an officer say that the pastor of the village must be carefully watched: that these gentry were unfortunately apt to be spreaders of contagium, the guards often allowing them to pass as favored persons, and then they innocently, of course, must go to the stable, see things, and afterward go to another neighbor to mention the loss of neighbor So-and-so. This has often been the case, I am told, in Germany. The manure, the stall, and all things about the stable, are carefully cleansed and disinfected under the supervision of veterinary officials. I was surprised to see numerous military about the fields and streets, apparently with no purpose, yet carrying rifles; their duty, it seems, was to shoot every dog, cat, or valiant chanticleer, which they might see straying abroad or leaving the proper quarters. Doubtless the Prussian course may seem tyrannical and severe—all the cattle are killed, not only the diseased, but all belonging to the infested farm or stable—but the law is, to my mind, essentially democratic; it is for the good of the whole, and the cattle killed and utensils destroyed are paid for by the state at market prices.

The remarks of Haller upon certain contagious animal diseases, more especially the pleuro-pneumonia of cattle, which is of such vital interest to the people of this country at present, and which bids fair to become a most serious economical problem to American statesmen, certainly more than warrants their introduction here. It is not, however, inappropriate to the subject of this book to give a short sketch of the life of a man who has wielded such a mighty intellectual influence in the world's progress.

"Albert von Haller * was born at Bern, Switzerland, in 1708, and in early youth demonstrated a systematic spirit and a strong scientific tendency. He began to make for himself a private dictionary as soon as he was able to write, in which he entered all words hitherto unknown to him, with their meanings. He also made a dictionary of a similar character as soon as he began the study of foreign languages, and when he began the study of history he followed the same course. He often said that in his later years he found valuable information in these works of his youthful days. When ten years old he had already shown his taste for poetry by writing ludicrous verses about his teachers, his poetic talent at this time having a special bent to satire, which he, however, entirely gave up in later years. In 1723, when he was fifteen years old, he went to the University of Tübingen, to study medicine under Duvernoi and Camerarius. In the next year he wrote a polemic against an anatomical assertion of Professor Coshwitz at Halle. He did not remain long at Tübingen, as he, with other students, had made a shepherd so drunk with high-wine (Branntwein) that the latter lost his life. In 1725 he removed to Leyden, to study under the guidance of the immortal Boerhaave. At eighteen years of age he acquired his degree of doctor of medicine, visited England and France, but had to flee from Paris, because it was found that he had made dissections of human bodies at his residence. From Paris he went to Basel and studied mathematics under Bernoulli; but in 1729 he returned to the place of his nativity, Bern, in order to practice his profession; at the same time he studied botany with great earnestness. In 1734 he became director of the hospitals of his city, and also had an amphitheatre built in which he gave anatomical lectures. Most of his poems were written at this time. In 1735 he had control of the City Library, which he himself used with the greatest diligence. In 1736 he was called to Göttingen as Professor of Anatomy, Chemistry, and Botany; he also explained the 'Institutions' of his master, Boerhaave, which he himself published with commentaries in 1739. At this period he still busied himself with botany, and published several works of classical importance upon the subject; he also wrote a large number of important anatomical papers, besides publishing an atlas of anatomy. But it is for his contributions to physiology that Haller is as much noted as for any other of his mani-

* "Geschichte d. Medicin," Wunderlich, Stuttgart, 1859.

fold accomplishments. His first appearance in this branch of science was a polemical work on respiration in 1727. He demonstrated that there was no air between the pleura costalis and lungs, against the contrary assertions of Professor Hamberger. Haller's fame, and with it that of the Göttingen University, increased each year; he laid the foundation of the Göttingen Scientific Society, and a periodical, which is still in existence, devoted to science. After seventeen years of unceasing activity his health broke down, and he was obliged to return to Bern in 1753, where he took an active interest and part in the government, and published numerous works upon botany, anatomy, surgery, the practice of medicine—all of them of classical importance. During the last years of his life he scarcely left his library—sleeping, eating, working, and receiving his friends and visitors there. His wife, children, pupils, and friends were all kept busy aiding this wonderfully gifted man in his work; only in this way was it possible for a human being to give to the world the almost incredible amount of literary work which he did. Haller died, beloved and respected of all, at the place of his birth, on the 12th of December, 1777." In 1877 his native city fitly celebrated the one hundredth anniversary of the death of this her greatest son, whose name and fame will be held immortal so long as memory lasts and mankind continues to reverence the noblest among the children of the world, who, though dead in form, still live that immortality which is given but to the selected few.

I have previously mentioned that among the most important contributions to veterinary literature in the eighteenth century was a writing by Haller upon an epizoötic disease of the cattle of Switzerland, an edition of which appeared at Bern in 1773, entitled "Mémoire sur la Contagion parmi le Bétail."

"In this year (1745) * the immortal Haller published his investigations into the nature of an epizoötic which had several times been observed in Switzerland. The great physician supposed it was the 'cattle-plague,' but no one can read his description of this Swiss malady without surmising that it was a different disease, in all probability the bovine contagious pleuro-pneumonia. Such an authority needs no apology for being quoted here, especially as his preventive measures are worthy of notice, and would probably have saved this country a great loss had they been adopted in recent years:

"1. The first thing necessary is to determine the nature of the disease. This knowledge is not easily acquired, for frequently it

* Fleming, *loc. cit.*, p. 446.

does not manifest itself by any perceptible symptoms for a long time. The veritable cause of death is the work of nothing but corruption, which often infects the intestines—corruption, which is the consequence, not the cause, of the disease. The ravages which this disease caused among the cattle of the most enlightened nations, before they knew its terrible character or the means to prevent its progress, are without doubt to be attributed to the great difficulty which is frequently met with in correctly recognizing it. In a general way, it is described as manifesting itself by a violent fever, shiverings, staring coat, by loss of rumination; but all these symptoms do not appear until the malady has already made deadly advances in the interior of the animal. We are told that, for a certainty, a beast taken out of an infected stable and transported to a perfectly healthy atmosphere does not become sick until a month after it has been removed from the diseased locality, and that it perishes from the veritable contagion which, without doubt, had been concealed during the whole of this month in the body of the animal. It is also a fact that the diseased cattle jump about for some weeks with vivacity; that they give their usual quantity of milk; that they eat their forage with avidity; that they work in harness, and yet that they carry death in their intestines. The only indication of pneumonia (*pulmonie*) which is to be noticed from the commencement is a slight cough, which affects the animal, notwithstanding every apparent indication of good health. It is not for some days or weeks after the animal has become infected that the disease shows itself by fever and horripilation. The cough now augments, the animal moans, its strength diminishes, it can not stand, and lies down very often; it has a difficulty in breathing; the pulse is frequent; the fever becomes intensified. It is now that the appetite and rumination cease. The disease prevails for some days, the fever increasing daily; the veins (?) beat with a force and quickness which is astonishing; a viscid froth escapes from the mouth and nostrils; the tongue is hot, the breath heavy and labored, and its odor insupportable; the eyes are withdrawn in their orbits, the horns cold; a diarrhœa of a bad odor, sometimes tinged with blood, and a thorough total sinking terminate the beast's days. Diarrhœa does not always take place."

"2. When we open the cattle after death we find the lungs constantly and infallibly affected. We might know this from the cough and the difficulty of breathing which precede death. In all the contagions which have reigned at Sulens, Grandson, Crassy, and elsewhere, the lungs have always been inflamed and attached to the pleura, and abscesses often form between the lungs and this membrane. I find the same observations in the best authorities who have written upon the contagion, and particularly in the writings of M. Bourgelat, who has made the treatment of these animals a particular study. In many cows the lungs are found gangrenous; in others, they are filled with abscesses; and in others, again, there are vesicles filled with water, mixed sometimes with pus; it is more rare to find tartarized or cretaceous matters. There are constantly inflammation and gangrene of the pleura, and we have never yet killed infected animals and found the lungs in a perfect state. The cough being the first symptom of this disease, it is present in every animal affected. The lungs being constantly diseased, it is evident that the disease of these organs is the essence of the contagion, and that it is with perfect justice that the people of France and Germany term it pneumonia. The alterations in the other viscera are not so essential as those in the lungs. It is common, nevertheless, to find the stomach inflamed and gorged with food. It is scarcely altered when the animals are killed shortly after the commencement of the disease; but, when they have been slaughtered at the last stages, or when they have died, the first compartment is inflamed, the food is found but little affected by digestion, or it may be rotten. The second compartment is equally inflamed, and filled with forage which is undigested. The third compartment suffers the most, and is often found inflamed and gangrenous, the food in it being extremely compact and dry, and sometimes rotten (*pourri*). The fourth or true stomach is frequently inflamed and gangrenous, but the food is not hardened.

"From the first days of the malady the beast has eaten and ruminated; and, as it would not be able to maintain either of these functions if the stomach had become inflamed, it is very evident that the disturbance of the stomach is a consequence of the fever, and the putridity of the juices of the beast, and that it is not the cause of the disease. The animal has been infected and the stomach maintained its health for a number of days, and it is only by a corruption of the humors that it is found vitiated.

"3. The true nature of a disease is known by the accidents which accompany it in its duration, and by the changes which we observe on the autopsy of the animal, when compared with the organs in health. But the essential features of the disease ought to consist in the symptoms which are manifested from the beginning, and which have continued during life, and in the marks of corruption in the interior, which are the actual causes of these symptoms. It requires care not to be deceived by these accidents, which are a consequence of the corruption of the humors, and are only most apparent in the latter stages of the disease. It is believed that the contagion among cattle is an inflammatory fever, a malignant fever—a fever accompanied by an eruption of the skin—as well as an inflammation of the stomach. It is evident that it is a disease of the lungs, which commences by an inflammation, running often into gangrene; at other times into abscesses, and which terminates in phthisis. It is very astonishing that among the number of modern doctors who have written on a contagion existing for so many years, scarcely one has observed that the seat of the disease exists in the lungs, or even that these were attacked.

"4. The doctors have established their remedial measures to cure this disease on the notion that they knew its nature. Those who look upon it as an inflammatory fever recommend bleeding, and remedies of a soothing and cooling kind; those who admit a corruption of the blood have ordered febrifuge and stimulating remedies; and those who consider it a putrid fever counsel the administration of acids; and, in Brandenburg, wild apples have been recommended as a specific. Others, again, have proposed quinine, and others mercury, while the people have had recourse in general to incongruous compositions, and to old-fashioned recipes. The ancients looked much to setons passed through the skin, in order to establish a long-continued suppuration. But it has been discovered, by sad experience, in Holland and England, that these remedies are impotent; all hope of curing this disease has been lost, and people are content to mitigate it by inoculation. *We pass in silence the pretended preservatives by which it is supposed animals are insured against the contagion, and to which no man of sense would give any confidence, seeing that they are useless against the plague, the small-pox, and other contagious diseases.*

"5. A long experience has taught us that remedies are useless against the contagion. The beginning of the disease is nearly imperceptible, and when the symptoms are manifested the cure has become almost impossible. The use of remedies is otherwise dangerous, for the infection is really communicated by the breath and exhalations. We have a proof of this in the foul smell attached to the clothes of people who look after the diseased beasts. We can not hope to cure in a day a disease of so serious a character; and thus the diseased creature, which lives in the same stable with other cattle, and feeds and drinks with them, may infect them during the time we are unsuccessfully attempting to cure it. These same exhalations may also lodge in the clothes of those who go about them, and thus become dangerous to the animals yet in health.

"We can not, then, hope for any good from remedies. For more than two thousand years an infinite number of the most learned men have given their constant attention to observing the effects of medicines on mankind. We know well enough the value of simples, the properties which they have of stimulating or evacuating, and their dose. But we have not nearly the same knowledge to guide us when we deal with animals: few talented persons have observed their diseases; the art of curing them has been left to men of low condition, who have no knowledge of the anatomy of the lower creatures, and who have not informed themselves by the study of nature or of good authors. The cattle-doctors invariably follow the same routine traced out by the ancient veterinarians, and their science (art) consists of divers receipts which they have found among the papers of their predecessors.

"The structure of the stomachs of cattle is very different from that of man; in general, the envelopes of their nerves are much thicker, the sensations less active, the pulse less frequent, the arteries more hard, the heart less irritable. All these peculiarities change the effect of remedies in animals, in a way quite different to man; and it is only within a few years that convincing proof has been afforded of the differences between the effect which a given remedy has on man and the animals. The saffron of metals is a violent emetic for man; in the horse it only increases the transpiration; a dose of glass of antimony, which produces violent vomiting in mankind, simply purges the horse; no poison will make a horse or cow vomit. Because the effects of medicines, therefore, on the lower animals are so little known; because scarcely any one has observed closely enough the diseases of cattle, or given definite rules for the exhibition of the proper remedies; because the use of remedies can only tend to spread the contagion—for all these reasons it is prudent to abstain from a dangerous tentative which promises but little, and which may have the worst effects; it is infinitely preferable to oppose the disease by means which are more certain and commendable.

"6. *We begin by disabusing the public of the idea that the pneumonia (la pulmonie) is not a contagious disease.* This outrageous idea even comes from some *savants.* There are those, too, who rob the plague of its contagious power. I do not pretend to say that the skin of an infected beast preserves its contagious properties for a long time after death; experiments upon this matter, which deserve attention, have been made in France. It is necessary, nevertheless, to remember that the plague attaches itself by preference to the wool and the hair of animals, that it may be transported by these materials, and that they will spread the contagion to other towns and countries free from the contagion. It is, then, possible that the poisonous exhalations of the diseased beast attach themselves to the hairs of animals which go near it. It is at least certain, in our country, that as often as the disease is manifested among cattle, and when it has been traced to its source, it has been found that a beast which has been purchased in the market of some suspected place, or which had been brought from some suspected locality, has carried the contagion with it to a new center. Sometimes, also, the cattle of our regions have been pastured with those of a neighboring infected country. It is very probable that at other times the air of the infected mountains has spread the dangerous exhalations over the country. We believe that we have observed that healthy cattle which had smelled of those that were diseased have shown, a few hours after, traces of the contagion. It is known that the ship from Sidon brought the plague to Marseilles, and that the bull which was taken from Hungary to Padua, in 1711, took with it the fearful contagion which first ravaged Italy, and then nearly the half of Europe. It thus appears that the plague of man and the cattle-plague take their origin in hot countries, that they can infect temperate regions, and that they are gradually destroyed during the cold of some rigorous winter. That which is yet a better proof that the pneumonia is perpetuated by infection, as the plague is, is the manner in which we can confine it in suspected places, and by cutting off all communication between the stables which are infected and those which are not. If this malady were generated spontaneously, like the ordinary fevers of man, we would in vain barricade stables, in vain would we slaughter the cattle of a village, and it would be useless to isolate the mountains by barriers and guards. All these precautions would not keep away a disease which has its origin in the blood itself of the healthiest cattle. ... The contagion, however, does not spread very far, and it does not infect a column of air for any great distance. If the air were infected, if it was able to carry afar the poison of the disease, the barriers and other precautionary measures of man would be unavailing. In this there is the greatest resemblance between the disease of cattle and the plague of man. The monks and nuns of Marseilles were saved because they kept their convents closed. The air was not, then, the cause of the disease, else the closing of the convents would not have prevented the pestilence from entering. The police have often confined this disease of cattle to a stable, or a small number of stables, and so prevented others being attacked.

"*It follows from all this that, on the one side, the disease arises from infection, and, on the other, that there are no hopes of a cure.* There only remain, then, those resources which we may employ to prevent infection, and for confining to the smallest possible limit the loss which might happen when animals are first attacked by this poison. These efforts should be directed to prevent the infection being communicated from foreign countries to ours; or, if it should have penetrated, then to stop its extension from diseased to healthy cattle. Above all, then, we should hinder the entrance of cattle from a country where the pneumonia nearly always reigns, sometimes in one district, sometimes in another, and these precautions ought to remain in force at all times, and be perpetual in regard to those countries where the police is not strict, and from which the disease might be carried to ours. *The danger will always be great if the trade in cattle is carried on without inspection.* This precaution is all the more necessary against the countries whose rulers care little for the welfare of the people, and in which the people have no confidence in the administration. The poor people of a country, despairing of being aided by the Government, conceal with extreme care the existence of the contagion; to evade more onerous consequences, they even inter their cattle in the stables; and it is very natural that they should endeavor to sell at modest prices beasts the keeping of which would only cause the extension of the disease among other cattle. In the countries where the ruler has a paternal feeling for his subjects, where he is always disposed to soften their losses, where he generously takes into account the expenses necessarily attending precautions, and where he gains the confidence of the people, the inhabitants at once denounce the disease, submit to the necessary restrictions, and rely on the wisdom of their king for their preservation and the amelioration of their hardships. *A wise government ought to prevent the contagion, and not wait until it has invaded the country, but check it at its frontiers, where it is easy to do so. The police ought, then, even in times of the greatest security, to take care that no animal shall become diseased without responsible people being informed. Even in ordinary times every animal purchased or sold ought to be vouched for, and should be marked on the horn with a particular stamp for each village, which mark should be renewed whenever it becomes effaced; so that by this proof we may know what village it comes from, and assure ourselves of the health of that village. For the same reason no cattle should be admitted to fairs or markets, sold or exchanged, without a voucher being given of perfect health, impressed and signed by the authorities, testifying to the health of the animal and that of the place whence it came. For this purpose inspectors are necessary. They should destroy cattle which are brought without attestation and give the flesh to the poor; there are but few cases where less rigorous measures are needed.*

"8. Notwithstanding all these precautions, the extent of the frontiers, the want of care on the part of neighboring nations, the exhalations from the infected mountains where the disease is raging, the greed of gain, and the desire to purchase at a low price, as well as the other failings of a police so difficult to enforce in human society, are all causes which may aid the contagion in insinuating itself into some village or on some mountain. In this unfortunate case it only rests with us to smother the flame in its first commencement, and to prevent its extension. *Every person who may have any knowledge of the disease, or even any suspicion of its existence among cattle, should be held liable to a penalty if the nearest magistrate is not at once informed; also, when a non-suspected beast becomes diseased or dies, the proprietor or other instructed person should give information, and the proper authorities should then pass on the tidings. Whoever conceals any suspected case should be severely punished. Every precaution should then be taken to extinguish the disease.*

"9. The first of these precautions is the prompt separation of the diseased beast from healthy ones. So long as it is suspected, it ought neither to be allowed to drink, feed, pasture, nor dwell with the healthy. It should be kept in a separate stable, or in an inclosed paddock, and those who attend it should wear clothes appropriate to the purpose, never even approaching healthy animals. The trough out of which this animal drinks ought not to be used for healthy ones, the dung should not be spread on the ground or carried away, but should be buried in deep pits and well covered with earth, and these places should be surrounded with palings, so that no healthy beast may be able to smell it.

"When the infected animal has been killed, or when it has died, it is necessary to aërate the stable for three months at least, and to remove and burn the thatch, and all the wooden movable articles; to dig up the ground to the depth of a foot, and replace it with other earth, and cover the whole with lime. The healthy should not go near the forage which the diseased may have been eating, and which might be infected by its breath, though it may be given to horses. Every animal dying of the disease should be opened in the presence of proper persons skilled in the veterinary art, and a report of the *post-mortem* appearance should be made. If the disease is made out to be a non-contagious one, the owner may be permitted to use the flesh and remove the skin. But if there is found the slightest cause for suspicion in the lungs, the skin ought to be cut crosswise, and buried in a grave six feet deep, which should be filled with lime. Palisades should be fixed around it, so that no animal may come near it. If the disease is really *a pneumonia*, it is preferable not to doctor it, but to kill without delay the first animals which, from their cough, would lead one to suspect the disease, or those which have been in the same stable with the sick; because we may set down as lost, without exception, every animal which has been in a house with a pulmonic beast. Experience has only too often demonstrated that they take the disease one after the other, and all die.

"10. When many stables are infected in the same village, the danger is yet greater, and it is here that it is necessary to redouble our efforts to prevent the extension of the contagion. All the infected stables should be carefully closed and excluded from all communication with the watering-places and pasturage; in serious cases, to make more certain, we should kill all animals which have been in the infected places, no less those in apparent health than those in which the disease is manifest. We are driven to this severe course because we can never be assured that those animals which have come out of the suspicious places have escaped the contagion. This apparent cruelty is the only means to be employed for preventing the contagion from penetrating into other stables and into neighboring villages, and from spreading over the whole country.

"The case is yet more dangerous when the contagion manifests itself on a mountain where a certain number of cattle find their subsistence during the winter. It has happened that the cattle of the plains have remained in health, but those on the neighboring mountains have been infected, and thus the herds of the republic have been encircled by contagion. In these unhappy circumstances it should be recommended that the mountain-passes be closed, and all communication cut off from the infected pasturage. Inspectors ought to make a visit every fifteen days to the mountains, where cattle belonging to the subjects of the state are kept, in order to examine with great care if any beasts are in a suspicious condition, or if, without exception, they are healthy.

"In those instances where the infected mountains of our neighbors abut too closely on our own, these last should be most strictly guarded, and it should not be for less than a year after the disease has disappeared that any communication should be allowed; as experience has amply demonstrated that cattle not suspected of the disease have been attacked by the contagion by grazing on mountains in the neighborhood of those infected. Sometimes we are obliged to exercise a greater degree of severity by destroying the hogs which, according to custom on the mountains, feed with the cattle. The contagion which destroys the cattle does not affect either pigs, sheep, or horses; but it is always to be apprehended that these may carry some of the contagion or their infected breath to these animals, and may thus spread the disease.

"It is only by these precautions, which should be constantly in force, that it is possible to confine the contagion to a village or mountain, and to keep the country free from infection."

That these explicit instructions of the great Haller have not been without their proper appreciation, may be seen from the following:

Professor Putz* (of the Veterinary Institute at Bern) says: "It is not difficult to determine what regulations are indicated, from a truly scientific stand-point, to suppress the contagious lung-plague of cattle. In order to effectually eradicate the generation of infectious material, the sole generator of the pest, there is no more radical method than the complete killing out of the infected herd. A view of the questionable conditions in Switzerland satisfactorily demonstrates how advantageous it would be were all the nations of Europe to adopt this plan. In the canton of Bern, noted for its richness in cattle, for about one hundred years (since Haller) this scientific procedure has been successfully carried out, and it has finally become universally adopted by the numerous cantons of the Swiss Republic. The law (of February 8, 1872) for the suppression of contagious animal diseases, especially the contagious pleuro-pneumonia of cattle, says, article 24, 'In Switzerland no cattle that *have* been diseased with the contagious lung-plague (Ansteckenden Lungenseuche) can ever again be allowed to become an article of traffic.'" In Massachusetts the same course was adopted, at a cost of some seventy-five thousand dollars to the people of the State, but the result has been, that while the disease has prevailed, and still prevails, in neighboring States, not a single case has again appeared in Massachusetts.

* "Die Lungenseuche," etc., by Professor Putz, "Vorträge für Thierärzte," Series i, Heft 6, v. 7.

As is well known, England has been repeatedly invaded by the rinderpest, which has caused the people to lose millions of pounds in valuable cattle; while legislation has been wofully imperfect in this regard, owing to the unfortunate influence exerted by the London Veterinary School in times past; still Britain has not been without patriotic and excellent advisers. Among the most noteworthy was a Mr. Bates, surgeon to George I, who wrote in 1714, but his advice seems to have fallen upon barren ground in later years. Bates was appointed by the Government to study the disease, and to devise means for its prevention. He writes, after examining a large number of diseased animals: "We then ordered some of the sick cows to be housed, and several sorts of cattle to be kept with them, to see whether the contagion would affect any other species. The next day I made a verbal report to their Excellencies of all the several opinions and discourses which I have had about it, and left them debating what method to take; at last I was called in, and ordered to consider it again the next day, and to deliver them in writing what would be proper to be done. Accordingly, I drew up and gave them the following proposals:

"1. That all such cows as are now in possession of Messrs. Ratcliffe, Rufford, and Pullen, be brought, killed, and burned; or, at least, that the sick be burned, and the well kept secured on the grounds where they now are, that such of them that sicken and die of the distemper may be burned.

"2. That the houses in which the sick cows have stood be washed very clean, and then smoked by the burning of pitch and wormwood, and be kept empty three months, at least, before other cows be put therein.

"3. That the fields where the sick cows have grazed be kept two months before any other cows are suffered to stand or graze upon them.

"4. That persons looking after such that are ill should have no communication with those that are well.

"5. That the same methods be observed if any other of the cowkeepers should get this distemper among them; and that they all be summoned, and told that as soon as they perceive any of the cows refuse their food, or have any other symptoms of this distemper, they immediately separate them from the others, and give notice to such persons as your Excellencies shall appoint, that they may be burned; and the places where they have stood or grazed ordered as before.

"6. That the cow-keepers be required to divide their cows into small parcels, not more than ten or twelve in a field together; and that they be allowed such satisfaction for complying with these proposals as your Excellencies shall think fit." *

These suggestions were accepted and acted upon, forty shillings per head being allowed for the sick cows killed by the authorities.

"Some of the cow-keepers appeared not content with this arrangement, and, believing that the disease would become general, *designed to have their cows sold at some distant market,* which the gentlemen having notice of, appointed several butchers to watch near their grounds, and count their numbers every morning, with orders to follow such as were sent to market, and to prevent their being sold by telling the people what they were.

"Another great obstacle at first was the cow-keepers not admitting the disease until they had lost several cows, for, as soon as it was known that any man had but one sick, no one would buy his milk, and to those who kept many cows the loss was considerable.

"*Nor was there ever wanting one or other who gave them hopes of cure.*

"It was endeavored to impress upon the cow-keepers that they would receive remuneration for their losses: '*This had a pretty good effect, but here in England, where every man is at liberty to dispose of his cattle as he pleases, nothing but making them sensible that it was each man's particular interest to comply with these methods, could do.*'"

The entire loss by this invasion was estimated, including expenses, at £31,174 1*s.* 1*d.*

In 1717, John Morley, of London, published a satirical poem of this invasion, which may not be without interest:

"As soon as Britain had sustained
That fatal loss which heaven had gained,
And parties squabbled to a madness
About their sorrows and their gladness,
A plague unprophesied succeeded,
That only reached the horny-headed,
And like a fatal rot or murrain
Turned all our bulls and cows to carrion.

"The farriers now their skill employed,
But still the cows in number died,
And with their horns and hides together
Were burnt, without reserve of leather.

* "Animal Plagues," p. 211.

"Some cunning hucksters, who had cows
Old, dry, and lean, not worth a souse,
Though sound in health, but scarce deserving
Of pasture, to prevent their starving,
They wisely knocked 'em on the head
By night, when neighbors were in bed.
Next day assigned their extirpation
To this new fatal visitation:
So bore 'em to some distant pit
Or ditch, for such a purpose fit;
There, to the terror of the isle,
Consumed 'em in their funeral pile.
Then like true hypocrites, put on
A mournful look, as if undone,
And claimed the sum of forty shilling
For every cow of heaven's killing—
A generous bounty, that destroyed
More cattle than the plague annoyed."

THE ESTABLISHMENT OF THE VETERINARY SCHOOLS.

There is no doubt that many of the nations of antiquity had some kind of hospitals for the care and treatment of diseased animals. We have stated, in a previous part of this work, that veterinarians were appointed to watch over the health of the animals used at the circus of Rome, but in this regard the Oriental nations took a high rank from their great veneration for all forms of animal life. Wise says: * "The peculiar humanity of the small and despised community of modern Buddhists, in the country of their ancient greatness, induced them to keep up brute hospitals—Pingra-Pol—which are still to be found in different parts of Hindostan. Trevinnier informs us that he found three or four such houses in Amandabab in 1772; and Scavoneur gives an account of the Banian hospital which still exists at Surat.† "This curious institution is supported by one anna per cent on the rupee of the merchants' clear gain, to which are added the fines for certain venial offenses, under the supervision of the chief Banians. In 1770, when trade had decayed, the revenue was upward of six hundred pounds a year; and so careful were they of the animals, that bread and milk were provided for two that could not crop the grass. The hospital grounds extended over twenty-five acres, and were surrounded by a high wall, and supplied with sheds and wards for the accommodation of the animals.

"At the present time there are no hospitals for the cure of human beings when sick, or maimed, or old, because they were supposed to be provided for by the Government; while places are prepared and persons engaged to attend the sick and aged of the inferior animals—proving how much the essential is sacrificed to an

* *Loc. cit.*, vol. ii, p. 395.

† "If proper inquiry were directed to this building," writes Princeps, "I dare say it would be discovered to be a living example (the only one that has braved twenty centuries) of the humane arts of Asoka, recorded, at no great distance, on a rock in Guzerat."

affected refinement of feeling. Niebuhr found the hospital containing horses, mules, cows, oxen, sheep, goats, monkeys, a variety of sick and maimed beasts, poultry, pigeons, and birds; also an old tortoise, which was known to have been there seventy-five years. In sickness the animals are attended by properly instructed individuals with the greatest care, and here they find a peaceable asylum for the infirmities of age. When an animal broke a limb, or was otherwise disabled, its owner brought it to this hospital, where it was always received without regard to the caste or nation of its master. There they remained for life, and the only work they were required to perform was drawing water for the patients of the hospital. Above-stairs were depositories for seeds of many sorts, and flat, broad dishes for water for birds and insects.

"In 1823 Sir Alexander Brown visited the brute hospital at Surat. It is situated in the suburbs, between the inner and outer wall, surrounded by houses and a dense population. It occupies a court fifty feet square, to which is attached a large area to admit cattle to roam about, and is strewed with grain and straw, to prevent the inmates wanting either food or bedding. They receive animals of all descriptions, from all countries, as the more numerous they are the more they increase the reputation, happiness, and prosperity of those who support them. In the hospital Sir Alexander found the old, lame, or disabled animals consisted of buffaloes, cows, goats, sheep, cocks, and hens; some of the latter had lost their feathers. There were cages to protect the birds, but most of them were empty, and a colony of pigeons were fed daily. One of the houses, twenty-five feet long, has a boarded floor elevated eight feet, under which the Buddhists throw a quantity of grain (the oftener the better for themselves), as a work of charity, which in the hot and stagnant air gives life to a mass of vermin dense as the sand of the sea-shore."

The Veterinary Institutions of France.

It is impossible for me to give more than a very incomplete account of the veterinary institutions of Europe, there being no modern history of veterinary medicine; hence I have been obliged to collect such information as I could from different articles in magazines in my possession, though I have derived great aid from the article entitled "Vétérinaire" in D'Arboval-Zundel's "Dictionnaire de Médecine," etc., Paris, 1877. I have also been fortunate in possessing two reports of German veterinarians of unquestionable ability, Hertwig and Müller, who visited France at different times in the interest of their own Government. I have myself visited several of the German schools, and also that at Alfort, France.

The Continental schools for the study and development of veterinary medicine were not founded by the respective governments so much to educate men to practice their profession, as to provide men capable of studying the nature of those fearful pests which had repeatedly brought poverty to the people, and even threatened nations with ruin, and to discover means for their prevention.

In this regard the French schools took a slightly different course from those of Germany, giving more attention to the practical at the expense of the scientific in their education; this reproach is not, however, applicable to the French schools of our day, especially those at Lyons and Toulouse, although that at Alfort has contributed no insignificant amount of scientific work, especially that of the veterinary physiologist Colin, and M. Bouley, the inspector-general of the schools. At the time when the first veterinary schools were established in France, that nation was approaching the proud position of leader in medical science and culture, which she held for half a century. Bichat, a giant among giants, founded a new system of anatomy, and died at the early age of thirty-one, a martyr to the cause of science and a benefactor to the world. Cruveilhier, the author of a noted work upon pathology; Laennec, the author of percussion and auscultation; Broussais, the vampire of medicine, so called on account of the extent to which he advocated bleeding; and many others, all tended to make Paris a haven toward which men desiring knowledge in this branch of science longingly turned; longing, not like some American women to go to Paris to die, but for that wisdom with which her intellectual fountains were so repletely filled.

It was but in the order of things that the first veterinary school of the world should be started by a Frenchman, and in France. This honor belongs to an "advocate," Claude Bourgelat, 1712–'79. This young man was educated to follow the profession of law, and studied at Toulouse. Having by his talent won a case which afterward appeared unjust to him—we wish some of our young American lawyers would follow his example!—he resolved to retire from that profession, and, having from early youth nourished a passionate fondness for the horse, resolved to encourage this taste; in order to do this, he became an officer in a cavalry regiment for a short time, and then chief of the riding academy at Lyons, which soon acquired great notoriety under the guidance of its enthusiastic teacher. The earnest spirit of the young riding-master could not content itself with studying the outward forms of his equine favorites alone—he must know more; he must know of the inner powers, the machinery of which this wonderful whole was composed. He therefore gave himself most diligently to the study of equine anatomy as well as physiology, these studies being encouraged by his friend Pouteau, one of the most eminent surgeons of Lyons. At the same time he devotedly studied the writings of earlier veterinarians, and published two works—"Nouveau Newcastle," 1747, and the "Elements of Veterinary Medicine," 1750. Bourgelat has mistakenly been called a *reformer* of veterinary medicine; on the contrary, his was the spirit which gave cause to the birth of scientific research in a branch of medicine which until his time had been nothing but the crudest empiricism. The real science in veterinary medicine did not find birth till many years after Bourgelat's death. He broke the bonds of quackery and superstition to a degree, and gave science room and opportunity to develop. In one thing Bourgelat was indeed wiser than Lafosse, in that he extended his studies beyond the horse, seeing the necessity of studying the anatomy, physiology, and pathology of all the domestic animals; but Lafosse was his superior in intellect, in that freedom of mind which evinced itself in his taking an active part for the freedom of his countrymen in the Revolution. On the 5th of August, 1761, through the influence of his friend Bertin, he received permission to found a school in Lyons, the aim of which was to study the diseases of all the domestic animals. The Government supported him with the assistance of 50,000 livres, payable in equal portions for six consecutive years. This school was opened to students the 2d of January, 1762, in a small house, formerly used as a hotel, in a suburb of Lyons called "La Guillatière." It soon acquired Continental celebrity, and among the students of its first year we find the names of three Danes, three Swedes, three Austrians, three Prussians, three Sardinians, and ten Swiss, all sent to study the elements of the new medicine by and at the expense of their respective governments. The branches at first taught were zoötomy, especially that of the horse (exterior), horsemanship, pharmacy, special pathology, surgery, and the principles of sanitary police.

Scarcely was the foundation of the school successfully accomplished, before France was again the seat of the ravages of the devastating animal plagues, which gave its students an opportunity to display the value of systematic education, crude as it then was, over the still cruder but futile attempts of a puerile empiricism. The students, guided by the teachings of their master, were so successful as to attract the attention of the king, Louis XV, who in an order dated June 30, 1764, gave to the institution the title of a "*Royal Veterinary School.*" A month previously the king had honored Bourgelat with the title of "Director and General Inspector of the Veterinary School at Lyons," and all other such institutions which should be founded in France. The intimate relation which Bourgelat bears to the early history of the first two veterinary schools of France and the world, makes it almost impossible to treat them separately. Such was the success above alluded to, of the students of the Lyons school, in combating the ravages of the animal pests, that the French Government determined to establish a second institution of a like character. It seems ever to have been the aim of the French Government to make Paris the center of French learning and civilization; hence it was but natural that a point in the vicinity of that city should be selected as the site of the second school. Therefore, on the 27th of December, 1765, a tract of land in the village of Alfort—opposite what is now called Charenton, at present connected with Paris by a horse-railroad, and also by steamboats on the river—was purchased for the sum of 32,000 livres, and Bourgelat called to be its director, which position he occupied until his death. Like the majority of men who give their lives for the development of science, and in service to their countrymen, Bourgelat died poor, but not unforgotten, as is attested by the immortality with which his name is reverenced in France, and the monument lately erected to his memory by his veterinary successors in France and other parts of the world. From the first, the Government did more for the support of the school at Alfort than that at Lyons, for, while the latter school received but 8,333 livres per year for a period of six years, we find the Alfort school receiving some 12,000. The Abbé Rozier succeeded Bourgelat in the direction of the school at Lyons, which for many years underwent all sorts of vicissitudes, but finally received its full share of acknowledgment, and is at present a most dangerous rival to that of Alfort for the honors with which fair Science *wreaths the brows of her successful children.*

Havemann,* afterward teacher and director of the Royal Veterinary School at Hanover, was sent by that Government to study veterinary medicine at Alfort at this time. While there he wrote the following letter, describing the condition of things, to the master of the Royal Horse at Hanover:

* "History of the Veterinary School at Hanover, from 1777 to 1877," p. 45.

"ALFORT BY CHARENTON, *August 29, 1777.*

"The Royal Veterinary School has, besides the director, M. Bourgelat (who, however, does not instruct any more, but resides generally in Paris), three teachers. The first, who is known as director and professor, educates in practice and pharmacy; the second teaches materia medica and botany, and the third anatomy. The majority of the students complete their course in three years, and take them in the following order:

"*First Summer.*—Exterior of the horse.

"*First Winter.*—Osteology and myology.

"*Second Summer.*—On the selection of horses, their care, etc.

"*Second Winter.*—Splanchnology.

"*Third Summer.*—Materia medica and botany.

"*Third Winter.*—Neurology, angiology, and adenology.

"Those students who are blessed with a good memory, and who are able to learn anatomy in two winters, end their course in two and one half years, while many require four. *Here no other books are in use than those Bourgelat himself has written upon the subject.* The books must be learned *verbatim* from beginning to end; in order that this may be complete, one of the older students, who is selected by the director and bears the title of 'chef,' reviews the students each week, and explains and illustrates the various points. When the course is ended, the whole is again repeated before the director, and he who can rattle his books off best receives the premium of a case of instruments valued at fifty livres.

"Those who have ended their course practice operative surgery upon the horses which are to be used for anatomy, and also practice horseshoeing in the forge. When not confined by the hours devoted to study, the students may practice in the forge at pleasure. In making shoes and farriery the instruction is given by a 'chef.' Scarcely any instruction is given in pathology, or the director does it in a very cursory manner when treating of other subjects; the director seldom detains the students by the sick horses in order that they may study the patients, or to explain their diseases to them, which can have no other result than that the students do not learn to diagnose diseases, and but few appreciate this great necessity. The medicines are prepared by the students and given by them to the patients. This is done by those who have ended their course, four such being weekly appointed to this purpose. At present there are about seventy sick horses in the hospital, and for each the daily fee is thirty-five sous (forty cents) for medicine, care, and feeding. The director has exceedingly little to do, and one person can as surely give as good instruction to the students as all three professors. The students are controlled very strictly. Aside from Sundays and Thursdays, no students can leave the grounds of the school without permission from the director. Everything is arranged by the ringing of a bell—getting up, study, attending to patients, eating, and retiring. Each student must be in the dissecting-room at 7 A. M. in the summer, and 8 in the winter. A chief calls the roll and reports each one who is absent. Each student must remain in this room, or at least on the grounds, and before 11 no student can go to his room. At 2 P. M. the same course is gone through with, and at 6 the studies are ended. The students are kept under severe military regulation, and the 'chefs' arrange the service of the sub-officers. There are about eighty students here, of whom twenty are destined for the cavalry regiments; these have special barracks outside the school, and are under their own officer; the rest are lodged in the school, and, inclusive of meals, pay yearly 360 livres. The king pays the professors. Each student, when he goes into the court-yard, must wear the school uniform, which consists of a blue frock with yellow buttons, upon which is a lily surrounded by the words 'École roiale vétérinaire.' The uniform of the 'chefs' is distinguished by a double golden 'tresse' upon the collar. The botanical garden is prettily arranged, and contains 6,700 plants. Nothing seems to have been forgotten which can add to the comfort and beauty of the school."

In 1795 the French Government considered the erection of a school at Toulouse for the south of France, but it was not until 1825 that the idea came to realization, Dupuy being its first director. This school was intended to give especial attention to the study of diseases of cattle, and if one may judge from the efforts of Toussaint in reference to "charbon," this intention has been most successful.

"Alexis Casimir Dupuy * was born at Breteuil, the 27th September, 1775, and died September, 1849. He was the son of the postmaster of his village. It is without doubt that his intimacy with horses and other animals in his youth was the cause of his devoting himself to the science which he so faithfully served. His first education was received at the college at Beauvais, and later at the college of 'Louis le Grand,' at Paris. In 1792, when seventeen years old, we find him, with many other young Frenchmen, in the ranks of the revolutionists; he took part in the battle of Je-

* Schraeder-Hering, *loc. cit.*, p. 111.

mappes, where he displayed so much courage as to be honored with the standard of his regiment. In 1795 he retired from the army and entered the veterinary school at Alfort. Having passed the requisite examination successfully, we find him, in 1798, acting as assistant at his Alma Mater, and, after passing successfully the required competitive examination, received the professorship of Botany, Chemistry, Pharmacy, and Materia Medica. In 1805 he acquired the title of Doctor of Medicine, after having devotedly given himself to the study of the necessary branches; his dissertation treated upon 'Purulent Abscesses and Tumors.' At this time he was very intimate with Dupuytren, so well known in the history of French medicine at this period. He gave his chief attention to the study of pathological anatomy, recognizing the fact that all talk about disease is but mere words, unless one knows intimately of what disease consists. The first product of his investigation in this important branch of medicine was a work which gave rise to much discussion, upon 'Tuberculosis, which is generally called Glanders,' Paris, 1817. Dieterichs, who studied with him in Paris, says that he 'sought to find tubercles everywhere, though no one with healthy eyes could see them, and that he would gladly have seen every disease classed under this one name, so enthusiastic was he in this direction.' His own countrymen seem to have recognized his zeal in this direction."

With the opening of the Toulouse school, he was called to be its director, but his mind was so exclusively scientific that he does not seem to have had the attributes necessary to successfully fill such a position, for in 1832 he was discharged, even without a pension. He then removed to Paris, and engaged in practice and the publication of books, but his endeavors do not appear to have been rewarded by success, for he left his family in such a destitute condition that the Central Veterinary Society of Paris felt themselves obliged to institute a collection for their benefit.

During the extension of the empire under Napoleon I the establishment of three other veterinary schools was considered, but only one came to a positive result—that at Turin, Italy, which is still in existence.

The French schools have from the beginning enjoyed a creditable independence from those of medicine, though not without attempts aiming to unite these two branches of medical education. At first they were under the control of the Minister of the Interior, but later have been controlled by the Minister of Agriculture, Commerce, and Industry, assisted by an inspector-general, that position being occupied by the accomplished M. Bouley, member of the Academy, etc. In the year 1777 the French Government published very detailed regulations for the guidance of the schools, which have suffered but few modifications to the present day, although their organization as part of a common institution of the land was not fully completed until May 19, 1873, when a decree to that effect was issued.

In accordance with this decree, the students are classed as "élèves internes," or regular students, "élèves externes," and "auditeurs libres"; of these, the first form by far the greater majority. On account of the similarity of organization, a visit to one of the three national schools will give an observer a very good idea of them all.

The number of professors is the same at each of the three schools, being six, and an irregular number of "chefs de service," or assistants. The professors and assistants receive their appointment from the minister, after having demonstrated their ability by public competition for the vacancy in question. These competitions are made known to the public in appropriate publications, some six months before they are to take place. Each competitor must be a Frenchman by birth or naturalized, and a graduate of one of the national schools. If the competition is for a place as assistant, the person must bring a certificate that he is free from military duty, or that he has permission to present himself for the purpose.

The competition is generally divided into five sittings or parts: at the first, the competitors have to present an essay upon some subject in connection with the vacancy which is open; in the second and third, they have to deliver oral dissertations of a like character; in the fourth, in connection with any subject belonging to veterinary medicine; in the fifth, they must show their practical ability in different branches of the profession. The tasks for the second, third, and fourth sittings are made known to the candidates twenty-four hours before each sitting. The candidates for the positions of "chefs de service" must make known their intention of competing one month previous to the date fixed for competition. In the year 1871 the budget ordered for the support of the veterinary schools was 673,000 francs; and in 1873, 656,500. No perquisites are allowed the professors for examinations, the money received for the same being added to the school funds; in the place of this the professors receive 500 francs a year in addition to their regular pay. At Alfort, all officers of the school have free lodgings found them, each professor having six rooms, two being situated on each story of a three-storied building. Each assistant has three rooms at his service.

In 1876 the corps of professors at Alfort were as follow:

M. Reynal (since retired and pensioned), Director and Lecturer on Veterinary Jurisprudence; M. Gouboux, Lecturer on Descriptive and General Anatomy, Histology, Physiology, and Exterior; M. Baillet, Lecturer on Breeding, Hygiene, Zoölogy, and Botany; M. Saunier, Lecturer on Physics, Chemistry, Materia Medica, and Pharmacy; M. Colen, Lecturer on General Pathology, Therapeutics, Surgery, Parasitic Diseases, and Horseshoeing; M. Trasbot, Superintendent of Clinic, Lecturer on Special and Surgical Pathology. The "chefs de service" were M. Baron, assistant to and repeater upon those subjects upon which M. Baillet lectures. He also conducts the excursions to the model farm situated about a mile from the institution, as well as to the cattle and horse markets of Paris, and botanical excursions; M. Barrier, assistant to and repeater of the subjects lectured upon by M. Gouboux, also teacher of histological microscopical practice; M. Nocard, assistant in the clinic and surgery, and demonstrator of autopsies; M. Baillet, assistant in clinic and surgery.

The course of study occupies four years, the lectures lasting one hour and a half each. The sessions are divided as follows:

First Session (Winter).—Anatomy, physics or chemistry, botany or zoölogy. These subjects are reviewed by M. Barrier during the session.

Second Session.—Chemistry or materia medica, exterior or general anatomy. Reviewed by M. Barrier.

Third Session.—Anatomy, physics or chemistry, botany or zoölogy, general pathology, and therapeutics. Reviewed by M. Barrier.

Fourth Session.—Physiology, general anatomy, botany, microscopy, and chemical analysis. Reviewed by M. Barrier.

Fifth Session.—Special pathology, therapeutics, hygiene, general pathology, agriculture; clinic is held three hours each day on week-days, and two on Sundays.

Sixth Session.—Special pathology and surgery, hygiene, pharmaceutical practice, general pathology, therapeutics, parasitic diseases, theories of operative surgery, and agriculture. Clinic as before. These subjects are reviewed by assistants Baron, Nocard, and Baillet.

Seventh Session.—Practice in operative surgery, special pathology and surgery, parasitic diseases, agriculture, forensic medicine, sanitary police, and excursions to the cattle and horse markets. Clinic as before. Subjects reviewed by MM. Nocard and Baillet.

Eighth Session.—Practice in operative surgery, special pathology and surgery, parasitic diseases, breeding, agriculture, toxicology. Excursions to the model farm. Clinic as before. Subjects reviewed by appropriate assistants.

The lectures on agriculture were then delivered by M. Heuzé. The subject of dissection has not been mentioned in the above course, because of the irregularity of the hours devoted to it.

The above plan is open to some criticism: one is at a loss to understand why the word "or" is placed between so many branches, except that the lecturer will dilate upon one "or" the other subject at the lecture in question. Pathological anatomy is not mentioned, but is treated at the same time with general pathology. Surgery and special pathology are united in one series of lectures, and the important branch of obstetrics is not mentioned, although we have reason to know it is not neglected. Professor Müller says that "when one adds the number of hours devoted to lectures in the four years' course of the French schools, he is surprised to find that they are exceeded by the number required by the (former) three years' course at Berlin." The number of professors at the French schools is insufficient to do the work well that is required of them, and they should be relieved by the addition of a greater number of specialists. We shall see this plan better carried out when we come to speak of the school at Berlin, although there is room for still further improvement there, so far as the clinic is concerned. At the French schools the distribution of the studies over the educational term is not conducive to the best interests of the scholars, too little being required of them during the early part of their studies, and too much toward their completion. This is equalized by the great number of repetitions to which they are subjected by the assistants. Clinical practice and surgery assume an undue prominence in the French system, to the cost of pathological anatomy and the fundamental elements upon which medical science rests. It should ever be remembered, in establishing a school for the education of men in the principles of medicine, *that the highly-prized practical man never advances science an iota; he is a money-getter, not a servant of his race; this has been most emphatically emphasized by the schools of Britain, where practice has been the one desideratum, and science almost totally neglected. The union of both in one person makes the perfect practitioner in veterinary as well as human practice.* One might suppose that the clinic of the Alfort school would suffer from its being so distant from Paris, but this does not appear to be the case, the country around being well populated. At the time of Müller's visit, which was during the vacation in the summer of 1876, the clinic was restricted as much as possible on account of the absence of students, yet there were forty horses and twenty dogs in the hospital. A free clinic is also held daily at the school, and is visited by fifty or sixty patients each day. The stables have room for about fifty horses, and the dog-hospital accommodates the same number of patients. The school is provided with a special room for operations, with raised steps, arranged in a semicircle, for the students to stand upon. The pharmacy dispenses the medicines used at the schools, and gives abundant opportunity for the students to become expert in the knowledge and preparation of drugs. The stables are excellently arranged in the form of a horseshoe, the operating saloon being the center or toe; two forges also join it, one on each side, the full clinic being held in the space between the wings. The collection of surgical implements at this school is very complete and well arranged. The school fails in not having the ambulatory clinic, common to the German schools, by which students obtain an acquaintance with much outside, especially herd practice. This is in a measure made up for by the visits which the French students make to the governmental model farms in the vicinity of the schools. The two rooms devoted to the practice of dissection are of middling size, high, and well lighted and ventilated. The anatomical lectures are held in one of these rooms, and there is an amphitheatre for the students to stand upon. Between these rooms is the room of the professor, overlooking both by means of windows. The students at Alfort belonging to the first and third sessions have separate rooms for anatomical practice, and also have different lectures. Those of the first session hear lectures upon osteology, syndesmology, and myology, and those of the third the remaining parts of anatomy. The practice of anatomy by the students of the first session is not begun until they have heard lectures on osteology, the dissection practice being limited to muscles and ligaments. The contents of abdominal, thoracic, and cranial cavities are passed to the students of the third session. The students of each class are forbidden to visit the rooms of the other. Both classes are divided into sections of twelve to fifteen students, half of the students of the first and third classes practicing dissection for one week, when not attending lectures, and then the other half, and so on alternately during the winter months. Each section has at its disposition one cadaver, and they are distributed to students of each section as above mentioned. During the week eight cadavers are generally given to the students, and one is used by the professor. Besides these, some twelve to fifteen cattle are purchased each year for the study of anatomy. Forty to fifty horses and ten or twelve cattle are also purchased each winter for the study of operative surgery, and the practice is also kept up in summer. In the course of the year some two hundred and fifty horses are used for these purposes at Alfort. They are bought by the school—the students paying no additional fees or buying themselves—and are supplied by a company in Paris, at about forty francs per head, the same company again receiving the remains after the school is done with them. The amount appropriated by the Government for these purposes alone is some eight to nine thousand francs per year, exclusive of the amount paid for cattle. During the fourth session the study of microscopical anatomy takes place; for this purpose the students are divided into sections of twelve, and practice one week at a time, the specified hours and turns coming round about once a month. The school possesses six microscopes, so that, unless a student possesses one himself, two students must be appointed to each microscope. The anatomical museum does not make the favorable impression which one might expect from the long existence of the school; it fails in richness of material and systematic arrangement. The number of normal skeletons is very small, scarcely six being observable. Among them is the skeleton of a thorough-bred horse, which was killed on account of having its forearm shattered by a ball at the time Fieschi made an attempt upon the life of Louis Philippe. The collection contains numerous dried preparations of muscles and ligaments, among them that of a horse upon which is seated what was once a man and groom at Alfort, who desired that his body should be preserved in this way. The most interesting and instructive collection is that of the teeth of the domestic animals, arranged so as to show their condition at each year of the animal's life. There are also many interesting artificial preparations of papier-maché and wax. The pathological collection contains a very extensive array of preparations illustrating those processes as they take place in rinderpest. Not more than ten specimens of monstrosities were observable. The individual preparations are tastefully mounted, but the systematic arrangement is poor. A zoölogical collection is being begun, owing to the distance of the school from the museums at Paris. A large, well-arranged botanical garden helps to make up the appurtenances of the school. The institution has also excellently arranged stables for some twenty-five cows, two hundred sheep and swine. The library of the school contains over ten thousand volumes, mostly French works, however; it was greatly enriched at the death of the noted veterinary author, Huzard, whose library of some forty thousand volumes was pretty well distributed among the three French schools. The school has a special librarian, who also serves as curator of the museum. Students are allowed to read the books at certain hours, but are not permitted to leave the room while there, or to take books to their rooms. None but the professors can take books to their residences. The school also possesses a well-arranged riding academy, having some twenty-five horses, and a riding-master for the instruction of the students. It also has a room fitted up for the students to practice music.

The Students.—It has been previously mentioned that the students are divided up into three classes, viz., the internal or regular students, the free students, and those known as external students, who come and go as they please. In the summer of 1876, Müller reports that there were at Alfort 275 regular students, 35 external, and 12 free students—the latter being mostly foreigners. The "élèves externes" are generally students that did not present themselves at the end of the fourth year for examination, and are studying, of their own free-will, the fifth, or those who have been put back one year and lost the support of the Government. For admittance, a student must not be under seventeen or over twenty-five years of age. Each student must present a certificate of birth, and the attestation of a doctor that he has been properly vaccinated, or has had the small-pox, and that he possesses a healthy physique, especially that he is free from scrofula; also an attestation from the superior officer of his locality—mayor or prefect—that he has a good moral character. Students over twenty years of age must also bring a certificate that they have fulfilled their military duties, or been freed therefrom. Their acceptance is dependent upon the consent of the minister having control of the schools. The students present themselves at the schools for the first time about the beginning of October (6th?), and are then subjected to a matriculatory examination, which consists in writing on dictation something in the French language, and analyzations of portions of the same; in arithmetic they must have a knowledge of its principal elements, of the decimal system, and arithmetical and geometric proportion; in geometry, a knowledge of its principal elements; in geography, a general idea of the geography of the world, and a special knowledge of that of France. They also have to write an essay, or something like it, upon history and geography. Special favors are given to those applicants who possess the title of "bachelier ès lettres et sciences." For a certain number of students, the "élèves internes," the Government supplies lodgings, the school at Alfort affording accommodation for 275, and generally all these places are occupied. These students pay a yearly fee of six hundred francs for education, lodging, heating, light, board, washing, etc., and the other two classes pay a yearly fee of two hundred francs.

Those students that have passed the necessary matriculatory examination, and for whom there is not the necessary lodging-room, have the right to enter as external students, not being then subjected to internal regulations of the school; but few, however, take advantage of this privilege, most of them preferring to wait another year for financial reasons, rooms, etc. The exclusion from the "internat," or school boarding-house, is considered the severest punishment which can come upon a student. Only one third of the "élèves internes" pay this six hundred francs from their own means; two thirds of them are the recipients of so-called "demi-bourses," or stipends, which equal the fees paid by the other third. To receive them, however, the student must first have been at the school six months, and have demonstrated his worthiness by appropriate conduct, diligence, etc. These stipends are paid every half-year, and as a rule are enjoyed by the students during their whole course of study, being only withdrawn in case of gross misconduct or want of proper knowledge, in proportion to the time the recipient has studied.

There are three sources from which these stipends come, viz., the prefects of departments, the Government, and the military funds. Each department has two stipends to pay toward the support of one of the veterinary schools. There are certain regulations to be complied with for the reception of the military stipends. The "élèves boursiers militaires," or military students, receive, aside from the benefits of the "internat," clothing, rent, the necessary books and instruments, and a small amount of pocket-money, in addition to which the Government pays the examination fee of one hundred francs; whereas the other students having the benefit of the "internat" have to pay all such expenses. The military administration provides for sixty stipends, all of which were enjoyed by Alfort previous to 1876, but they are now so divided that Alfort receives thirty and the schools at Lyons and Toulouse fifteen each. The military students, after becoming twenty years of age, are required to sign agreements by which they promise to serve in the army for five years, but are, during their course of study, generally free from military regulations. The number of students at Lyons and Toulouse is somewhat less than at Alfort. The whole number of students at these schools is, in general, about 600, so that each year would give to France somewhere about 150 newly graduated veterinarians. (The number of civil veterinary surgeons in France was in 1860, 2,760; in 1871, 3,036; in 1875, 3,019.) Every two or four students at Alfort have a room in which they sleep only, otherwise they are in the study or lecture rooms the whole day; each year-student having a separate study-room appropriated to his use, except that the third and fourth year students have a study-room in common. They are allowed certain hours for recreation, in which they are permitted to visit one another in the different study-rooms, or to roam over the court and garden of the institute. The meals are taken in a common room (*réfectoire*) at fixed hours, and are good and sufficient. Each Sunday a "bill of fare" is posted in this room for the ensuing week, which has been inspected by the director, and indorsed by him. The students are continually under the eye of certain officers—"surveillants"—who have their discipline in charge during the hours of study. On Sundays the students are permitted to go outside the school, the roll being called at 11.30 P. M. On the first Sunday of every month they are allowed to remain out until 12.30, that they may attend the theatres in the city. They are only allowed to receive visitors at certain hours, and in rooms near the gate appointed for the purpose. On entering the school one is immediately struck with the peculiar blue frock worn by all the students, which would, however, give a far better appearance of uniformity were they obliged to wear the same form of hat or cap.

There is no state examination at the French schools as in Germany; on the contrary, the students are subjected to repeated examinations by the assistants, and at the end of each session by the professors in their respective branches. The result of these sessional provings is, that students found unsatisfactory are put back for a year in their course, and lose the advantages of the "internat," or are sent from the school. The final examination for the diploma of the French Government is simply a more extended sessional examination. Of late, the professors have been ordered by the Government to prove the students in the branches of the first two sessions of their course. This examination is further distinguished from the ordinary sessional in that each student must attend to two sick animals in the hospital and perform three operations. (It should be mentioned here that in the French schools, other Continental schools also, the students have a certain number of patients under their entire charge during the whole course of their hospital practice, being simply guided and questioned by the clinical teachers. This amounts to the same thing as being in practice while studying, and offers the great advantage of a competent adviser and consulting assistant.) Aside from an anatomico-physiological essay, the examination is entirely oral. Each professor hands in an account, with reference to each student examined, in the form of a number, which is inclosed and sealed; these numbers are then added together in a somewhat complicated manner.

Hertwig, who visited the French schools in 1871, in speaking of the veterinary condition outside the schools, says that the civil veterinarian is entirely dependent upon his practice for a livelihood, there being no civil official veterinarians, as in Germany, occupying positions for which they are paid by the Government. Müller, who visited the school in 1876, and whose report I have mostly followed, also says the same thing; "but that in some departments there are so-called 'arrondissements' which receive from the communal funds from three to six hundred francs per year, but they are not connected directly with the Government, and their pay is yearly resumed." A revision of the "Laws and Regulations of France for the Prevention and Suppression of Contagious Animal Diseases" has lately been made by the Government (1879), but I have failed to see any indication of the division of that country into departments and districts, with its appropriate government veterinarian, as we shall see is the case in Germany when we come to speak of the veterinary institutions of that country. Such may be in contemplation, however, and will be a great gain for the profession in that country. There are, however, municipal and local veterinary officials stationed as inspectors of markets, horse-fairs, and the like. Notwithstanding most earnest remonstrance on the part of the veterinary profession of France for many years, the Government has not yet taken the steps it should for the protection of the holders of its own diploma, by enacting laws for the suppression of quackery, which renders the task of gaining an honest living unnecessarily difficult for the graduated members of the profession, for the quack is ever ready with infallible cure-alls, and is ever such a glutton and an unprincipled wretch that he will work for any fee, no matter how small; and, on the other hand, frequently gets fees for services rendered which a graduated man would scarce have the effrontery to ask. All that the Government does is to make known in a public print that the veterinarian is the holder of a government diploma when he settles in a district to practice. These conditions are made still more onerous by the large number of graduates which are yearly turned out from the schools. "In 1871 the department of the Seine, inclusive of Paris and the school at Alfort, and several military veterinarians, had 115. Of these, four were attached to the Ministry of War, two to the omnibus companies, one as inspector of the horse-market, two as inspectors at the slaughter-houses, one to the market-police, and one to the court stables.

"The military organization is, on the contrary, well arranged, and the army veterinarians are well placed, both in regard to their rank and pecuniarily. According to the decree of 1860, the French army had in all its departments 337 veterinarians, who enjoyed the following positions: 4 principal, 120 first class, and 128 second class, and 25 assistant veterinarians. The yearly pay of the chiefs was 4,000 francs, and that of the assistants 1,800. When the chiefs were retired, they received a pension of 2,340 francs, which could be increased to 3,744. Two of these veterinarians were members of the commission 'd'hygiène hippique' at the Ministry of War, and a third was veterinary to the Guards, and resided in Paris. A fourth was stationed as superior veterinarian at the cavalry-school at Saumur, and a fifth in a similar position with the troops and royal stud in Algeria, under the rank of 'état major.' The other three classes have also the rank of officer, with corresponding pay: for the first class, 1,700 francs as minimal, and 2,760 as maximal; the second class from 1,400 to 2,800 francs; and the assistants from 1,300 to 2,112 francs. On the other hand, the value of veterinary science has been from the early days of schools well acknowledged by the members of the Academy and other scientific societies in France, and members of the profession have taken no second rank among the scientists of France and the world. At the present day the literary-scientific horizon of France has no more refulgent lights than Chauveau, Toussaint, Bouley, Colin, Megnin, and other members of the veterinary profession."

The Veterinary Institute at Vienna, Austria.

With the termination of the school-term for 1877, this institution began a second centennial existence, and it is to be hoped its prosperity and usefulness will go on increasing as the years pass on. The school is known as the "Royal Military Veterinary Institute of Vienna." Professor Dr. Roell, its late director, gave a complete sketch of its history for the first hundred years of its existence in the "Oesterreichse Vierteljahrsschrift für wissenschaftliche Veterinärkunde," vol. xlviii; to which are added lithographic illustrations of the grounds and buildings. This periodical (quarterly) has been issued by the faculty of the institute since the year 1851, and contains many articles of value. The establishment of this school was preceded by the opening of a school for the treatment of the diseases of the horse and operative practice in 1764, with the consent and support of the Government, by an Italian named Luigi Scotti, who, in company with an apothecary named Mengmann, was sent by Maria Theresa to Lyons to study the principles of veterinary medicine. During this visit to France Scotti received 420 guldens each year from the Government. On their return they presented the Government with a proposal for the erection of a school, and recommended a course of two years, considering the study of anatomy as the most important subject. They recommended that the students be taken from among the experienced smiths of the army, that could read and write, and felt confident that they could make competent veterinarians in the time mentioned. According to their plan of instruction, general anatomy, osteology, and exterior, were to be taught in the fall, as well as horseshoeing, upon which great stress was laid; in winter, myology and practice in horseshoeing; and in spring and summer, a knowledge of the useful plants, their preparations and use. The second year was little more than a repetition of the first, with the exception that the students were made acquainted with disease and its treatment by hospital practice. There were but two teachers attached to the school, which was opened January 12, 1767, the whole being under the supervision of a military official, who attended to the general order, cleanliness, and deportment of the students. The purpose of the school was limited to the education of better qualified smiths for the army, and only army horses were treated therein. The students were taken for the full two-years' course, and only at the expiration of the same were new students taken.

While this horse-school was still in active operation, J. Gottlieb Wolstein, surgeon, and a selected military farrier by the name of Schmid, were sent by the Minister of War to Alfort, to carefully study the principles and practice of veterinary medicine as there taught. Both of them were paid by the Government, as well as having an allowance for the necessary expense, in return for which they were obliged to bind themselves for life to serve the Government, and on their return Wolstein was named as professor and Schmid as assistant.

Schraeder* says: "Joh. Gottlieb Wolstein, Doctor of Medicine and Surgery, was born at Flinsberg, in Silesia, March 14, 1738, and died at Altona, near Hamburg, July 3, 1820. He at first gave his attention to the study of surgery for nine years at Vienna, and

* *Loc. cit.*, p. 476.

in 1769 was sent to France by the Austrian Government to study veterinary medicine under Bourgelat and Chabert, where he at the same time studied human medicine in the Paris hospitals, as well as taking an active interest in the work of Lafosse between the years 1772-'73. In 1773 he visited London, and, on his return to Austria, Denmark, Mecklenburg, Holland, and in 1779 took the degree of Doctor of Medicine and Surgery at Jena. The school at Vienna bore witness to the practical abilities possessed by Wolstein. In the year 1795 he received his discharge from the Vienna school, but it is not known whether it was owing to his free-thinking tendencies (for he was the first Protestant who received an appointment in the state service of Austria), or to other circumstances. Wolstein was a most extensive author, nearly all his works bearing testimony to his clear-headedness and practical ability. Among other things, he was the first to establish the causal connection between an accumulation of fluids in the lateral ventricles of the brain of the horse, causing the condition known in German as "Dummkoller"; French, "immobilité"; Latin, "amentia." He also wrote a book upon the "Scientific Breeding of Human Beings."

On his return to Austria he gave the Government his ideas with reference to the formation of a veterinary school, and on the 23d of July, 1777, he received from the Government 13,740 florins toward the erection of the school; and on the 26th of December, 1877, the Government issued the instructions for the regulation of the school, which was soon opened.

The *personnel* of the school at this time consisted of one professor, one superior assistant, two assistants, and a number of half-invalided soldiers, necessary to the care of the animals in the hospital; also one inspecting officer, and one farrier. The school and hospital were placed under the control of the Minister of War, and the supervision given to a brigadier. In the buildings were provided lodgings for the teachers of the school, and seventy army farriers, as students. To the school belonged a botanical garden, an anatomical saloon, a lecture-room, dispensary, laboratory, and library; a smithy with four fires; four stables, with room in each for seven horses; fifteen separate stalls (probably boxes), and a small stable for cattle and sheep. The instruction was divided as follows, and extended for two years:

Professor Dr. Wolstein lectured upon the theoretical and practical application of the principles of medicine to the diseases of the horse.

First Assistant Schmid lectured upon horseshoeing, and demonstrated and supervised operative surgery, and represented Wolstein when the latter was unable to be present.

Assistant Toegl (1779) demonstrated anatomy, and Mengmann controlled the pharmacy, and lectured upon medical botany and pharmacy. The military students came either from cavalry regiments or were selected by the school from among young smiths who displayed unusual ability. The students must be under thirty years of age, unmarried, natives of Austria (Hungary also?), of perfect physique and good moral education, and be able to read and write in the German language.

The admittance of civil students was dependent upon the judgment of the teachers, who were made responsible for the ability and character of the same.

From 1778 to 1799, 178 military, 137 civil, and 144 foreign students graduated at the school.

During this period, 4,208 army horses were treated, of which 3,665 recovered, 291 were discharged uncured, and 252 were killed. In 1806 numerous changes were made in the buildings and some in the curriculum, the intention of the school being to educate superior and ordinary farriers for the army, "Kurschmieden" (farriers educated in the principles of medicine), veterinary surgeons, and ordinary farriers. The course was still continued at two years: in the first year, horseshoeing, anatomy, pharmaceutical chemistry, physiology, exterior of the horse, breeding; in the second year, therapeutics, pharmacology, and veterinary police. The military students were compelled to work from 6 to 11.30 A. M. and from 3 to 6 P. M. in the forge. The *personnel* of the school was increased by a professor of pathology and another of anatomy. The school was limited to forty military students—thirty-five from the cavalry regiments, and five for the royal studs. *In 1809 it was ordered that all must be taught which belongs to veterinary medicine, and not limited to the horse alone.* In 1812 the school was united with the university at Vienna, the military inspection being limited to supervision of the military students. In the year 1823 a revision of the school was again undertaken, which remained unchanged until 1849, and suffered but few modifications until 1857. The aim of the institute was to give full instruction in the principles of veterinary medicine.

The form of instruction was appointed to the necessities of the different kinds of students:

1. *Common farriers*, i. e., such who, after completion of their course, were considered educated for the profession of horseshoers.

On their admittance they were obliged to certify that they had already served a practical apprenticeship, and be able to read and write. The course of study extended over one year, during which they received instruction in the theories of horseshoeing, and upon the anatomy and physiology of the horse's hoof, the materia medica and special therapy of the horse, and were obliged to visit the school hospital.

2. *Agriculturists.*—The conditions of their admittance were a good knowledge of reading, writing, and arithmetic, and proof of having attended the necessary lectures at a public school of agriculture. The course was limited to one year, in which they heard lectures *upon the natural history of the domestic animals, the principles of breeding, the care of the domestic animals, and upon the animal pests and their prevention.*

3. *Officers, Riding-Masters, and Masters of the Horse.*—Officers had to be furnished with certificates of permission to attend the school; the others with certificates of faithful performance of their duties, and of their ability to read and write. The course also lasted one year, and was limited to natural history, breeding, equine hygiene, theory of horseshoeing, anatomy and physiology of the horse, the management of breeding studs, exterior, and equine jurisprudence.

4. *Future Physicists* ("Künftige Physiker"), who could only become practitioners of the third, and doctors of the second year's course of the medico-surgical branches. The lecturers were limited to the theories of animal plagues and veterinary police for one session.

5. a. *Inspectors of Animal and Meat Markets.*—Ou their admittance they had to bring certificates of ability to slaughter well, and be able to read and write. The course was limited to twelve hours, during which they received demonstrations of the chief parts of animals used for food, and of the diseases which made them unfit for that purpose, and lectures upon the laws and ordinances regulating such business.

b. *Cattle-drovers and Shepherds.*—The course extended over two months, and consisted of instruction in the care and feeding of animals, upon those things which could incite disease, of their prevention, and upon the common diseases, and the first principles of treatment necessary in case a veterinarian could not be had.

c. *Hunters.*—The instruction consisted of a popular form of education upon the dog and its diseases, with especial reference to rabies.

6. "*Kurschmiede*" (*Farriers with authority to treat certain diseases of the horse*).—The course was two years, and all applicants had to bring certificates of ability to shoe horses, and as to their having faithfully served their allotted time in the army, and be able to read and write. In the first year they attended lectures upon the elements of physics and chemistry, equine anatomy and physiology, and therapeutics and materia medica; in the second, the special pathology and therapy of equine diseases, surgery, operative surgery and obstetrics, exterior, breeding, forensic equine medicine and practice in relation to the external and internal diseases of the horse; further, anatomy and physiology were again repeated.

7. *Veterinary Surgeons.—None but graduated doctors or wound doctors were admitted.* The course also lasted two years: the first being devoted to natural history, dietetics, breeding, hygiene, anatomy and physiology of the domestic animals, general pathology and therapeutics; the second to special pathology and therapeutics, theoretic and operative surgery, exterior, breeding, forensic equine medicine, contagious diseases and veterinary police, literature of veterinary medicine, practical exercise in the hospitals, and repetition of anatomy and physiology.

The faculty consisted of five professors, receiving 2,000, 1,500, 1,200, and 1,000 florins each, with free lodging and other perquisites; also four assistants, receiving 700, 600, 500, and 400 florins.

On the 17th of November, 1823, the corner-stone of the new school was laid with appropriate ceremonies, and in the presence of many of the nobility and noted personages. In this year the commencement of a library was begun in earnest by an appropriation of three thousand florins, but at the present day a yearly sum is appropriated to the purpose. In the year 1835 an institution for experiments with reference to the variola of sheep was added to the institution and continued until 1864. *In the year 1849 the institution was separated from the university, and has since remained independent, subject to the control of the Ministry of War.* In 1871 the curriculum again suffered revision, and was placed in its present form; the purpose of the school being to educate *civil and military veterinarians, and also civil and military horseshoers; aside from this it must do its utmost to forward veterinary science, and is the highest technical authority with reference to contagious animal diseases and their suppression.* The director also acts as adviser in all things with reference to the military veterinary institutions at the Ministry of War. The guidance of the school is dependent upon the director and the military supervisor. The latter is directly subservient to the Minister of War, and conducts the institute in its relation to the military organization, supervising the internal arrangements and the discipline of the servants and students. The director controls the scientific-technical parts of the institution. The teachers are represented by professors, docents, adjuncts, assistants, and a teacher of horseshoeing. The number of professors is limited to six, one of whom is director. The subjects taught are as follow, divided among the following professors and assistants:

Director (1877), Moriz F. Roell,* and Lecturer upon Animal Pests, their Causes and Prevention; also Conductor of the Inner Clinic.

Professor Franz Müller, Lecturer on Zoötomy, the Theories of Shoeing, Exterior, and Conductor of the Dog Hospital.

Professor Andreas Brückmüller (recently deceased), Lecturer on Breeding, Obstetrics, and Zoöphysiology. Professor Brückmüller is the author of the only text-book extant on "Animal Pathological Anatomy," which is too largely founded upon Rokitansky to be uncritically followed at the present day, however.

Professor Franz August Armbrecht, Lecturer on Veterinary Surgery and Operative Surgery, and Conductor of the Surgical Clinic.

Professor Leopold Förster, Lecturer on Special Pathology and Therapeutics, Pharmacology, Pharmacognosy, Botany, Instruments and Bandages, their Uses and Application.

Professor Franz Zahn, Lecturer on General Pathology, Pathological Zoötomy, and Forensic Medicine.

The lectures in Chemistry are delivered by Professor Dr. I. Moser, of the Agricultural Academy.

Adjuncts.—Max von Paumgartten, Assistant Lecturer on Zootomy, Exterior, and Theoretic Horseshoeing.

Raimund Koezil, Assistant Lecturer on Path.-Zoötomy, Forensic Medicine, and Cattle and Meat Inspection.

Franz Konhäuser, Assistant in the Medical Clinic, and Teacher of Special Pathology and Therapeutics.

Josef Bayer, Assistant in the Surgical Clinic, and Teacher of Veterinary Surgery and Operations; also Lecturer on Veterinary Literature and History.

Johann Csókor, Assistant-Lecturer on Breeding and Zoöphysiology.

Assistants.—J. R. von Froschauer, to the Medical Clinic.

Josef Stengel, to the Surgical Clinic.

* Since retired and pensioned.

Franz Wildner, on Descriptive and Pathological Zoötomy.
Over-Veterinarian F. Schuller, Teacher of Horseshoeing.
Inspecting Veterinarians.—Ferdinand Wicher, for the Hospitals.
Anton Janich, for Horseshoeing.
Accountants.—Franz Mühln, Superior.
Heinrich Lázló, Assistant.

Other Persons.—One gardener, two official servants, one porter, three saloon-servants, one apothecary's servant, one watchman, two drivers, three smiths in forge, three corporals, and forty-one soldiers as servants in the stables.

The ground of the school covers a territory of 42,514 square metres. It is plentifully supplied with fresh water. The stables contain room for eighty horses, besides twenty-two boxes, with grain magazines, rooms, and all necessary appurtenances. There is also a stable for fourteen cattle, and the dog-hospital is fitted up with cages for forty-four dogs. There is also a quarantine-stable for the isolation of suspected or diseased animals, with five boxes. The school has a fine botanical garden, lecture-room, laboratories, museums, forge, grazing-ground, and everything necessary to such an institution. The number of works in the library is 4,132, or 9,630 volumes, six to seven hundred florins being allowed for its repletion each year. The books are all arranged, according to the subjects treated, upon appropriate shelves.

At the end of the year 1876 the anatomical museum contained:

Stuffed mammalia and monstrosities	160	specimens.
" birds	59	"
Skeletons: Mammalia	190	"
Birds	62	"
Amphibia and reptiles	10	"
Fishes	9	"
Individual bony specimens	366	"
Teeth	428	"
Ligaments, cartilage, and muscle preparations	95	"
Intestines	156	"
Nerves	27	"
Blood-vessels	160	"
Lymphatics	8	"
Monstrosities in spirit	110	"
Embryos	129	"
Varia	115	"
Total	2,084	"

The pathological museum contains 2,762 specimens. The collection of surgical instruments is very complete, 224 new ones being added to it in the last twenty years.

The collection of herbs, minerals, etc., used in medicine, and all other appurtenances of a school of like nature, are kept full and in perfect order.

During the years between 1823 and 1877, 100,558 animals (of these 87,436 recovered, 8,787 died, and 4,281 were killed), with the exception of dogs, were treated at the school, being 1,845 for each year.

From 1857 to 1877, 20,241 dogs were treated in the dog-hospital, of which 14,023 recovered, 4,725 died, and 1,463 were killed.

The Students.—The students belong either to the civil or military professions. The first are either students of veterinary medicine *per se*, or of horseshoeing. Neither the Minister of War nor his representative, the military supervisor, exercises any control over them, they being subjected to the control of the directors, and all regulations concerning them emanate from the "cultus" minister. The conditions for admittance are:

1. At the military veterinary school the students are educated in the entire principles of veterinary medicine.

2. Whoever intends to become a student must subject himself to a matriculatory examination. This examination is not required of students that are graduates of the sixth class in a "gymnasial" or "real" school.

(The matriculatory examination is limited to the following subjects: German language, physics, chemistry, natural history, geography, history, and algebra.)

In the *German language* the student must write an essay in good, clear orthography and good grammar, upon a subject of natural history.

Physics.—He must explain and demonstrate upon instruments the ordinary phenomena.

Chemistry.—The elements of inorganic and organic chemistry, with simple tests.

Natural History.—General knowledge of the classification of the three kingdoms.

Geography.—Physical geography in general, and the climatical and geographical conditions of all parts of the world, and a special knowledge of Central Europe, and Austria in particular.

History.—A knowledge of the chief historical events of the world at large, and Austria in special.

Algebra.—Elementary.

This examination takes place in the first week of October of each year by a special commission named by the "cultus" minister, three members being professors of the school, and one each representing a gymnasium and real school. The examination costs five guldens, and goes to the examiners. Students must not be over twenty-six or under eighteen years of age; consideration is sometimes taken in case of students whose studies have been unintentionally interrupted in a scientific or agricultural academy. The course extends over three years, of two sessions each, as follows:

First Year (*First Session*).—Introduction to the study of veterinary medicine for two weeks, three hours each week; zoötomy of all domestic animals, weekly, five hours; general chemistry, weekly, three hours; breeding, weekly, three hours; theoretic horseshoeing, weekly, two hours; dissection and practical horseshoeing, arranged in the hours not taken up by other branches.

(*Second Session.*)—Topographical zoötomy, weekly, five hours; organic chemistry, with especial reference to physiological and pathological chemistry, weekly, three hours; breeding, five hours; medicinal botany, weekly, two hours; dissection and practical horseshoeing, as before.

Second Year (*Third Session*).—General pathology and pathological anatomy, weekly, three hours; physiology with microscopical practice, weekly, two hours; pharmacognosy, materia medica, and art of writing prescriptions, weekly, three hours; clinic, daily; dissection, and the preparation of two anatomical subjects, in hours to be fixed at convenience; autopsies; practical horseshoeing.

(*Fourth Session.*)—Pathological zoötomy, weekly, three hours; physiology, with microscopical practice, weekly, two hours; obstetrics, weekly, two hours; theoretic use of instruments and bandages, weekly, two hours; clinic, daily; autopsies; practice in chemical laboratory; horseshoeing.

Third Year (*Fifth Session*).—Medical and surgical clinic, daily; special pathology and therapeutics, weekly, three hours; veterinary surgery, weekly, two hours; practice in operative surgery, weekly, three hours; exercise in making reports of forensic cases and in reference to veterinary police; animal pests and veterinary police, weekly, three hours; cattle and meat inspection, weekly, one hour; horseshoeing.

(*Sixth Session.*)—Clinics, and other branches as before; history of veterinary medicine, weekly, one hour; horseshoeing.

The school also has a special course of two years for medical men and wound-doctors.

The Examinations.—The examination takes place at the end of each year in the subjects which have been lectured upon or demonstrated. The results are designated as "excellent" ("sehr gut" *), "good," and "middling." Students who have received the last censor may apply for a second examination, but those who have received it in two or more branches are obliged to repeat the full course for the completed year.

The professors are free to make examinations on any subjects during the session.

Students who desire the state diploma as veterinarians must, among other things, make an autopsy and correctly dictate the results; also prepare certain anatomical specimens, and give in to the appropriate professor certain written documents upon cases in connection with forensic medicine and veterinary police.

Aside from this, the final examination consists in the student attending a selected patient (a tough case selected by the teacher) in both the internal and surgical clinic for three days, of which the student has to make, unaided, the diagnosis, and attend to and direct the treatment, and write a full description of the case, its history, treatment, and prognosis. Further, he must make several surgical operations upon a living animal, and demonstrate a subject in anatomy.

The partial examinations take place under the special professor in each branch, with changes of professors, the last examination in the presence of the whole examining body. All members of the examining commissions are free to ask of the candidate any questions they please in connection with veterinary medicine or its collateral branches. The examining commission consists of the professors and a person named by the Minister of the Interior. If a candidate has failed in one part of his examination, he may again present himself at a time fixed by the commission, which can never be in less than three months. If he has failed in two divisions of the examination, he must be examined again in all parts of his studies, but never in less than six months. The final examination costs fifty-four florins. Foreigners are admitted by the consent of the direction, and have a right to an examination for a diploma, *but not to practice in Austria when not naturalized citizens.* Foreigners have to pay twenty guldens fee for each session before it begins. Single courses of lectures may be arranged with the director. Certain rules of conduct must be observed.

* The German "*sehr gut*" is not correctly interpreted by the English "*very good*," it being spoken with a peculiar emphasis, and used only in a sense of the English "*excellent*."

Some fifteen years ago the school at Vienna enjoyed a very high reputation in Europe. Brückmüller was then a first-class authority. Roell had made himself famous by his clinical ability, especially with reference to pulmonary disease, and is accredited with being the first to systematically introduce auscultation and percussion of the chest into veterinary practice; but all things must fade: the professors have grown old and lost some of their youthful energy, and at present their places have not been filled by "young blood," so that this once famous school is in a sort of semi-torpid condition. Nearly all schools of medicine and science have to undergo these changes, so that we may be sure that the Vienna school will ere long assume its old rank among the bright sisterhood of European veterinary institutes.

Short Notices of the Veterinary Schools at Brussels, Belgium, and those of Russia, Sweden, and Norway.

The small kingdom of Belgium was by no means to be outdone by her larger sisters, and ranks high among the Continental nations in reference to its veterinary institutions. The Royal Veterinary School was instituted in 1832, but not organized until 1835, and is situated in the environs of Brussels; one of the streets bounding it on one side is named after Brogniez, one of its most distinguished professors, who added many valuable instruments to the veterinary cabinet. Among other noted professors who have been attached to this school we find the names of Thiernesse, Wehenkel, and Dupont; and, among the practitioners, Willems, the introducer of inoculation as a prophylactic against pleuro-pneumonia in cattle. The Brussels school is modeled after those of France; the fee for the regular students (élèves internes) is fixed at 700 francs per year. The preliminary education demanded of students is higher than in France, the consent of the minister being necessary to their admittance. Many young men study the natural sciences at this school, who intend studying medicine at the university, thereby enjoying the advantages of the "internat." The number of teachers is larger than at the French schools, there being eight professors and four assistants. The number of lectures is also greater. There are two examinations—one at the end of the first two years, and the other at the completion of the course, which extends over four years. The hospital has room for about thirty horses, each one paying a fee of two francs daily. The school has a visiting clinic, but no school conveyance, the visits being made, however, at the expense of the institution. Three horses are weekly used for anatomical and operative practice by the students, and one for the anatomical teacher; they cost some eighty francs each; about eighty animals are used in this way each year. The anatomical museum is very rich in specimens, and they are better arranged than at Alfort.

The four-year course is arranged as follows:

First Session.—Anatomy, dissection, physics, botany.

Second Session.—Botany, physics, repetition in anatomy, and the two former subjects.

Third Session.—Anatomy, dissection, physics, chemistry, with reviewings upon the two latter.

Fourth Session.—Anatomy of the domestic animals aside from the horse; physics, histology, chemistry, horseshoeing.

Fifth Session.—Clinic, pharmacy, general and special pathology, anatomy, operative surgery, therapeutics and materia medica; theory and practice of horseshoeing.

Sixth Session.—Clinic, general and special pathology, anatomy, pathological anatomy, therapeutics and materia medica, pharmacy, with practice, operative surgery, horseshoeing.

Seventh Session.—Clinic, surgical pathology, horseshoeing, breeding, topographic anatomy, operative surgery (theoretical and practical), pharmaceutical practice, forensic medicine, and sanitary police.

Eighth Session.—Clinic, surgical pathology, breeding, obstetrics, meat-inspection, pharmacy, horseshoeing. Numerous repetitions or reviewings of each branch of study take place during each session.

The regulations for the control of the Government veterinary officials are about as follows—I say "about," for they are taken from the law of 1851, and some changes may have since been made:

ARTICLE 1. According to the requirements, there shall be one or more Government veterinarians in each agricultural district.

These veterinarians are named by the Minister of the Interior, on the proposal of the permanent deputation of the provincial council, and the agricultural commission; the minister fixes their residence, and the territory over which they shall exert control.

ART. 2. The Government veterinarians are generally selected from among those who have passed an especially satisfactory examination at the school.

ART. 3. Each appointment is at first made provisory for a period of three years, and only at the end of this term can the appointment become permanent.

ART. 4. In those districts where the rewards of practice are insufficient, the minister may allow the veterinary official a support which shall not exceed three hundred francs yearly, in addition to that allowed by the local authorities.

ART. 5. The duties of the Government veterinarians are: 1. To exert a careful supervision of the hygienic conditions of the animals in their district. 2. To watch over the healthy condition of the stallions used for breeding, and to see that they are adapted to the provincial regulations for the improvement of stock. 3. They must carefully investigate all animals in their district with reference to contagious or infectious diseases. 4. At the requisition of the governor of their province, they must visit public markets and fairs and watch over the health of the animals.

ART. 6. Such veterinarians as are members of the provincial agricultural commission control, when required by the governor or said commission, the official duties of the other Government veterinarians of the province.

ART. 7. It is their duty to notify the commissioner of the "arrondissements," and the members of the agricultural commission, of the presence of contagio-infectious diseases in their province. The governor of the province receives his notification from the above-named officials. In important cases the Minister of the Interior is also to be notified by the General Inspector of Hygiene, who is notified directly by the veterinary official.

ART. 8. The Government veterinarians are also obliged to observe the conditions of agriculture in their respective districts, so far as their other duties will permit of, and to make reports to the Minister of the Interior.

ART. 9. These officials must make official returns within the first ten days of each quarter to the governor of the province, with reference to each case of an infectious or contagious animal disease that has taken place during the past quarter in their district, and also with reference to all other facts which are of importance to the Government. These reports are collected by the Provincial Agricultural Commission, and sent by them to the governor, who in his turn sends them to the minister. The General Inspector of Public Hygiene must return a yearly report of all cases of contagious animal diseases which have occurred in the kingdom.

ART. 10. The Government veterinarians have exclusively the control of the infectious animal diseases, and must always be called upon to make such examination by the higher officers of the Government.

ART. 13. Such officials can only order the peremptory killing of an animal when it is affected to an incurable (?) degree with the following diseases:

Horses.—Glanders.

Cattle.—Anthrax, rinderpest, and pleuro-pneumonia.

Sheep.—Variola, and in all animals when complicated with rabies.

The rank and advancement of veterinarians in the Belgian army are as follow:

The veterinary inspectors rank as major; the first-class veterinarians as captain; the second-class veterinarians as first lieutenant; the third-class veterinarians as second lieutenant.

In order to become a third-class veterinarian, the applicant must have graduated well for a civil veterinarian; must be twenty-four years of age, and a citizen, or naturalized. No one can become second class without having served creditably in the third for at least two years. To become first class, he must have served in the second for at least two years to the same degree. As inspectors, three years' first-class service is necessary. To be first or second class, the applicant must also stand a practical examination. The inspectors are appointed by the king. Veterinarians of all grades receive, after ten years' active service, one fifth more pension than army officers having a corresponding rank.

*Russia.**

We are somewhat inclined to look upon the Russians as a sort of half-civilized people, but the reverse is much more near to the truth, at least so far as it has reference to the support given by the Government to the advancement of science. In no way is this more true than in relation to veterinary science, the need of which made itself apparent very early in this century, on account of the wealth of the nation in domestic animals, especially cattle, horses, and sheep. As should be known to every one, rinderpest, the most terrible and devastating of all animal plagues, makes its home upon the steppes of Southern Russia, causing yearly a loss of thousands of cattle, and frequently extending its ravages to neighboring countries. In 1877 the official returns of the losses caused by rinderpest are given as 217,768 cattle and 1,884 sheep; and the same authority gives as the number of cattle in the empire, 25,918,600: the loss from this cause amounting, therefore, to 0·82 per cent.

Russia has three veterinary institutes, one each at Kharkov, Dorpat, and Kazan, all supported and regulated by the Government; the degrees given are doctor and magistrate of veterinary science. The

* Müller, "Russische Veterinär Institut Magazin," vol. xxx.

regulations for these schools suffered a complete reorganization soon after the veterinary congress at Frankfort in the year 1872, the aim of the Government being to make them second to none in Europe *from a truly scientific point of view.* The new regulations bear date May 8, 1873. The schools are subjected to the control of the cultus minister in the first place, and directly under the curator of the educational district in which they are situated. The immediate direction, however, consists of the director and council of the school. At each institute there are three regular, one extra professor, four docents; of the last, one for pharmacy, one for agriculture, one prosector who is also a docent, and an extra prosector and a teacher of horseshoeing, with various assistant teachers. The director receives, aside from a free residence, 3,300 silver rubles yearly; the regular professors, 3,000; the extra, 2,000; the docents and prosectors, 1,200; the assistants, 700; and the teacher of horseshoeing the same, with residence. The director, professors, docents, and prosectors must all have the qualification of a magistrate of veterinary science. The docents of pharmacy and agriculture must likewise be of the same grade in their respective branches, but the teacher of horseshoeing may have only the ordinary veterinary diploma. Private docents are also permitted to lecture upon any branch of veterinary science which they may select. To these last the qualification of doctor of veterinary medicine is necessary, but each aspirant must write an essay upon a selected subject, which must be publicly defended, and also stand two test-examinations upon themes selected by the council of the institute. The private docents have no certain pay, but the same is regulated by the council, and they have before them the privilege of adding to their education by study in foreign countries at the Government's expense. The natural sciences—mineralogy, botany, zoölogy, comparative anatomy (not zootomy), physics, physical geography, and chemistry—are taught at the schools by special professors, appointed for the purpose from the university. The students also receive lectures upon religion on appointed days. A high grade of preliminary education is demanded of the students. The course is extended over four years. Three thousand silver rubles are at the disposal of the council for each school, as stipends for desirable students. The general censors are excellent and satisfactory, which give the student the diploma of doctor, but in case of extraordinary ability the council may give the diploma of magistrate of veterinary medicine. A foreigner may also obtain them by standing the same examination. The director also possesses the grade and rights of a dean of a university, while the professors, docents, and prosectors rank with those of the universities. The teachers are appointed by the council from candidates who have distinguished themselves in scientific research, but must also demonstrate that they have the gifts necessary to becoming proficient teachers. The allowance for each veterinary institute, to pay the teachers, and other educational expenses, is yearly 35,700 silver rubles. To each institute is added a school for veterinary assistants, the course being three years, and is limited to practical instruction by the teacher of horseshoeing, two clinical assistants, a pharmaceutical assistant, and special teachers appointed for the purpose.

*Organization of the Royal Veterinary College at Copenhagen, Denmark.**

The Royal Danish Veterinary School was founded in 1773 by the talented veterinarian Alildgaard; it was again reorganized in 1858, and changed to a royal veterinary and agricultural high school, and removed to the suburbs of Copenhagen. By this arrangement, veterinary instruction can be directly carried out at one school, and in it are also taught agriculturists, surveyors, gardeners, and foresters, though the education of the latter is chiefly theoretical. Owing to the number of departments or sections in the school, there is a better opportunity for more classes, and particularly for special instruction of each class in its own branch of study.

This school is under the control of the Minister of the Interior, and is presided over by a director, who does not teach, but who is a member of the Privy Council. The present director is Dr. C. E. Fenger. An agriculturist is also connected with the school as associate director.

The number of teachers is eighteen, ten of whom are appointed by the Government for duty only in the school; the other eight belong, more or less, to the university, the polytechnic, and other schools. The assistants are in addition engaged in teaching the various sections, and there is also a pharmaceutist in the dispensary. The following are the branches taught the veterinary student:

Anatomy, including dissection and physiology, by Dr. Bendz.

Internal pathology and clinical instruction, by Professor Bagge.

Chemistry and pharmacy, by Professor Barfaed.

Exterior zoötechny, hygiene, and theoretic farriery, by Professor Prosch.

* "Veterinary Journal," ii, p. 123.

Operative surgery, obstetrics, and surgical clinics, by Professor Stockfleth.

Botany, by Professor Langs.

Physics and meteorology, by Assistant Fjord.

Zoölogy, by Professor Schiödte.

Veterinary jurisprudence, by Assistant Bay.

Practical farriery, by Assistant Green.

The average number of students attending the school since 1858 has been yearly about two hundred and fifty, being mostly veterinary and agricultural students. The students must provide their own maintenance and lodging. A free education and scholarship can be obtained if the student enters his name; moreover, it is necessary that he has received a certain specified general education, which is considerably less than is required for matriculation at the university. Latin is not required.

The scholastic year commences on the 23d of August, the annual period of instruction consisting of two sessions of six months each. Although the student is at liberty in the matter of attending lectures, yet the instruction is so arranged that these may occupy a period of six sessions; as a rule, the period of study is four years if the following plan is pursued:

First Session.—Physics and meteorology, six hours per week; inorganic chemistry, four hours ditto; zoölogy, four to six hours ditto; shoeing practice, twelve hours ditto.

Second Session.—Physics and meteorology, two to three hours per week for the first two months; organic chemistry, three to four hours; botany, two to five hours; anatomy and physiology, five hours; zoötechny, five hours; practical botany, one hour; practical farriery, twelve hours; practical grooming, twelve hours a week for a month; clinic, twelve hours per week.

Third Session.—Botany, seven hours per week for a month; anatomy and physiology, five hours per week; zoötechny, four hours; theoretic farriery, two hours; pharmacy and pharmacology, two hours; pathology and therapeutics, three to four hours; surgery, three to four hours; veterinary jurisprudence, two hours; practical botany, one hour per week for a month; practical farriery, eight hours per week; dissection, exterior, one hour; clinic, twelve hours; practical pharmacy, twelve hours.

Fourth Session.—Anatomy and physiology, five hours weekly; zoötechny, five hours; pathology and therapeutics, three to four hours; surgery and obstetrics, three to four hours; veterinary jurisprudence, two hours; dissection, operative surgery, four hours;

practical farriery, eight hours; clinic, twelve hours; practical pharmacy, twelve hours.

Fifth Session.—Pathology and therapeutics, three to four hours weekly; surgery, three to four hours; dissection, operative surgery, four hours; practical farriery, eight hours; clinic and pharmacy, twelve hours each weekly.

Sixth Session.—Ambulatory or visiting clinic; veterinary jurisprudence.

The veterinary examinations take place in April and October, and are divided into two parts: the first of these is in pure natural science only; the second, in the other branches of veterinary medicine.

*Veterinary Medicine in Sweden.**

The first veterinary school in Sweden was founded by Hernquist, born in 1726. After passing his examination as a doctor in philosophy at the University of Upsala, Hernquist went in 1763 to France, and, more especially at Lyons, studied veterinary medicine. In 1774 he established the veterinary school of Skara, Sweden, and was designated professor of it in 1778, remaining in it until his death, 1808. He was a writer and practitioner of very high order. One of the best of his pupils, Norling, took his place in 1814; and in 1820, by order of the Swedish Government, he organized the veterinary school at Stockholm, remaining director of it, as well as that of Skara, until his death in 1855. The Skara school served as a preparatory one for that of Stockholm, where the student, after a stay of two or three years, underwent the examination for the degree of veterinary surgeon. At that time, as now, the students came from Sweden, Norway, and Finland, and during this period a great number of men belonging to each of these countries graduated at the Stockholm school.

In 1867 it was fixed by royal ordinance that before a student could enter that college he must have obtained the diploma of graduate in letters from the university. This excellent measure for the elevation of veterinary instruction was due to the initiative of Professor Landberg; and, instead of diminishing the number of students, as some had predicted, it led to an increase. In requiring from candidates for admission to this school an amount of preparatory knowledge not demanded by any other veterinary school in Europe, the Swedish Government has taken care to protect the interests of its graduates and increase their income; the consequence is, that the number of graduates has correspondingly aug-

* "Veterinary Journal," vol. ix, p. 266, 1879.

mented in quantity and quality. The candidate, twenty or twenty-one years of age, being a graduate in letters, is received into the veterinary school, and there he has to study for four or even six years.

The school has four professors, each with an annual salary of about £230; a lecturer, with a salary of £168; an assistant, or adjunct, and a teacher of farriery. Two of the professors, the assistant, and the instructor in farriery, reside at the college; the others have a yearly lodging allowance of £28. The course of teaching at present is as follows:

Anatomy, physiology, zoölogy, and pathological anatomy—Professor Kinnberg.

Zoötechny, sanitary science and police, and the ambulatory clinic—Professor Morell.

Surgery, obstetrics, farriery, and clinical surgery—Professor Sjostedt.

Pathology, therapeutics, epizoötics, pharmaco-dynamics, pharmacotechny, and special clinic—Professor Lindquist.

Botany, physics, chemistry, pharmacology, and pharmacy—Lecturer Ericsson.

The assistant aids in the clinic, and the other official instructs in the farriery.

In Sweden there are thirty Government veterinary surgeons, who receive an annual allowance of £80 and traveling expenses. The regiments in garrison have a regimental veterinary surgeon, with a yearly pay of £170; and a battalion veterinary surgeon with the rank of sub-lieutenant, who receives annually £112. Regiments of the line have regimental and squadron veterinary surgeons, having the grade of non-commissioned officers, and a pay of £56 yearly. The number of civil and military veterinary surgeons under the Government is 170, and all, so far as their technical duties are concerned, are under the direction of the medical authorities.

The Schools of Germany.

*The School at Stuttgart.**

This school was the last established among the German schools. It was built on territory which had previously been occupied by the Zoölogical Garden, the royal order for its establishment being dated August 21, 1796. Walz, Hördt, and Haussmann were prominent

* "Die Königlich. Würtemberg. Thierarznei-Schule." Historically considered by Hering. 1847. Rueff, 1871.

among the veterinarians of the state at this time, and were called upon to advise and take part in it. The former was by far the most influential of the trio. He was born in Stuttgart, the 7th of December, 1771, and died there, February 4, 1834. He received his first education in the gymnasium of his native city, and then in the Karls School of Philosophy, where he studied natural philosophy and the general principles of medicine, at the same time acquainting himself with pharmacy in the shop of his father. Having selected veterinary medicine as his means of livelihood, he went to Vienna, for a time enjoying the teachings of Wolstein; then visited the breeding establishments in Austria and Hungary; thence his travels brought him to Dresden, where he tarried at the Veterinary School for a while; then visiting the Universities of Jena, Erfurt, Leipsic, and Halle, and finally at Berlin, where he remained for nine months at the School of Veterinary Medicine. The reputation which the school at Copenhagen acquired under Abildgaard drew him to Denmark; at the same time he studied medicine in the hospital of the city under Bang and Winslow. After three years' absence he returned to Stuttgart by way of Hoya, Hanover, and Göttingen, and on the 9th of September, 1794, received the position of an official veterinarian, having the supervision of the entire veterinary system of the dukedom. He soon became a member of the sanitary commission, and of many scientific and public associations. Walz was one of the first who asserted that the cheapest and best way to stamp out the rinderpest was to kill all diseased animals, as well as those exposed to infection. The invasion began in 1795, but so many difficulties presented themselves to the proper execution of these principles that it was not until 1801 that the pest was finally got rid of, at a cost of some 40,000 cattle. His treatment of the scabies of sheep has become one of the fundamental elements of the veterinary practice. He took a most active part in advocating a governmental veterinary school, his efforts being finally rewarded by success; his life was eminently successful, and he died respected by all and mourned by many.

The conditions of admittance to the school were at first very easy, requiring applicants to be—

1. Twenty years old.
2. A healthy physique, with sufficient strength.
3. Free from military duty.
4. The necessary educational qualifications.
5. Of good moral character.
6. Must know some trade.

7. Must have means enough to pay the expenses of their education.

The school supplies sleeping apartments for quite a number of students, and residence for a number of the teachers. It is fitted up with the auxiliaries to instruction, the same as other schools, but the collections of skeletons and specimens in the anatomical department are wonderfully large for so small an institute. The course of study was at first fixed at one year, many students, however, remaining over one, two, or even three sessions, themselves seeing the necessity of a more complete education. In this regard, it may be well remarked that the first year in any medical school can do nothing more than introduce a student to his work; and if, at the end of a four-years' course, he has progressed so far as to get a general view of the field before him, and has himself *really learned how to study*, how to select the chaff from the wheat, he may consider himself as among the few who enter in at the strait gate which leadeth unto knowledge. All this talk about "completing an education," or "he has a complete education," with reference to graduates from schools, simply shows the ignorance of the speaker; for, as I have previously said, it is only the Virchows, the Franklins, the Darwins, and Hallers among men who get so far as to obtain firm hold of the keys which are to unlock to them the treasury of knowledge in the future, but not without untiring work and unceasing self-sacrifice, however. The rest never even get hold of the keys; they are and always remain pettifoggers, dabblers, or mere routiners and followers in the path of the true lights which lead on to the perfect day.

The example of the students finally led to an increase of the term of study to two years, after a lapse of twenty-five years from the opening of the school.

The school had at first four professors (a vast improvement over that at Hanover, which at first had but one, and for a long time but two) and a teacher of horseshoeing. The course begins every year on the 16th of October and ends the 31st of August the following year. Vacations come at Christmas and Easter, but such a number of students must always remain at the school as is requisite to attend to the patients in the hospital. The library contains 2,128 books, and is open to the students under certain regulations, which are very easy to comply with: "They can keep a book out for four weeks at a time, and are allowed all books except such as are very rare or costly, which can only be used in the rooms of the library."

Patients treated by the Students from 1821 to 1871.

Horses:		
In the school hospital	18,091	
Visited by students outside the school	5,896	
Used for anatomy and operative practice	684	
Asses and mules	45	
		24,716
Dogs:		
In school hospital	5,270	
Brought in by police	755	
		6,025
Cattle:		
In school	270	
Outside	16,794	
		17,064
Other animals		2,652
Autopsies		2,722
Whole number of animals treated in school for fifty years		53,179

Whole number of students in same period, 2,140. Of these, the following are recorded as having emigrated to America:

L. Bickard, 1841–'42; Alois Ebach, 1865–'67; Will. Eberhardt, 1838–'39; J. F. Erpf, 1831–'32; A. Fritz, 1841–'42; B. Fussenegger, 1844–'45; Aug. Gleich, studied winter of 1860; J. Haussler, 1840; G. Hahn, 1842; L. D. Hess, 1824; Chr. Hörz, 1849–'50; A. Ibach, 1866–'68; G. F. Lütze, J. E. Mack, 1864–'65; J. Ritters, C. Shock, J. J. Schwarz, J. Stiefel, Chr. Tröscher, C. E. Wolff.

The school at Stuttgart is, I hope, soon to be among the "have beens." At one time it enjoyed quite an exalted reputation, but since the retirement of Dr. Hering, Sr., it has steadily been going into decline, and the students becoming fewer and fewer. This is in part owing to a very injurious stand adhered to by some of its teachers, and which was once quite general in Germany, viz., that a school should give two different forms of education, and graduate first and second class veterinarians—the first for the use of the state, the latter for the people. The nonsense of such an idea should be apparent to any one, but to no one so quickly as to a veterinarian. Of one hundred students graduating from a given class and a given school, and enjoying instruction uniting to the fullest possible degree a scientific foundation and practical execution, not all will be successful practitioners, and but few suitable for state work, and still fewer for the highest state work—perhaps one of the hundred may make a really gifted and capable teacher. Let the education be as perfect as possible: the world's test will do the winnowing.

It will not do to leave even this brief notice of this school without duly noticing the man who did more to give it fame than, in all probability, all the others combined who have taught within its walls. About the thirtieth year of this century really marks the birth of the scientific tendency in veterinary medicine. At this time Germany was far beyond any other country in the quality of the work she was giving to the world, so far as veterinary medicine was concerned. Gurlt, Haubner, Hertwig, and Hering were the four, among others, who took part in this work. Of these four, Eduard Hering was by no means the least. He was born in Stuttgart on the 20th of March, 1799. Dying recently, he enjoyed the well-merited fruits of his years of labor, as pensioner of his Government, but a free man, nevertheless, for the services of such men are not to be counted by a few dollars paid yearly in supporting them in comfort in their old age. It is impossible for me to give even a brief account of the literary work of this man. It covers three finely printed pages in the historical sketch I am now using. He was the best historian living on veterinary literature, and in this respect may be ranked with Schrader, Huzard, and Ercolani, the four being the only men who have been especially noted in this regard. He also edited the "Repertorium der Thierheilkunde," 1840 to date, a journal in which he endeavored to give to German readers a digest of all important matters and articles which came to pass in connection with their profession in other lands. His "Special Pathology and Therapeutics," and his "Book for Horsemen," are still well worthy of study; the latter is beautifully illustrated by the celebrated Baumeister, also professor at the school, and is bought up so closely as a work of real art that it is impossible to get a copy, it being out of print for many years. His work on operative surgery should be translated into English, it being much more practical and condensed than the two-volume verbose and indistinct work of Peuch and Toussaint; a compendium, critically revised, would be a grand thing, but deliver us from the original! But the one act which has given Hering the most fame, the one act which did more for the elevation of veterinary medicine into a science than all the work of all the other professors at the school, the one act which has made his name immortal as a discoverer of a new fact, was that Hering was the first to experimentally demonstrate the velocity of the circulation in the living organism, published in "Tiedemann und Trevirarnus Zeitschrift für Physiologie," Heidelberg, 1828.

*The School at Hanover.**

On the 15th of April, 1777, the first steps toward the erection of a veterinary school were taken into consideration by the king, or rather elector, who was at the same time George III of England, and Kersting, the superior veterinarian of the court at Cassel, a neighboring province, was invited to visit Hanover to advise about the opening of the school, and take charge of it. Kersting's popularity was so great at the court of Cassel that he could not obtain permission to leave for Hanover, and was obliged to run away. As Kersting was by all means the most important German veterinarian of his day, a short sketch of his life is not out of place here:

"Johann Adam Kersting was the descendant of a Huguenot family, and was born at Liebenau, in Lower Hesse, in 1726, and died at Hanover, March 2, 1784, from the effects of a wound caused by the kick of a horse, at a time when he could ill be spared, being but fifty-eight years old, and full of bodily vigor and mental activity. His father was a farrier, wound-doctor, and veterinarian. At fifteen years of age the son went into the forge of his father at Cassel, where he soon displayed unusual abilities. Among others, he became acquainted with a clock-maker, and took so much interest in the work of the latter that he himself constructed a clock and hung it up in his father's forge, which so incited the wrath of the latter that he knocked it in pieces, declaring he would have no such nonsense interfering with the proper work of his son. The son also busied himself in studying the diseases of the horse, and practicing their treatment; and we find him, in 1745, as farrier accompanying a squadron of Hessians into Scotland in favor of the Stuarts. He accompanied the Hessian prince of the day during several wars as farrier, and at the close of the Seven Years' War studied medicine in Göttingen for a time. During the war in Silesia (1757) he was thrown from a baggage-wagon, with such force as to lose both sight and hearing, the former not returning for a period of two years. During his blindness he attended to the publication of the first edition of his book, "Sicherer und wohlerfahrener Huf und Reitschmidt" ("Sure and Well-experienced Farrier and Rider"). During a winter's quarters at Brunswick he again studied medicine diligently. At the end of the war he settled at Cassel, as farrier veterinarian to the court, where he busily pursued his studies, espe-

* These remarks are taken from "Die königliche Thierarznei-Schule zu Hannover," during the first hundred years of its existence, by K. Günther, director and professor, to which the reader is referred for all minute details.

cially of anatomy, and soon acquired a reputation which extended into neighboring provinces. That he acquired no inconsiderable skill in anatomical dissection may be divined from the fact that he discovered and very minutely described the membrane of Decemet in the horse, on the inner part of the cornea, and communicated the same to Haller in a letter which is among the collections at the Hanover school. He soon received students from the adjoining provinces, other governments sending young men to study under his guidance at their expense. It was but natural that, on opening the discussion for the erection of a veterinary school at Hanover, the attention of the Government should be directed to him as the man best fitted to successfully conduct the venture. Kersting's sudden departure for Hanover, against the will of his elector, gave rise to a most interesting discussion between the two Governments, that of Cassel declaring him to be a deserter, and demanding his return, which was not, however, conceded, Kersting declaring himself to be no slave but a free man, and in debt to no one. Kersting was a man of irreproachable character and lively temperament, an indefatigable worker, sharp and logical thinker, and close observer of the phenomena of disease. In this regard, a remark which he makes upon glanders is not without public interest, when we consider how long ago it was made, and how ignorant many people still are with reference to this disease, thinking that when no nasal outflow and ulcers are present there is no glanders. Kersting says, after giving the usual characteristics of the disease: 'I must concede, and it is true, that a glandered horse *ean* present these phenomena, but not in the beginning of the disease. For a horse may have glanders for a whole year, and, according to circumstances, still longer, without its having ulcers in the nose, and at the same time have a good appetite, smooth hair, and be in good condition.'"

Kersting received 300 thalers ($225) pay, a free residence, and the title of superior veterinarian to the Hanoverian court.

Havemann, who had been sent to Alfort, at the expense of and by the Government, was appointed as assistant teacher, at the same pay. There seems to have been an extreme prejudice existing among the people at this time against those persons who had anything to do with cutting up animals, for the king was obliged to issue a royal order, by which any slurs or other ill-treatment of the teachers, students, or servants at the school for this cause would be punished. The course at the school under Kersting was limited to one year, though many of the students remained through two, hearing the same lectures a second time. It was as follows:

WINTER SESSION. *Before noon.*—8 to 9, horseshoeing, daily; 9 to 10, instruction upon the internal and external diseases of the horse, four days each week; 10 to 11, clinic.

Afternoon.—1 to 2, dissection, daily; 2 to 3, anatomical lecture, four days per week. General examination upon all subjects twice weekly; 3 to 4, dissection.

SUMMER SESSION. *Before noon.*—8 to 9, horseshoeing, daily; 9 to 10, internal and external diseases, daily; 10 to 11, clinic.

Afternoon.—2 to 3, osteology, exterior, physiology, hygiene, obstetrics, materia medica, pharmacy, bandaging, etc, one day each per week.

On Kersting's death, the direction of the school passed to Havemann, who had for a time been stationed at one of the royal studs, which he left with great regret. He was a man of extreme modesty, but nevertheless proved himself to be a competent and pleasant teacher. There was but little change in the course or manner of instruction. Havemann was requested to give his views upon veterinary education to the Government; and this man of the last century embodies some ideas therein which are not unworthy of appreciation in this country, which, to-day, in spite of self-conceited Americanism, is no further advanced, so far as veterinary science is concerned, than Hanover was then: "According to my ideas, *veterinary medicine would receive a much more rapid development if the education were made entirely free to the children of the land, as there are so few veterinarians to be had.* Applicants must not only be able to write legibly, but must give reason to hope for their future success by diligence and a natural adaptability to the profession. Those who have not these two necessary qualifications must be dismissed the schools, for, while it is an undoubted truth that capable veterinarians are of much benefit to the public, so is it beyond all doubt that empirics and quacks are nothing else than lashes to the land, even though they be supplied with letters of apprenticeship, saying that they have studied in a royal veterinary school an art of which they have not acquired the least idea." In answer to the question, "How long would it take a gifted and industrious man to become an educated veterinarian?" he says, "One learns quicker, another slower, but to all are necessary great capability, much work, and these all demand time, and three years are none too little." But, in spite of all this good advice, the course was not much extended by the Government, or the conditions to admittance made much more severe.

Hausemann succeeded Havemann as director in 1819, and had

for assistant the veterinarian Frederick Günther. Little change was made in the plan of instruction until 1828, except that the courses were made longer. In 1828 Günther introduced into the curriculum forensic medicine and veterinary police, materia medica, and the art of writing and making prescriptions, with several other essential improvements. A teacher for horseshoeing was also added to the school. The period of study was extended to two and a half years, although Günther worked earnestly to have it three years. In 1847 Günther became director, and with it began a new era in the school. There is no doubt that he was one of the most eminently practical men that has ever graced the veterinary profession in any country; perhaps it would not be going too far to say that the scientific and practical were united in him to a degree which has been but rarely met with in the members of our profession. He was an earnest experimenter, a close observer, and his greatest failure seems to have been too much delay in publishing his results. No better hippo-anatomist has ever lived; his work on the "Myology of the Horse" has never been equaled, and has been a source of assistance to all succeeding authors. He was the first to discover the chief cause of roaring, if not the only one, in atrophy of the laryngeal muscles, upon which opening of the glottis depends, especially of the left side, and connected it by experiment with diseased conditions of the left recurrent nerve. He gave us the first book of any moment upon the horse's teeth and their diseases, and invented numerous *practical* (not useless) instruments for their extraction, etc. No one has followed him in this direction, and we remain just where he left us in the middle of this century. His work on obstetrics was for a long time the best which we had. Through his earnest endeavors and untiring energy, the school-term was finally fixed at three years, at which it continued until 1877, when with all the German schools it was extended to three and a half, and the conditions to admission and receiving the diploma of the empire were fixed alike for all.

Gerlach succeeded Günther as director, and under him the school attained a still greater celebrity, but, as we have to speak of him in connection with the school at Berlin, we will defer further remark till then. The grounds of the Hanover school are quite extensive, the library replete with books and many valuable manuscripts and works of early German and other Continental veterinarians. The buildings are many of them new, and all have recently suffered renovation. The hospital is roomy, airy, and well lighted; in fact, the school has all the requisites necessary to such an institution of a smaller variety, except a special physiologist and physiological laboratory. The above-mentioned historical sketch, from which I have taken these few facts, gives a list of all the students, their place of birth, time of entrance, and whether they received a diploma or not, from the year 1820 to 1877; from which we see that during that time 1,269 students were recorded upon the books: many of these never stood their examination; among the latter will be found, in all probability, quite a number of "graduates of a German school" (?) now practicing in this country.

The present corps of teachers is as follows (1877):

Medical Councilors.—K. Guenther, Director; Professor Begemann, Professor Dr. Dammaun, Dr. Harms, Dr. Lustig, Dr. Rabe, Dr. Brücher, Dr. Eichbaum, Vet. Ernst (assistant).

The School at Munich.

Instead of offering an imperfect historical sketch of this institution, it seems more conformable with the purposes of this book to offer to your consideration a translation of the following address, "*Upon the Necessity for the Reform of Veterinary Education in Germany, as proved by the History of the Munich School,*" by my friend Professor Johann Feser, of that institution, delivered August 6, 1873; the more so as there is much contained therein of unquestionable importance to the people of this country, and further, that the author is one of the most advanced thinkers as well as accomplished scientists in the veterinary profession of our day:

"The veterinary schools have assumed no less a task than the education of completely qualified veterinarians, for their graduates have a manifold service to perform to states interested in the breeding of domestic animals, which can only be well done by a complete scientific and practical education, united to great diligence and unceasing activity by the veterinarian himself.

"The veterinarian must not only be capable of performing the practical duties of his profession when called upon by the public, but he has much higher duties; he must at the same time act as counselor and protector of the state, and that portion of its citizens interested in the breeding and rearing of domestic animals, thereby contributing to the nation's welfare by keeping distant and suppressing those pests which carry death and desolation in their path.

"*The chief task of the veterinarian lies in keeping the domestic animals in health, and in exerting a favorable influence toward their perfection by aiding, as educated advisers, the progressive development of breeding in the land (to which may well be added, and in preventing many diseases of human beings caused by unsuitable animal products which would otherwise be offered for consumption as articles of food*). *The veterinary schools are not, therefore, founded for the education of mere curers;* they are not instituted to send raw empirics into the land, for in such cases the aims of veterinary medicine are by no means attained. Such empirics were plenty enough long before the foundation of the veterinary schools; and only because of their utter uselessness to the state were the veterinary schools founded, in order that veterinarians could be had suitable to the higher purposes which the public necessities demanded.

"In order to prove the correctness of this assertion, it is necessary to refer to the history of the veterinary schools. We must know why these schools were really founded, what necessity they were expected to fill, and how observing men thought this end was best to be attained.

"To this purpose nothing serves better than the address delivered by Cothenius, body-surgeon to Frederick the Great of Prussia, before the Academy of Sciences on the 21st of January, 1768, before there was any veterinary school in Germany. Cothenius first demonstrated from the records of history that in antiquity, and following down to his time, devastating animal plagues had always existed, which produced immense misery to the people, and concluded with the advice that only veterinary schools had the power to give the means of freeing the nation from these plagues; but he placed great emphasis upon the necessity of an exact fundamental education, giving a plan for their establishment which is well worthy our present consideration, though elucidated over one hundred years since. He knew very well that at that time there was no thorough plan of education, no veterinary science, and no teachers, and that for the last purpose men of great ability were necessary, for they were to teach subjects of which they knew nothing, and upon which there were no suitable books of reference, or other assistance. He said: 'The first teachers must not be ashamed to be themselves students; their greatest honor must be the public admission of their own ignorance. The less they at present know, and the more they feel the necessity of learning, the more have we reason to hope that they will in time attain to that degree of perfection which they so much desire.' Thus we see that Cothenius well appreciated the only way by which veterinary science was to be successfully developed. He looked upon this task from a purely scientific stand-point, and well knew that progress was only to be attained by the methods and assistance of scientific research. To this end he demanded not only macroscopic but microscopic anatomy, a physio-pathologic, therapeutic method of exact investigation, and recognized the necessity of a well-ordered chemical laboratory. He laid emphasis upon the necessity of several teachers for such schools. He recommended paying especial attention to the study of the animal plagues, and laid great stress upon the value of exact observation and experiment. He says: 'In the study-room one can make no such observations. The teacher must, at the time such pests prevail, go out into the country, and hold his dietetic, pathologic, and therapeutic discussion in the afflicted stables; he must observe the situation and character of the stables, and cause better ventilation, cleanliness, and care of the animals; he must visit the fields, meadows, and drinking-places, in order to ascertain if in them are not to be sought either immediate or mediate causes of infection, and what in every case is necessary to propose for the better protection of the animals. He must gather all forms of dew, and make therewith chemical and physiological experiments, and must also have recourse to the microscope in order to see if he can not discover some poisonous insects, which, either of themselves or with their semen, so pollute the vegetation as to cause the generation of the pest or other infectious disease.' (In reading this one almost forgets he is passing over words written more than one hundred years since.) 'The teacher shall study the animal in all its parts, its mode of life, procreation; and, when necessary, shall have recourse to the crucible and distillation to increase his knowledge. He must separate things into their minute parts, unite and make new bodies, and seek to attain a sort of despotic power over nature.'"

This is what was thought in the last century by the founder of veterinary medicine in Germany. *The schools must be useful nurseries of science, and not produce mere empirics.*

Let us see if the schools have fulfilled their task, and, if not, seek to discover what has prevented them from doing so.

It is all the more our duty to do this, as the popular judgment with regard to the results at the schools seems to be at present unfavorable. Not only the organs of the state and agriculture, the interests of which are to be served by the educated veterinarian from an economical point of view, but also the graduates of the schools, concur, more or less, in this opinion, as was sufficiently demonstrated at the Frankfort congress of German veterinarians in 1872.

It is especially the duty of the teachers at the schools to acknowledge these evils, and to seek for their removal, and I doubt not that the governments will respectfully listen to our demands for reform.

I pledge myself to have the strictest regard for the truth in the task I have undertaken, even though it may be unpleasant to some, and to bind myself to facts; and, in proving the questions we have to consider, to do it according to the strictest methods of science, and to keep in mind only the attainable and practical parts of the question.

With reference to the history of the Munich school, we shall most speedily atain our end if we consider those causes which have, at different times, interfered with the production of good veterinarians. Then I will show that even in our day evil conditions still exist, the complete removal of which is beyond the power of the best teachers, notwithstanding all diligence and perseverance. The proposals for improvement will then receive their consideration.

The school at Munich has passed through two epochs since its foundation. The first extends from its establishment in 1790 to the year 1852, and the second from that date to the end of the school year 1872.

Nothing satisfactory can be said about the condition and results at our school during the first epoch. Empiricism obtained a greatly extended duration in Bavaria, while at the other veterinary schools (German) it extended only to the second decennium of our century. Many of the learned gentlemen present studied at our school during this period and must confirm my judgment, that our institute had until then never filled the place of a scientific veterinary school as portrayed by Cothenius. Nothing but schooled "routiniers" were produced, nor did they dare to produce anything else. They *hid* themselves under a deceptive cloud, by boasting of their abhorrence of speculative theories and of their great respect for practical things, which by no means should be neglected, but by this means they nourished an imbecile empiricism and sought to keep distant from all true science. It was made exceedingly difficult for young men of better preparatory education to gain entrance to the school; in fact, they appear to have been intentionally avoided, so that any external incitement to scientific work became impossible. The experimental method suggested by Cothenius as absolutely necessary to the schools had no place in the programme. The great reforms in medicine in general, and every natural science, were passed heedlessly by, by the Munich school of that period. Instruction in natural sciences, the foundation of the study of medicine, was so neglected that one feels almost ashamed to mention it. The few students who gained admittance from the "real schools" were astonished thereby, and scorned to make notes upon the nonsense which they heard from the lecturer at the desks of the school. There was neither chemical laboratory nor physical cabinet, but every "real school" had these long before 1852, and all the attributes necessary to good elementary instruction in natural science.

Let it remain so! We will not follow this sad relation further. You will believe me, however, that with the exception of anatomy, the conditions were no more flattering with reference to the purely veterinary branches than with the natural sciences upon which they are founded. One would naturally assume that, although the scientific side of our education was so much neglected, the students at least received a good practical education. On the contrary, that was not the case.

Let us see if we can not discover the causes of this neglect of the teachings of Cothenius.

To this end we must again have reference to the general history of the schools, and bear in mind the extravagances of the first French schools, to which many evil influences may be justly attributed.

Two schools (Lyons and Alfort) were organized in France some years before the foundation of any in Germany. The Alfort school was larger than that at Lyons, and received from the beginning great attention and care from the Government. The fittings of the school exceeded those of the German schools, even in our day, and every condition was present to attain the ends which should be required of a school except fitting teachers and promoting veterinary science. *Suitable teachers are and ever will be the chief desideratum; without them all donations of money are useless.* This was soon experienced by the French schools. Instead of proceeding in the manner indicated by Cothenius, and first paying their attention to the development of proper teachers, they sought at once to make the world wise by a display of superficial knowledge. The students were educated in a manner to produce superficial but ready talkers, but not to become methodical and educated veterinarians. The Alfort school especially sought to gain an acknowledgment of superiority from other nations, which was, indeed, attained, but not without great injury to herself. Chairs for agriculture, comparative anatomy, natural sciences, animal painting, etc., were even then attained, although the raw empirical material at command had by no means been sufficiently culled out. The students must at once be educated to be obstetricians, wound and eye doctors, coroners, etc., in order to fill the wants of the country in this regard. They founded a menagerie filled mostly with exotic animals, and gave great attention to the breeding of sheep, rabbits, fowls, and even silk-worms. To the formation of the so-called "royal cabinet," students and teachers were sent at great expense to the sea-coast to gather examples of different sea-animals. They studied the anatomy of the dolphin and ray, and forgot that of the domestic animals. This superficial learning of a little of many things was especially cultivated by Bourgelat to the cost of a true scientific method, and found, fortunately, little imitation in Germany. But instead of passing quietly by these French extravagances, and copying them in what good things they had, we fell into the opposite extreme of developing one-sided empirics, the so-called "Rossärzte" (horse-doctors) and "Kurschmiede" (farriers). Every attempt of individual men at the schools to introduce the true scientific method was energetically combated, and the French schools quoted to strengthen the ground of the opponents. Bojanus, medical councilor in Hesse, enjoys the unenviable reputation of having most successfully opposed all improvement. I can not refrain from telling you how Bojanus would have the veterinarians educated and the schools conducted. He had a controlling power at the Munich school until 1852.

Bojanus looked upon the education of *practical* men as the sole task of the schools. They would fail of our purpose were they educated to be scientific veterinarians. (The English have most religiously followed in this direction even to our day, and here in America a good practical ignoramus is in general more prized than the man of genuine scientific attainments; let it be understood, I claim, a *truly* scientific man can never be aught else than practical.) Certain axioms were to be learned as articles of practical belief, the students being reduced to mere mechanical machines. The state needed only veterinary hand-workers (in some parts of France the veterinarians are still spoken of as "artistes vétérinaires"), who would follow the rules learned at school with blind confidence. Such a practitioner never asks the cause of the phenomena which he sees presented to him by a diseased organism; he does not seek to enter into the real nature of the disease, but is contented to know that disease is before him. He does not seek to arrange a special method of treatment, but uses that which he has learned as something discovered for all time. He is all content when the patient recovers, and asks not why, nor under what necessary laws, it has taken place. He enters public life as a common artisan, and must always be classed as such; he never feels the power in him that is given to the scientifically educated man, but is content with the bounds and bars which surround him. The school was to take only such students from the masses as were fitted to go back again to the same. Their knowledge was to be limited to what was necessary to their livelihood, and to read and write sufficient to support the memory. No other preliminary knowledge was considered necessary. They were entirely wanting in a preparatory scientific education or spirit.

You will permit me to describe to you the method of instruction which Bojanus would have introduced into the schools, especially as two teachers of modern times (Director Rueff, of Stuttgart, and Professor Plug, of Giessen) would have us follow in the same direction.

Bojanus writes: "It is the duty of the practical veterinarian to cure the sick animals belonging to the public. His office, which does not belong to the most respected, brings him constantly in relation with the commonest people, to whose ideas and conceptions he must adapt himself if he will not endanger his success and let it pass over into the hands of quacks and herdsmen. He busies himself with disgusting work in dirty stables, and all his endeavors and privations are rewarded with but a scanty income which scarcely covers his necessities, and, at the most, permits him to enter society as an ordinary artisan." Bojanus then goes on to say that "the scientifically educated veterinarian is unsuited to such work, and could not lower himself to the necessary level, and is therefore never looked upon by the people as a *practical* man, and, therefore, it is the duty of the schools to educate practical, not scientific, veterinarians." These words of Bojanus justify us in concluding that he knew right well the qualifications of a scientific veterinarian, but he intentionally put all he could in the way of their education. On the contrary, Bojanus would have the teachers scientific men in order that they might discover new methods of treatment and give them to the students, who were supposed to follow implicitly in these ruts in practice. To the end that the state may have such teachers, Bojanus would have another form of school, a higher, scientific school. In these were to be taken the candidates for teachers' positions, with a complete scientific education from the lap of the academy. Bojanus either did not see, or passed intentionally by, the fact that the state needs scientifically educated veterinarians for the purposes of veterinary police and forensic medicine, and for the perfection of the breeds of the domestic animals. The second class of veterinarians were there only to be curers, and a very small class of scientific veterinarians to develop cure-methods for the benefit of the former. In this way there came to pass the idea that two classes of veterinary schools were necessary, which occasionally finds an advocate even in our day, although it must be remarked that these people go higher in their demands for a veterinary academy, and propose that not only teachers but a small number of scientific veterinarians also shall be educated for the purposes of the state.

If we return to the conditions in Bavaria, we shall find that only the poorest proposals of Bojanus came to fulfillment, and that no one bothered himself about the education of scientific veterinarians. According to the edict of 1810 for the organization of the veterinary institutes of Bavaria, that only went out of power in the last few years, it was found very convenient (at first, doubtless, necessary) to promote the forensic M. D.'s to veterinarians of the first class, falsely assuming that the doctor, from his education, was well adapted to be the highest veterinary authority, and that a short visit to the lectures at a veterinary school would completely equalize any want of knowledge he previously might have. The lectures for this purpose in Munich lasted eight days. In two or three hours were completed the lectures upon nutrition in the horse and ruminants; in one hour those upon operative surgery; and in one to five hours the elements of animal pests, or veterinary police; one to three hours were given to gaining practical knowledge in the clinic. Only an idiot could assert that this kind of education would suffice to the production of scientific veterinarians, for even in 1790 the full course of study for second-class veterinarians at Munich extended over three full years.

The above description sufficiently indicates the hindrances in the way to the education of scientific veterinarians in the first epoch of our school, and no one need wonder that our science stood still impotent in comparison to human medicine and that it could not develop to that position which it was expected would be the case with the foundation of the schools. Notwithstanding the difficulties which they had to overcome, it must be said, to the credit of the profession, that even during this period many men of acknowledged ability were to be found in the land; but it is impossible to place this to the credit of the school, but to the great diligence of the individuals, who overcame the failures of their school education. A not less praiseworthy service of these men was the fact that they mercilessly exposed the weakness of the school, and finally succeeded in bringing about the reform which took place in 1852.

After the Government of Bavaria had seen the failures in the manner in which the school was conducted, and after it had repeatedly heard the grumblings of the agriculturists that *mere empirics were useless*, a reform was decided upon, which, however, failed of a scientific basis. The germ of the failure was that the school still remained patterned after those of France, and was left free from every connection with the medical faculty. It was assumed that all scientific foundation in the preliminary education was unnecessary, save what little was gained by students in a low class of a "real" school, and the two lowest classes in Latin. The teachers were too few, and, taken mostly from the old empirical school, were not adequate to the education of veterinarians suitable to the purposes of the state. They were so poorly paid that they were obliged to have outside occupations in order to live, so that teaching and self-improvement became a matter of secondary importance.

"I myself had the misfortune to study three years (1857–'60) under this *régime*. The conditions at the school then were sad indeed, for I will describe to you a time when we should have seen something of the development of the scientific spirit. The school did not then have the least scientific character; even the good of the old school, the instruction in anatomy and dissection, was neglected. The physiology which we heard was nothing else than what Schwab had written many years before for the instruction of empirics. Not a single experiment illustrated the lectures. There was no practice in the use of the microscope. The instruction in natural science, over which so much talk was made, consisted in nothing else than in learning by rote a few pages of poorly compiled chemical analyses from Gorup-Besanez's work upon that subject. There was a chemical laboratory which had just been erected, but only for the agricultural experiment station, and exclusively for the use of students of agriculture and forestry from the university. The instruction in botany was very poor. Physics was not taught. The formulas for the preparation of medicines passed as traditions from student to student, and I do not say too much in stating that not a single one was correct. Pharmaceutical chemistry was lectured upon by an assistant, but a second one coming after one lecture had been delivered, we did not attend them further, for we knew more chemistry than he did. The pharmacognostical collection was poor, old, moldy, and unsuitable for study or demonstration. The teaching upon the action of medicines was nothing more than a mere phraseology, which served to hide the ignorance of the teacher, but did not help to instruct the students. The balance of the instruction bore the same character. The dependency and insufficiency of the institute is well illustrated by one fact, which amply shows the requirements which were necessary. In order to make a correct necroscopical diagnosis, for instance, of Bright's condition of the kidneys, it was necessary to call in the assistance of a professor of pathological anatomy from the medical faculty of the university, and numerous valuable and instructive specimens sent to the school by practicing veterinarians perished for want of proper appreciation. It is no wonder that the congress of veterinarians at Würzburg, in 1860, pronounced it a waste of time, trouble, and money, to allow the institute to continue its existence. I will cease, at this point, enumerating the sins of the Munich school during the first half of this epoch, as it would not be courteous to extend it to the present teachers."

Let us turn our attention for a moment to the other schools of Germany, for I have endeavored to get at the true facts, so far as was in my power. With the exception of Berlin, which, notwithstanding a brilliant external reputation, had fallen into a stage of semi-torpidity, its teachers having become old, and new power being needed, and the school at Stuttgart, the schools at Dresden and Hanover were in many instances worthy of being considered as models. Dresden had suffered a complete renovation, and Gerlach worked in Hanover. (In both these cases it was, however, the work of single individuals which gave these schools what little advantage they had. Haubner in Dresden, and, as Feser says, Gerlach in Hanover; there was nothing general about it.) But neither of them went beyond the education of clever empirics—in proof of which may be noted the fact that, after the reformation of the plan of the Dresden school, of which so much was spoken and expected, it was found impossible to find veterinarians suitable for teachers, and the chairs were only finally filled by going outside of Saxony, and at great expense. (Here is a proper place for me to remark that, notwithstanding the high position which I have claimed for the German schools and other veterinary institutions, no one unacquainted with the true conditions can realize how few men there are among the graduates of the German veterinary schools at all fitted to become teachers, and every one of these few, and every man who has gained fame before them, have been obliged, at great cost to their physique and demands upon means which in no case are too plenty, to fill the great gaps in their education by studies at the medical schools of German universities. The number of men of real value to the scientific advancement of veterinary medicine at the schools of Germany is not more than sufficient to make a faculty for one school. There are unquestionably men of practical ability at these schools, but they are of that empirical character that does not advance science an inch, but, with a terrible reverence for the traditions of the past, stand obstinately in the way of progress, and by a great display of verbose repetition of other people's work, make the world think they know more than they really do. If there is a man I fear, as an enemy to my profession, though personally he may be a good friend, it is *the man of great experience, of great reverence for the past, of good talking abilities, but without a particle of originality or scientific spirit.* Such men are more fitted for political intriguers than teachers at a scientific school.)

After this diversion, let us return to Feser's remarks:

"Under the above retarding conditions, it is no wonder that progress was checked, and all sorts of complaints found ready utterance. The agricultural papers and the organs of the state opened up the subject continually, complaining of the insufficiency of the veterinary profession in comparison with the demands which were made upon it. The reflecting Bavarian veterinarians again joined hands with the above-named forces, and loudly demanded reform both in the manner of instruction and a more exacting preparatory education. The battle for the improvement of the school finally found its way into the Chamber of Representatives (1861), and resulted in a free offering of means to help on the purpose. But, instead of making a thorough reform, they contented themselves with all sorts of corrective regulations. They burnished up the roof of the school and whitewashed the façades, instead of beginning anew and laying a solid and enduring foundation. New professors were added to the old, until the school had eight, which was more than any other school in Europe. The clinic was improved, and many other innovations made. Finally, the director was changed, but not the system of instruction. The matriculatory examination still remained the same; the entire weight of instruction in the natural sciences had to be borne by one man, who was at first without assistance or sufficient material support, and at the same time had to lecture on other strictly technical subjects. Physiology, the very foundation of scientific medicine, was lectured upon in only two sessions, before even the lectures on the natural sciences were ended, and therefore lacked the necessary basis. Empiricism in the hospital still continued. Microscopic practice was begun, but very imperfectly, and so was it with everything at this school as well as the other German schools."

The cause of all these difficulties is easy of discovery. Professor Carl Voit has done this in a very thorough manner. According to him, it is not so necessary to consider the improvement of individual evils which are evident to us, but above all a change is necessary in the direction of the school, without which great exertions of both teachers and pupils can never lead to promising results. The causes why the Bavarian school has not developed into the institution which it was expected it would, are to be sought, mostly, in the absolute neglect of those basal conditions upon which such a school can alone thrive. *Such a school, to thrive, must be placed upon a scientific foundation.* The first means by which this end is to be attained is a general and exact preparatory education of young men before they enter the school. The preparatory education of the students up to this time has been totally insufficient for them to be able to comprehend well the teachings of their technical teachers. To the study of veterinary medicine the same degree of preliminary education is necessary that is required for entering upon the study of human medicine, and without this the best teaching will be resultless.

"The second condition to improvement is, that all students must be well grounded in the necessary natural sciences before entering the school. It is absolutely certain that this should also be of the same grade as for the students of medicine. The study of the natural sciences in the school itself must be completed before the technical branches of the profession are entered upon. It is impossible for the student to comprehend the teachings in physiology without a thorough anticipatory education in physics and chemistry. The thorough study of the natural sciences is the only means by which the student can learn to become a good experimenter, or learn to think logically, or understand the processes of diseases and their products" (Voit). The present students *have never learned to think*, because of the want of a thorough drilling in scientific methods; it is this reason, and not because of want of discipline, that has made the results of teaching at our school so futile. "Or is it to be looked upon as a favorable result that out of twenty students, only five, and of these only two Bavarians, successfully passed their final examination after three years' study? The evil is to be sought in the system."

Only when a rigid education in the necessary branches of general science is required as a preparation, can the teachers hope for genuine success from the study of the strictly professional branches. From men thus educated can we alone hope to select those fitted for teachers.

These unhappy conditions can only be equalized when the educational chairs are filled with men whose education itself has been most strictly scientific, and when the students themselves have a similar exact foundation before entering the school.

"This has been well seen by the veterinary profession, as is illustrated by the following resolutions, drafted at the late Veterinary Congress at Frankfort":

I. With reference to the preparatory education of the German veterinarians:

"The same conditions must be exacted of students entering upon the study of veterinary medicine, as of those entering upon the study of medicine or special natural sciences."

II. With reference to the professional education of German veterinarians:

"1. To gain a good general knowledge of the elements of their profession, a four-year course is necessary and sufficient."

"2. The veterinary school must be an integral yet independent branch of the universities."

The immense importance of the last resolution can not be overestimated. The intimate relation which our domestic animals bear to human health; the value of the studies of comparative anatomy and physiology; the immense importance of the knowledge of general pathology and comparative pathological anatomy, are all things which have not yet had their due degree of appreciation.

Further, the value of such a union in lessening the expenses of veterinary institutions should by no means fail of earnest consideration. The natural sciences can be heard by the students of both branches of medicine in common, thereby doing away with the necessity of quite a number of special teachers at a veterinary school. Such a union is only practicable, however, at universities situated in large cities, for otherwise it would be impossible to fill the veterinary hospitals with the large number of animals necessary for the students to gain practical knowledge and dexterity.

THE VETERINARY INSTITUTIONS OF PRUSSIA.

THE purpose of these sketches of some of the veterinary schools of the Continent is to afford, if possible, the American people some idea of the causes which led to their foundation, and of their weaknesses as well as their many good points. While I have entered into details, as far as the means at my command offered me opportunity, of those of France and Austria, I have reserved those of Prussia to the last, in order to notice them more in detail: first, because many of the regulations which we shall at present consider are more or less common to the German Empire; and, second, because, taken as a whole, I believe these institutions better capable of serving as a model for us to follow after, with necessary modifications according to our peculiar conditions, than those of any other country. I do not claim for them perfection, as some people seem to think, nor do I desire to ingraft them wholesale and inconsiderately upon the institutions of this country, as some ignorant persons have affirmed.

THE VETERINARY INSTITUTE AT BERLIN.

This school covers, so far as I am aware, the largest tract of land of any of the European veterinary schools. It is situated on Louisen-strasse, opposite the noted Charité Hospital, and occupies some six acres of ground. It was founded in 1786, but was not opened until 1790. The causes which led to its foundation were the losses which the nation had repeatedly suffered from devastating animal pests, especially the cattle-plague, against which every endeavor of the state had been utterly powerless. In the address, previously given, from Professor Feser, of Munich, we have shown the part which Cothenius took in the matter, although the idea undoubtedly originated in the mind of the king, Frederick the Great; the school was organized, however, under his successor, Frederick William II. The school has been under the supervision of different officers of the Government, being at first controlled by the chief official of the royal stables, Graf Lindenau; in 1817 it was transferred to the Ministers of War and the Interior; in 1847 to the Minister of the Medical Institutions, etc., and finally, in 1872, to the Minister of Agriculture, where it still remains. The instruction at the school was at first very elementary, its purpose being to educate young farriers, quite in contradiction to the express purposes for which the school was supposed to be founded. Professors Neumann and Sick conducted the instruction, the first having been sent to Alfort, the latter to Vienna, to study veterinary medicine at the expense of the

Government. An apothecary, Ratzeburg, lectured upon materia medica, etc. The course extended over three years, the education having an essentially practical tendency, and, as Feser says, the scientific ideas of Cothenius seem to have fallen on barren ground here at Berlin as well as elsewhere in Germany. Few changes took place previous to 1817, when complaints began to make themselves unpleasantly common with reference to the total insufficiency of the school to the needs of the country, the graduates being nothing more nor less than somewhat better schooled empirics than the raw material which had preceded them. William von Humboldt, Minister of State to Frederick William II, and brother to the great naturalist, seems to have been well aware of these deficiencies, and to have proposed a plan which, if it had been carried out, would have placed this institution at an early day much further ahead than it even now is as a useful adjunct of the state: he proposed to unite it to the university; but, alas! the "*horsey* element" prevailed, and his advice was passed heedlessly by through the opposition of the Head-Master of the Royal Horse, Von Jagow. Other untoward influences were also exerted by the great naturalist Rudolphi, who afterward became director; it is said that he desired to use the school as a means of enriching the collections in the museum of the university; on the other hand, Thaer, the father of modern agriculture in Germany, used an influence in that direction, so that these, and probably other things, combined to nullify the sound ideas of a statesman like Von Humboldt.

Nevertheless, the discussion was not without benefit, for a revision followed and many improvements were introduced, among them the attachment to the school of one of the most important personages in connection with its history—Dr. Gurlt, afterward director. Gurlt was a scientist *par excellence*—a man wholly bound up in study, investigations, and in making collections for the museum. The school gained great fame from his presence, but the benefits he conferred upon it were not so much due to his powers as a teacher as they were to his literary productions and the magnificence and great number of his scientific collections. I believe I do not exaggerate in saying that Gurlt was in reality the founder of all our veterinary anatomy of the present day; he certainly introduced the true nomenclature of comparative anatomy, and more than any other man established the relation of given muscles in the domestic animals to those of man. He was also the chief worker in the field of the periodic development of the fœtus in animals, as well as that of the monstrosities, and his collection of animal parasites in the museum of the school is probably greater than those of any three schools combined. He also gave us the first book of zoopathological anatomy, which has only been followed by Brückmüller. His last work, on animal monstrosities, issued when he was nearly ninety years old, is an ornament to the profession, although Gurlt's only connection with the school was as teacher and director, he being an M. D. He gave as the number of anatomical specimens in the museum of the school in 1869—6,408, which were mostly collected by him, and mounted under his supervision; this number has been steadily increasing under his able successor in pathology, Professor Schutz, so that, although I have not the catalogue number, there must be at present in the museum some eight to ten thousand specimens. His collection of fetal specimens, illustrating their periodical development, is one of the ornaments of the school.

In 1823 another M. D., Hertwig, was attached to the school after studying veterinary medicine at the most prominent institutions of the world at the expense of the Government. It was these two men who raised this school to the high degree of renown which it enjoyed up to about 1850. Hertwig has been one of the greatest contributors to veterinary literature that has ever lived; he is a contemporary of Hering, Haubner, and, of course, Gurlt, who with Spinola, as practical author, served to make the German name so famous in the middle of this century. His studies of rabies, supported by numerous experiments, opened a new light upon the subject, and have never been much improved upon; these, with other contributions to canine pathology, in unison with those of Gerlach and Fürstenberg, have served to make up about all there is, or has been written upon the diseases of the dog, other than a few practical hints gained from experience. His work on materia medica was not excelled by any in human medicine in its day, and is founded largely on personal experiments. His surgery and work on operations are by no means antiquated. As the years increased with these men, the school slowly passed into decline; its wonted activity was no more, but no want is felt long in this world before the right man is found to fill it. Leisering most beautifully pictures this condition in his obituary notice of Gerlach, who was called from Hanover to fill this place: "Slower and slower went the machine, which was chiefly to be sought in the increasing years of her once active men, who were no more able to keep pace with the rapid march of science, and who also nourished the opinion that new things are not always the best. But the machine moved again with new fire, partly with permanent and partly with transient powers, for as well-organized a body as the Berlin school had been since Langermann's time does not so easily come to a complete stand-still; but that such an evil condition should not really occur a new fireman was necessary—and he came. He made fresh fire, and we soon saw the glistening sparks." As Gerlach was, in my opinion, the most important character, the most original genius that has ever appeared on the German veterinary arena, if not of the world, I may be pardoned a short sketch of his life. I do this the more willingly, as the memory of this man still waits due appreciation in his native land, probably because of the intense severity with which he sought to instill into drones the grand fire by which he himself was impelled to sacrifice life, health, and friendship for the good of his profession and country.

Andreas Christian Gerlach was born at Wedderstedt, in the Harz Mountains, the 15th of May, 1811. His parents were honest peasants, but had little means. His early education was received at the hands of some childless relations who resided near Halberstadt, who soon learned to love the pale, earnest boy as their own child. The child saw one day an old veterinarian in the village busied about some animals, which greatly excited his interest. He followed the old man from stable to stable, from patient to patient, and only returned late at night to the friends who had adopted him. This childhood's experience seems to have determined his future destiny. After his confirmation, his adopted parents sent him to Halberstadt to school, without, however, having sufficient means to cover his expenses. Here began a time which indeed proved the stuff the boy was made of, and which developed in him that character which drew little love toward the man in later years, but which enabled him to overcome obstacles and trample under foot an opposition as bitter as any man ever had to combat. He had first to prepare for his entrance into the gymnasium, and lived in the family of a poor artisan, who kindly gave him food. He sought with great perseverance the company of students in the higher classes, hoping to improve his knowledge thereby. Leisering, from whom the above remarks are taken, says: "A doctor, with whom he is acquainted, who lived at Halberstadt at this time, told him some years back, after Gerlach had already become a noted man, that it was not without much feeling that he recollected how the boy Gerlach had come to him in his peasant clothing and begged, with his eyes filled with tears, that he would give him free instruction in Latin. . . . He finally completed his school-days at Halberstadt, after enduring untold hardships and a continued battle for the food necessary to support life; but he had attained his end, and acquired the necessary knowledge for admittance to a veterinary school." He gained this knowledge at great cost, and therefore highly appreciated diligence in others. He was ever an advocate of higher education for veterinarians; ever on the side which tended to the advancement of his profession; from first to last he was a scientist and a student. He graduated from Berlin in 1833, and until 1844 practiced his profession at the place of his nativity in Saxony. He there published a pamphlet upon "Anthrax in Sheep," which soon attracted the attention of the Government, and led to his being called to Berlin, first as assistant and then as teacher. In 1859 he received the honorable appointment of Director of the Veterinary School at Hanover, which he came near losing, however, as he placed as absolute condition to his acceptance that he should have the title of "professor," which had never before been given to a veterinarian, and which in North Germany does not mean, as it does in these glorious and free United States of America, anything from a genuine man of genius at a university down to a shoeblack, dealer in old clothes, or vender of quack medicines. His promotion to professor was soon followed by that to privy medical councilor. "He was in Prussia not alone the first veterinarian who received the direction of the veterinary school (previously it had always been given to medical men of note), but also the first veterinarian who, without being also an M. D., received the titles 'medical' and 'privy medical councilor.'" Between 1859 and 1870 were made the greater part of those original researches, which have gained acceptance not only in veterinary but human medicine. He was the first to obstinately deny the abiogenesis (self-development) of glanders. To his investigations is also owing the excitement with reference to the transmissibility to human beings of the tuberculosis of cattle. To the extreme obstinacy with which he defended these opinions is due much of the opposition which he received from the profession. In 1870 he became director of the school at Berlin, and began, or rather went on, developing the work of his life—the further introduction of the scientific method into veterinary instruction. So far as the future of the profession in Germany is concerned, I think that Gerlach's last act was by far his greatest—that is, the introduction of a specialist as physiologist to the school, and the erection of a proper laboratory and experiment station. I myself lived through this, and no one better knows the bitter opposition which conservatism and selfishness put in the way of the purposes of this man, whose only desire was to improve the school and serve well his country.

Gerlach was said to be a very one-sided man by those who felt the power of his opposition; but this was only true in so far as it had reference to a man who was bending everything for the success of an ideal object. He was an idealist of the truest type. His entire character is expressed in the saying, "Be sure you are right, then go ahead." He was a hard and exact student of his position and responsibilities, and tried his best to fulfill them. He was not generous, as the world calls it, to the opinions of others. In persons occupying such positions, generosity, which in general society becomes a virtue, is nothing but a weakness. Gerlach was externally cold and autocratic, with the handsomest and cleanest-cut face I ever saw; but behind all this coldness was a heart warm and generous, which went out to the hard-working student with almost a mother's love. He paid but little attention to the opinions of others, seldom consulted with the other professors, but, like a king among men and like a Prussian as he was, ruled the school with an iron hand so far as his powers would permit. Naturally, men lacking ambition, in whom the sparks of science found no fitting material to ignite, felt ill at ease with such a man, and he felt discontented with them; hence, during his whole administration of the school there was a healthy excitement kept up between these two opposing forces. But, had Gerlach lived ten years longer, there is no doubt who would have won. He died at sixty-six years of age, at Berlin, August 29, 1877, of cancer of the stomach.

Gerlach died ten years too soon. At present, at the Berlin school, the practical education bears no proper relation to the scientific. The teachers are too bitterly opposed to one another, the one set being purely scientific, the other representing the scholastic-empiric school of which Feser speaks, which ruled absolutely until after the middle of the century. The German Government showed itself unequal to the occasion when Gerlach died. The manner of appointing professors, so far as the veterinary school is concerned, is not so just or good in Germany as in France. It is based too much upon literary reputation, without taking into consideration that ability to teach well, which is as necessary as extensive knowledge. Another great evil in Germany, which all countries share more or less, is fear of a young man. Other things being equal, the experiences of years have value, but men of genius often gain more experience in a few years than the average man does in a lifetime. The moment a man ceases to be progressive he is of little use to the world. In appointing a new director at the school, there was fully as much political wire-pulling as is exercised by candidates for mayor or governor in this country, and this in Germany, where Americanism is sneered at. There was this difference, the wire-pulling was done by men of unquestionable ability in some directions, but neither one of the candidates was fitted to carry on the work of progress. They were all good men, but unfortunately had too much of the old school about them to meet the demands of the time. The Government seemed to be entirely ignorant of the great failing of the school, which is the surgical clinic, and everything pertaining to it. An utter want of practical horsemanship runs through the whole thing. The treatment of internal diseases leaves nothing to be desired, but the external treatment, in many cases, may be truly expressed by the English word "botch." There had never been any real practical surgery taught at the school. A great many operations are made, but seldom handsomely. The opportunity to reform all this was placed at the disposal of the German Government. But there was no one to inform it, and how should the ministers know? The opportunity was there to reform the surgical clinic, but, what is still more to the point, the man was there also. Dr. —— knew that a school hospital is for the purpose of instructing students, and that the curing of patients, so long as the interests of the owner are respected, is a matter of secondary importance. The death-rate was perhaps a little large, but the number of recoveries in desperate cases more than counterbalanced it. Our clinical instruction was really magnificent. He knew, better than any one at the school, its greatest failure, and studied night and day as to the best means of overcoming it. One great mistake and waste of material at the Bèrlin school, one which clearly demonstrates that from the beginning the aim of education in a given direction was never understood (it is the same at the French school), is the way in which the students practice operative surgery. *It is plain butchery, not surgery.* What sense is there in merely cutting certain nerves, opening certain cavities, ligaturing an artery or two, upon a living animal, though it be chloroformed? The students learn *to cut, not to operate.* Is cutting the whole of surgery? In human medicine they learn *to cut* upon the cadaver, and it can be done equally well in veterinary medicine. But I none the less believe in taking advantage of our ability of practicing operative surgery upon the living animal in veterinary medicine, *when chloroformed.* But if this is limited to mere cutting, it is but butchery. *To be practical,* the necessary number of horses should be procured by the school, properly groomed and fed; the students to operate should be selected; they should be privileged to select their assistants from their colleagues; then they should deliver a lecture before the class as to the operation, its history, and ways of performing it, the reasons for its performance in practice, the teacher correcting or suggesting as the student proceeds. One such operation, and sometimes more, should be done daily throughout the year. The cutting exercise can be under the guidance of an anatomical assistant on the cadaver. These operations should be performed according to the strictest rules of surgery, and the different forms of treatment experimented with; the student operating should receive the animal operated upon as a patient, and treat him in the hospital as such; the wounds should be bound up, the same as in practice, and every endeavor should be made to improve the methods. All other operative surgery, either as practiced at Berlin or in France, is a "botch" and humbug, cruel to animals and degrading to the profession; but the above plan is dignified with a scientific purpose; it may serve two ends at the same time—properly exercise the student, and serve as an experiment by which general surgery may be benefited, and some new method find proof or contradiction. It is in unison with the true purpose of a school, the perfect union of theory and practice, which makes up the science of medicine.

Were this the only error of the Government in the management of this school, it would be fortunate indeed. But, not satisfied with making an error in one direction, they must equal it in another. At the school was a young man of marked genius, of genuine scientific spirit, who was ranked as prosector in anatomy, the only trouble being that he knew too much, and was not to be brought into the scholastic-empiric leading-strings. The non-progressive tricksters, unable to control, resolved to get rid of him. As in England incumbrancers have often been confined in lunatic asylums, or great men banished by imbecile governments, so they sought to send him to the Russian frontier to watch the rinderpest. A man of science to act as an ordinary policeman! was ever anything more ridiculous? Fortunately, other powers existed. Instead of banishment to the Russian frontier, our young assistant received government aid to pursue the study of comparative anatomy under Gegenbauer and Waldeyer. He was the man above all others to take Gurlt's place in veterinary anatomy; ay, more! he recognized the practical needs, and his lectures were models of scientific foundation applied to practical ends. One would think that such a man could not fail of appreciation; but such was not the case. He received a call to Dresden, and the Prussian Government, blind to its own interests, the direction of the school false to its duties to the profession, quietly let him go.

The Buildings.

As one approaches the school from "Louisen-strasse," he is struck at once by the imposing building which marks the entrance, and serves as a residence for most of the teachers. The front wall of that part of the building, which serves as entrance to the grounds in the rear, is embellished with busts of Aristotle, Absyrtus, Ramazzini, Lancisi, Lafosse, Pessina, Bourgelat, Kersting, Cothenius, Langermann, Wollstein, and Abildgaard, men intimately connected with the birth of veterinary science. The accommodations for the residences of the teachers are liberal in the extreme, and in many respects the suites are really magnificent. In this building are three lecture-rooms, and one for chemistry and physics, with appropriate cabinets. The fine library, of some ten thousand volumes, especially rich in valuable historical works, is situated in this building. The students are allowed to take books home and to keep them a reasonable length of time. On passing through the corridor of this building, the fine grounds of the institution, with their winding walks and grand shade-trees, make a most pleasing impression upon the visitor.

The anatomy building and museum is, strange to say, almost spoiled, so far as appearances are concerned, by being situated in a hollow, when sufficient commanding ground was and is to be had to show the truly fine architectural proportions of the building. It was drafted by the celebrated architect Langhans, and the main portion, which was built under his direction, is frequently pointed out as an example of his genius. In the basement is the dissection-room, with accommodation for two hundred students. Like many older German buildings, it is miserably ventilated, but it would be well lighted were it not for its abominable situation. The anatomical lecture-room, which is also used for the same purpose by the physiologist and pathologist, is without doubt the finest of its kind at any school. It can seat some three hundred students, the seats being arranged in an amphitheatre, the entrance being in the center; it is lighted entirely from above. The preparations are elevated upon a table from the room below.

The Physiological and Pathological Institutes, two fine buildings, costing with their appointments some $50,000, are something which no other veterinary school has in the world.

In the Anatomical Institute is situated also the microscopical laboratory, with microscopes for the class, and every convenience for work in this branch of study.

As we turn to go toward the horse hospital we pass that for dogs, with accommodations for about fifty, and fitted up with a small laboratory for chemical and microscopical examinations. The attendant resides in the building. The dog practice is very large at Berlin; one good feature is, that if a dog bites any one in the city, he can report it to the police, and the owner *must* bring the dog here to be watched for the requisite number of days with reference to rabies.

The horse hospital has room for about one hundred and thirty patients, many of the stalls being boxes; the stables surround a court, in which the free clinic is held. A new and handsome stable was added during Gerlach's direction. In this stable is the laboratory for clinical examination. The stables are fine and clean, but they need the genius of an English or American head groom to make them what they really should be. The fees for patients taken into the hospital are in general fifty cents per day, which includes every expense; operations are all performed free of charge. There is a special department for animals affected with contagious diseases, or in which the same are suspected; another for forensic cases, for which a fee is asked in addition, as well as for the exact examination of horses. In both cases a warrant is given, and the questionable animal must remain at least three days, during which time it is tested in every possible manner. Casual examinations cost nothing, but no warrant is given. There are also special stalls for animals with cerebral troubles, so that they can not injure themselves, so far as it is possible to prevent it. There are two large halls for operations. There is also a cow-stable, holding some forty head, besides sheep, goats, swine, rabbits, etc., which are to be used for experimental purposes. The servants of the school live in buildings on one side of the court. At one entrance of this inclosure is the pharmacy, treasury, and some teachers' and assistants' residences. The patients in the open clinic receive advice free, but pay for medicines prescribed at the regular price of the drugs, without the cost of preparation at the pharmacy. The students prepare all medicines, under the guidance of the assistant to the teacher of chemistry. The patients in the hospitals are divided equally among the senior students, each of whom directs and looks out for them as if in actual practice, being guided and questioned by the teachers. Each day the students hear a special lecture upon some selected patient, illustrating some special phase in the progress of certain diseases. From the large amount of material at command, the teacher is enabled to follow a certain course in these clinical talks.

Practice and lectures upon auscultation and percussion form a very strong point in the clinical instruction. There are, during the last half year of a graduating class, two classes of students in the hospital, those of the lower acting as assistants to their seniors. On the graduation of the latter, the others then have a full year to themselves, when the same course is again pursued. Everything necessary to absolutely perfect instruction is present at this school, the guiding genius to set things in the right direction being alone needed.

The following statistics will give some idea of the practical discipline which this school offers to its students, and which is not equaled by any other in the world.

In 1875 the following animals were received in the hospital, or treated elsewhere by the students:

In the clinic, 2,333 horses, 2 cattle, 2 sheep, 3 swine—2,340.

In the dog-clinic (dogs, cats, etc., mostly dogs)—3,368.

In the free clinic, 4,459 horses, 5 goats, 2 swine—4,466.

Visiting clinic,* 268 cattle, 49 sheep, 11 goats, 191 swine—519. Grand total, 10,693 animals.

The number of herds also visited was thirty.

The number of surgical operations performed at the school was 542.

In 1876 the number of patients taken into the clinic, or visited, was 11,537.

In one of the stables is the forge of the school.

The expenses of this institution, from the first quarter of 1878 to the end of the first quarter of 1879, were 157,670 marks, or $39,-417.50; derived as follows:

From the hospital and students' fees............	91,190 marks,† or	$22,797 50
" " state funds.........................	66,480 " "	16,620 00
Total..		$39,417 50

The money granted by the state is more or less, according to the needs of the institution; and we see that, during this year, when but little building was carried on, the expenses of the school exceeded the income by over $16,000.

All the teachers of the institution, as well as other officials and servants, have free residence found them. All the professors and

* The institution has four horses, and suitable vehicles for this purpose, and such visits are made daily, four students at a time going with a certain teacher.

† A mark is a quarter of a dollar.

teachers have a fluctuating income of from 500 to 600 marks ($125 to $150) per year, from the examination fees of the students.

The salaries of the teachers are as follows:

1. Privy Councilor and Director Roloff, 7,800 marks, or $1,950.
2. Professor Müller, anatomist, 5,100 marks, or $1,775.
3. Professor Schütz, pathologist, 3,900 marks, or $975.
4. Professor Munk, physiologist, 3,600 marks, or $900.
5. Professor Pinner, chemist, 3,600 marks, or $900.
6. Professor Dierkerhoff, special pathology, history, and clinic, 3,300 marks, or $825.
7. Professor Dr. Moeller, materia medica, etc., and dog-clinic, 3,000 marks, or $750.

Teacher, Mr. Eggeling, surgery, etc., 1,800 marks, or $450.

All the professors have besides additional incomes from positions held by them on the National Board of Health, or on the Veterinary Department of Prussia, or as lecturers at the University or Agricultural Academy, or as inspectors in the province of Brandenburg, or for a district in the neighborhood of Berlin.

There are a number of resident assistants, who receive each 1,200 to 1,500 marks, a portion of the examination-fees, and furnished lodgings, fuel, gas, service, etc. Aside from these, professors 2, 3, 4, 5, 6, 7, have each a junior assistant, being young graduates who have received their diplomas the year before. These assistants receive a stipend (granted for the half-year, but generally renewed for two to three half-years) of from 500 to 600 marks for each session, being from 1,000 to 1,200 marks per year. Two of these assistants have free lodgings at the school. The Professor of Chemistry has a special assistant, who receives 1,800 marks yearly.

Other Officials.

1. Two secretaries, with salaries of 3,300 and 2,100 marks each.
2. A treasurer, with a salary of 3,000 marks.
3. An inspector, who superintends the servants, with a salary of 2,400 marks.
4. A messenger, with a salary of 1,000 marks. *All these persons are royal officers, and are appointed for life, and can only be dismissed by verdict of the Court of Discipline.*
5. A gardener, with a salary of 1,000 marks, who holds his office by a contract with the directors.

Servants.—There are fourteen servants for the stables, the Anatomical and Physiological Institutes, and the pharmacy, receiving each from 60 to 75 marks per month. Also four women who do the cleaning, with from 18 to 24 marks' pay per month. They all live upon the grounds.

The Students.

The students are divided into two classes, military and civil, to which may be added certain "hospitants," who are agriculturists, graduates of other schools, foreigners, or other persons desiring to hear certain lectures.

The military students form by far the greater majority, and reside in a fine barracks, just outside the school-grounds, and opposite the military school for horseshoeing, in which they all have to study, and serve six months in practice, and pass an examination, before they can enter the veterinary institution. They do not dress in uniform, except at certain hours each week, or when called upon to appear on dress parade. Each class has a superior army veterinarian over them, who is responsible for their attention to their studies, and attendance at the lectures, and who questions them weekly in order to keep posted as to their progress. Students who are inattentive to duty are warned, examined, and, if their ill-conduct is persisted in, are turned over to the army to serve out their time as soldiers. This may take place at any time during the student's course, even after he has failed in the second final examination, unless he may have already served his appointed time in the army. Their general conduct is subject to the control of an army officer, and they are kept under very strict discipline, being sometimes punished with confinement. The Government supplies them with a small amount of pocket-money—30 marks per month, I believe—besides the necessary books, instruments, fuel, attendance, etc.; in addition to which their building has lately been supplied with a very complete medical library, costing some $1,500, so that the army students have not to go out of their building if they desire to read up any special subject, either in human or veterinary medicine. Each military graduate must serve two years in the army, as an army veterinary surgeon, for each year's schooling. Their pay is not large, nor do they rank so high, or receive the consideration which similar officers do in other armies, especially in the English, but their expenses are also smaller. They have the privilege, however, of studying, and enjoying a stipend by which they can again visit the school, and hear lectures and make the examinations for the high civil positions, so that on completion of their army service they can immediately apply for any vacancies which may occur. This privilege is only granted to those who have passed the first two grades in the examination; those having the best can undergo these examinations in two years, the next in three, respectively. I can not give the number of students at the Berlin school, but it is not far from two hundred. A private letter informs me that there are to be one hundred and twenty-five in the dissecting-room in the study of anatomy this winter. The fees are very small; for the three years I was there as a student, and the extra year, including the examination-fee, they were not over one hundred dollars. All material necessary for study is supplied by the Government free of expense to the students, including the use of the microscopes.

The course of study and terms of examination are the same for all the schools in the empire, and were revised and published March 27, 1878. I consider they can well serve as a model for the foundation of a school in this country, with but few modifications. There is no matriculation examination for foreigners, but they must stand the regular examination without change or favor. There is no need of a matriculatory examination for Germans, as they are only taken from classes of certain public schools, and the standard is fixed much higher than in nearly all other Continental schools. The school at Berlin will not, however, be what it should be until it is united with the university, which will give it a greater number of special instructors in the natural sciences, at but little extra expense to the Government.

The following are the regulations for the admittance and examination of the students, and are taken from the "Central-Blatt für das Deutsche Reich," herausgegeben in Reichskanzler-Amt, April 5, 1878:

I. *Central powers which can give the diploma to veterinarians:*

The diploma for veterinarians for the German Empire can only be given by the central powers ("Centralbehörden") of such states of the empire in which one or more veterinary schools are situated; consequently, at the present time, by the appropriate ministers of Prussia, Bavaria, Saxony, Würtemberg, and Hesse. (There is no independent school in Hesse, but the university at Giessen has a veterinary department.)

II. *Regulations with reference to the qualifications of candidates:*

The veterinary diploma is only to be given to such candidates as have satisfactorily stood the fixed examination.

The examination is divided into *two parts:* 1. In the natural sciences; and, 2. In the technical branches of study.

The examination must take place at a German veterinary institute.

The examining body consists of the directors and teachers of the institute, with such persons as shall be ordered to be present by the appropriate minister.

The composition of the examining commissions in the different sections of the examination is regulated by the ministers.

The director conducts the whole examination.

The Examination in the Natural Sciences.—1. Conditions for competing. The candidate must testify:

(*a.*) That he has had the requisite education. He must have the proper certificate of having been prepared to enter the first class ("prima") of a gymnasium, or of a first class "real" school, in which the study of Latin has been obligatory, or of such an educational institute as is recognized by the Government as of equal standing with the above.

(*b.*) After having acquired the requisite scientific preparatory education, he must have studied for three sessions (one and a half year) at a veterinary or other high scientific school of the German Empire.

The period for the examination in the natural sciences, as well as the notification of the candidate of his fitness to take part in it, is arranged by the directors of the respective schools.

The notification of readiness to participate in the examinations, and the certificate of his having fulfilled the above conditions, must be handed by the candidate to the directors and indorsed by him. (The schools have especial forms for this purpose, on which each teacher testifies to the regular attendance of the students at the respective lectures and demonstrations.)

The following are the branches in which the candidates are to be examined: Zoötomy, inclusive of histology, physiology, botany, chemistry, physics, and zoölogy.

The examination is oral, and public. Its aim is to ascertain if the candidate has obtained sufficient knowledge in the above scientific branches to warrant his proceeding with the study of the strictly professional ones.

Only four candidates can be examined at one time.

The examining commission consists of the director as chairman, and at least three associates.

A complete account is kept of the progress of the examination by each candidate in each section of the examination.

The examination in chemistry and physics, the "tentamen physicum" of the medical examination, or the pharmaceutical examination, may be taken as an equivalent to the above examination in the same branches at a veterinary school.

The results of the examination are to be indicated as follows:

A judgment is to be given on the results of the examination in each of the above branches. The judgments are as follows: "Sehr gut" (excellent), "gut" (good), "genügend" (satisfactory), "ungenügend" (unsatisfactory), and "schlecht" (bad).

The judgment in each branch is to be given by vote of the examining commission. In a tie-vote, that of the director (chairman) decides.

The candidate has passed his examination when he has at least received the judgment "satisfactory" in each individual branch.

The conclusive judgment "excellent" can only be given when the candidate has passed in the majority of the branches as "excellent," and in the remainder as "good."

The conclusive judgment "good" can only be given when he has passed in the greater number as "good," and in the remainder as "satisfactory."

The conclusive judgment "satisfactory" can only be given when he has passed in the majority as "satisfactory," and in no branch as "unsatisfactory."

The conclusive judgment "unsatisfactory" is given when the candidate has not passed in each branch with "satisfactory."

If the candidate has received the judgment "unsatisfactory" in more than two branches, or as "bad" in more than *one*, or in one as "bad" and another as "unsatisfactory," he can only receive the conclusive judgment of "bad."

Repetition of the Examination.—When the candidate has received the conclusive judgment of "unsatisfactory," he may be allowed a second examination at the expiration of three months; it is only extended to those branches in which the candidate has received the judgment of "unsatisfactory" or "bad."

When he has received the conclusive judgment of "bad," a second examination can only be permitted him at the end of one year, and is to be extended over all the above-named branches. A second repetition of the examination can only be allowed a candidate with the consent of the minister.

The Expense of the Examination.—For the first examination, twenty marks ($5); for a repetition of the same, ten marks ($2.50) more.

The Technical Examination.—For admittance to this examination the candidate must present his certificate of having successfully passed the examination in natural sciences; and, secondly, he must bring a certificate of having attended lectures for seven sessions at a German veterinary institute, or other German academy, and have heard lectures on the succeeding subjects, which must be testified to by the appropriate teachers: Zoötomy and histology, inclusive of practical study in both branches; physiology; botany (anatomy and physiology of plants, classification, and practice in determination of species; the Berlin school has a special professor of botany from the university); chemistry, inorganic and organic, with practical exercises; physics; zoölogy; general pathology and therapeutics; materia medica; toxicology; pharmacology, with practice; pathological anatomy, with necroscopical practice and attendance at the demonstrations; special pathology and therapeutics; surgery and aciurgy; theory and practice of horseshoeing; dietetics; breeding; obstetrics; exterior of domestic animals; veterinary police; hygiene; forensic medicine; history of veterinary medicine; clinical attendance, with practice; and visiting clinic.

Notification of the Examination.—The period for the notification, as well as for holding this examination, is fixed by the director, with the consent of the minister. The notification must be accompanied with the proper attests from the teachers of attendance at the lectures upon the above subjects, and a short description of the principal events of the candidate's life.

The director fixes the period for the examination in the different branches.

Sections of the Examination, and the Regulations for the same.—The examination is public, and is subdivided into the following sections: 1. In anatomy, physiology, and pathological anatomy; 2. In the medicinal clinic; in the surgical clinic; in operative surgery; in pharmacology (practical and theoretical); 3. The conclusion.

The examinations in the different sections follow in immediate succession.

No candidate can enter upon an examination in a section until he has passed in the previous one.

In the examinations in anatomy, physiology, and pathological anatomy, the candidate has to follow the following course: 1. To demonstrate and open one of the cavities of the body in the presence of the examining body; 2. To explain an osteological and syndesmological preparation; 3. To demonstrate and prepare an anatomical preparation; 4. To prepare and explain histological preparations in the presence of the teacher; 5. To give an oral dissertation upon a physiological subject; 6. To make an autopsy of a diseased animal, or one of the cavities of the same, or to demonstrate a pathological specimen, and in both cases to reduce the results to writing; further, to prepare and demonstrate pathological specimens with the microscope.

The tasks in anatomy and physiology are given to the student by lot. The commission for this examination consists of three members.

In the clinical examination the candidate has—1. To examine an animal having an internal disease, and to make the diagnosis and direct its treatment for three successive days; 2. The same with an animal having some surgical disease.

In both cases the candidate is isolated, and has to prepare a written history of his patients and their diseases, their pathology, treatment, and the probable results of the case.

The oral examination takes place in each case after the written descriptions have been handed in. The candidate must prepare the medicines exhibited to the patients.

The candidate has, further, to perform, demonstrate, and explain three surgical operations upon a living animal; also, to demonstrate two fresh or dried officinal vegetable preparations, as well as to recognize two chemical-pharmaceutical preparations, give their elements, formula, etc.; also, to stand an examination in materia medica, toxicology, etc.

The operations, as well as the above-named medicinal objects, are selected by the students by lot. The examining body in each branch consists of two members.

The conclusive examination can extend over all branches of study, so far as they have not been the object of special examinations in the above sections.

Only four candidates can be examined at one time, which must take place under the supervision of the director and at least three other members. Each member of the commission must occupy at least ten to fifteen minutes with each candidate.

A special written report must be made with reference to the examination of each candidate in each branch, and indorsed by each member of the commission.

The judgments are given in the same manner as before. The repetition must take place in the next year, and may extend itself to all branches of study.

A second repetition of the examination can only take place with the consent of the minister. The written part of the examination and the written attests of the examining commission must be placed before the minister for approval. The costs of this second examination are sixty marks ($15), and the repetitions fifteen marks each.

If a candidate retires from the examination, a proportionate part of the fees for the sections he has not been examined in will be returned.

(The fees for the examination of the military students are paid by the war department.)

Conclusive Judgment.—This is given after the examination in all the sections has taken place. It is given by vote, and is influenced by the judgments obtained in the sectional examinations.

The judgments are the same as for the sectional examinations.

The chancellor of the empire is empowered to absolve a candidate from single conditions of the examination upon reasonable grounds.

The names of the graduates are published in the official organ, from which these regulations are taken.

The military students are absolved from the examination in horseshoeing, having passed it before entering the school.

The course is extended over seven sessions (three years and a half), and, as the military students must first serve for six months in the military school for farriers, their course of study is in reality extended over four years.

The course of study at the veterinary schools of Germany is as follows:

First Session (*Winter*).—Introduction to the study of veterinary medicine; physics; inorganic chemistry; general zoölogy; zoötomy; dissection.

Second Session (*Summer*).—Organic chemistry; botany; zoölogy of the vertebrata; histology and embryology; physiology (1); chemical practice in the laboratory; practical histology.

Third Session (*Winter*).—Physiology (2); exterior of the domestic animals; breeding; dissection in anatomy; lectures; practice in the pharmacy; repetition of lectures in chemistry and physics.

Fourth Session (*Summer*).—General pathology and therapeutics; pharmacognosy; pharmacology, toxicology, and practice in the art of writing and combining prescriptions; practice in pharmacy; horseshoeing.

Fifth Session (*Winter*).—Special pathological anatomy; special pathology and therapeutics; special surgery; operative surgery, with practice; clinic for large animals; clinic for small animals.

Sixth Session (*Summer*).—Dietetics; obstetrics; animal pests, veterinary police; microscopical practice in pathological anatomy; clinics; visiting clinic.

Seventh Session (*Winter*).—Forensic medicine; history of veterinary medicine; clinics; visiting clinic; practice in writing legal papers with reference to veterinary police and forensic medicine; repetitions in anatomy and physiology.

There is room left for an eighth session in the schedule, which it is to be hoped will be soon added to the curriculum.

THE PRUSSIAN LAWS AND REGULATIONS FOR THE SUPPRESSION OF CONTAGIOUS ANIMAL DISEASES.

The first attempt at the organization of a veterinary police, and drafting regulations for the suppression of contagious animal diseases in Prussia, dates back to 1803. It has been the object of constant improvement, and it seems that a translation of the principal parts of these laws can not be without value to the people of this country. We have nothing in a condensed form to which our legislators can refer when drafting regulations for the *suppression* and *prevention* of contagious animal diseases; and as these questions are sooner or later to take no insignificant part in national legislation, their appearance here is justified.

The supreme supervision of the veterinary institutions of Prussia rests with the Minister of Agriculture, who is assisted by a resident director, and a board of assistants, composed of lawyers and eminent agriculturists. In addition to this there is a veterinary council, the duty of which is to give the decisive opinion with reference to all technical points in relation to veterinary questions. The active members are selected from the teachers at the veterinary school and the department veterinarian of Berlin, with Professor Virchow and other eminent medical counsel.

In Prussia there were (1879) 36 department veterinarians, 12 so-called veterinary assessors, who rank higher than the above, 16 frontier veterinarians, and 407 district veterinarians. These officers have fixed remuneration for their official work, and their traveling expenses; with the exception of the frontier veterinarians, they are almost all permitted to practice; the latter receive about $800 per year, and enjoy no very enviable positions, from the difficulties and exposures, as well as the comparative isolation of their positions. Each district is further supervised by an "imperial president." The department veterinarians are named by the minister, with the advice of the council, from among those district veterinarians who have especially distinguished themselves in the execution of their duties; the latter have to pass special and severe examinations, both oral and written, with reference to the duties required of them at the veterinary school: those graduates who have received the two highest judgments, "very good" and "good" as students, are allowed to present themselves for examination as district veterinarians in two and three years, respectively, from the time of their qualification as veterinarians.

Attached to the German army as veterinarians are 14 corps and 523 other veterinarians; of the latter, each horse regiment has a superior veterinarian ("Oberrossarzt"), the others being subject to him. The number of civil veterinarians in Prussia (1875) was 1,296; the territory over which they were each estimated to exercise control was 4·75 square geographical miles, and the number of animals over which they each were estimated to watch was 1,544 horses, 4,592 cattle, 14,421 sheep, and 2,192 swine.

Only those persons that have graduated at a German veterinary school are allowed to present themselves to the public as veterinarians. Persons falsely representing themselves as such are punished with a fine of 100 thalers ($75), but, if unable to pay this, with confinement in jail for a period of six weeks.

The Laws and Regulations for Rinderpest.

"When this disease breaks out in any of the states composing the empire of Germany, or in a country which is in direct connection with them, the individual governments of the empire are empowered and required to place in active execution all the regulations which are intended to prevent its introduction or further extension in the land, as follows:

"1. The restriction and prevention of the introduction or transport or commerce in living or dead cattle, sheep, goats, hides, hair, and other raw animal products, in fresh or dried condition; also raw feed, straw, junk, old clothes, harness, stable utensils; also the execution of a stringent frontier quarantine.

"2. Quarantining single farms, localities, or districts from intercourse with the surrounding country.

"3. Killing of all animals, inclusive of healthy ones, and the destruction of all things which may act as vehicles to the infectious elements, when disinfection will not be found sufficient for the purpose.

"4. Disinfection of the buildings, vehicles of transport, and other objects, as well as persons, that have been in any relation with the diseased animals.

"5. Expropriation of the necessary territory for burying the killed animals, and of such things as may act as infectious vehicles, and burying the same.

"Remuneration is given by the state for such animals as may be killed by the authorities, and for the land which has been taken, and also for the animals of those owners that have given a timely notice of suspicion of the disease among the cattle to the authorities; the price to be paid for the same is to be fixed by impartial assessors.

"This remuneration is, however, not awarded for animals which perish from the pest within ten days from the time of its introduction, or from the time when the animals introducing it have been driven over the frontier.

"It is the duty of every one who has gained knowledge of the outbreak of the disease among animals, or of the death of a single one, or even of the suspicion of either, to notify the police officials without delay. Any neglect in giving this notice by the owner of animals who may have the disease in his stables, shuts him off completely from all remuneration for animals which have died of the disease or have been killed by the authorities.

"The residents of pest-infested localities are obliged to support the Government officials in the execution of the laws.

"The railroad companies are obliged to disinfect all cars which have been used for the transport of cattle, or other animals, immediately after using, for such a time as the danger exists of the introduction of the pest *into* the land, or while it is present in any part of the empire itself. The companies are empowered to charge a special fee (twenty-five cents) to the shipper for each wagon used for such transport.

"The government *of each state* is responsible for the exact execution of the foregoing regulations. It is also bound to send in official reports to the central Government.

"The government of each state must at once notify the central Government and the other state governments the moment they are obliged to forbid the introduction of animals from other countries, or when they are obliged to change the regulations, or when they declare them ended.

"The restriction of traffic in animals between the different states of the empire is inaugurated when the pest has broken out in any single state.

"When the pest breaks out in a given state, the central Government is to be at once notified, as well as public notification given that the requisite regulations are in force, in an appropriate manner. The progress of the disease must be frequently reported to the central Government.

"It is the duty of the Chancellor of the Empire to watch over the proper execution of these laws. The chancellor is empowered to make such special regulations as the urgency of the case may demand, but must notify the different state governments of the same. The different state governments are obliged to support one another in the execution of these regulations.

"The military may be called in to help carry out the regulations. The central Government pays the expenses of the latter."

Special Regulations to prevent the Introduction of the Pest from Foreign Countries.

"When the pest breaks out in distant parts of a foreign country which is in connection with Germany, either by railroad or canal, so that animals could be transported in a short time into the land, then all cattle, sheep, swine, or other ruminants from those regions are strictly forbidden entrance. This regulation extends to all products from animals in a fresh condition, with the exception of butter, milk, and cheese. Traffic may be allowed in completely dried hides, wool, hair, and bristles, as well as melted tallow in casks, completely dried bones, horns, and claws, which must be entirely free from all fleshy parts.

"Ruminants from non-infested districts of the country in question may be allowed entrance at certain points, fixed by law, under the following conditions:

"(*a.*) An official attestation must be given that the animals came from a place which has been free from the pest for at least thirty days, and that no pest rages within a distance of twenty kilometres of the place whence they came.

"(*b.*) Their transport must have taken place through sections entirely free from the pest.

"(*c.*) The imported animals must be strictly examined at the frontiers by an official veterinarian, and have been found absolutely free from all disease.

"These regulations may be modified when the animals are destined for a city having a public slaughter-house, and when the railroad connects directly with the same. The importation can only take place in each individual case with the consent of the Government, and in each case is to be governed by special police regulations.

"All that has been said with reference to *importation* bears equal relation to transport *through* the land, or any portion of it.

"When the pest breaks out in a foreign country, but in the vicinity of the frontiers:

"If the outbreak takes place in a region within forty to eighty kilometres of the frontier, the importation of animals and animal products, as above, is to be strictly forbidden along the frontier for a distance corresponding to the threatened danger.

"Persons whose occupation brings them in relation with cattle, can only pass the frontier at certain places, and must there and then be subjected to disinfection.

"No exception to the above regulations can be made without the consent of the Government.

"When the pest approaches the immediate neighborhood of the frontiers, all transport is absolutely forbidden across the borders, and a military cordon may be formed for the requisite limit.

"The passage of passenger trains and posts can only take place subject to appropriate regulations.

"If the quarantine is broken, then all quarantined animals are to be immediately killed and buried, as well as articles which may serve to spread the disease.

"Such objects, as well as men, must be at once transferred back over the boundaries, if the quarantine has been broken, unless the authorities feel confident of the thorough disinfection of the same.

"The following regulations are to be enforced in all places along the threatened frontiers which lie within fifteen kilometres of the limits:

"A cattle-inspector is to be appointed in each village, who must make an exact register of all cattle present, and of every change in number or locality which takes place.

"These registers are to be revised weekly by the village authorities.

"The authorities are to be at once notified of any case of disease among the cattle of a village."

Regulations with reference to Rinderpest in Germany.

"As soon as a suspicion of the presence of rinderpest, or the death of an animal from it, takes place within the empire, or when two cases of death occur with suspicious symptoms within eight days, in any place, the regulations for its suppression come into force.

"Under such circumstances the owner of cattle can neither slaughter nor kill the sick animals, or bury or remove any that may have died, before the nature of the disease has been determined.

Until the latter has taken place, the dead animals are to be so kept that neither men nor animals can come in contact with them.

"The local police must call in the services of a competent veterinarian as soon as they have been notified of the existence of either of the above conditions, in order that the nature of the disease may be determined. If no cadaver is to be had, the authorities may kill an animal for the purpose. The results of such examination must be reported in writing.

"If the disease is ascertained to be rinderpest, every effort must at once be made to discover the way in which it was introduced. The General Government is to be at once notified, as well as the public. From this time all control regulations come into action.

"If there exists but a very strong suspicion of the presence of the disease, a temporary quarantining of the infested locality is to be ordered, until the presence of the disease is confirmed or the suspicion removed. In doubtful cases a high veterinary official must be called in.

"*The exhibition (offering) for sale, or recommendation of prophylactic or healing remedies for rinderpest, is to be severely punished.* Disinfection materials are not included in the above.

"On the outbreak of rinderpest, the holding of cattle-markets within a circuit of twenty kilometres of the infested locality is to be forbidden; and, if the circumstances require it, all cattle or other markets, or large gatherings of men, are to be forbidden; also all traffic in animals or their products. The animals necessary for food can only be sold subject to the control of the veterinary police.

"In the infested district or locality it becomes the duty of every one to notify the authorities of every case of disease, of whatever nature, among cattle, with the exception of external injuries.

"The place (farm or stable) in which the pest has broken out is to be isolated and controlled by watchers, who must not enter the grounds, or have intercourse with the residents, nor allow any one to pass in or out, except those especially legitimatized, nor can anything, living or dead, be allowed to leave the grounds. The guards must be matured individuals, and must wear appropriate badges.

"No one can enter the grounds except those employed in the suppression of the disease, or ministers, doctors, or nurses, when necessary to the fulfillment of their occupations. On leaving the premises such persons must be subjected to disinfection. Signs must be placed upon the boundaries of the premises with 'Rinderpest' upon them.

"A relatively local quarantine must be placed over the town or village in which the infected premises are situated. The residents of the place may have intercourse with one another, but can not leave it except with special permission, and this is only to be granted to those who have no connection with cattle.

"All animals, with the exception of horses, mules, and asses, must be confined to their stables; if found running about free, they are to be at once killed. Only the above animals can be used for draught or traveling purposes. The removal of all objects, such as hay, straw, manure, or other vehicles of infection, is forbidden.

"When the disease spreads over the greater part of any locality, an absolute isolation of the place is to be ordered. It is to be surrounded by guards (in this case military), and all forms of intercourse strictly forbidden among the inhabitants, except that of necessary persons about their occupations, such as doctors, etc. Schools and public meetings must be forbidden, the beer-houses and hotels closed. The streets leading through such a place are to be guarded. If the place is located upon a railroad, no trains can be stopped there, even though the place be a regular station, unless the latter is so situated outside the place that no communication with it is possible.

"All sick or suspected animals are to be at once killed. Cattle are always to be considered as 'suspected' as soon as they have stood in the same stable with diseased ones, or have had the same servants, drinking-utensils, etc., which have been used about the sick ones.

"The central powers can order the killing of healthy animals when warranted by the circumstances. In large cities, and in slaughter-houses which are under the control of the veterinary police, the sale of the skins and flesh of cattle which have been found healthy in both a living and slaughtered condition may be allowed. The slaughtering must take place under the supervision of the veterinary police, and only in special places. The flesh and inner organs can only be removed after they have entirely cooled off, and the skins when they are completely dried, or have lain in lime-water (1 to 60) for three days previously.

"The animals which have been killed by the authorities are to be buried in places distant from the public ways, and where no cattle can gain access. Such places are to be fenced in, and to be planted with a vegetation which grows rapidly and sends down deep roots into the earth. The excavation must be so deep that at least six feet of earth lies upon the cadavers. The persons employed in this service must be residents of the place, and such as do not own cattle themselves, or come in contact with them. When the work is completed they must be subjected to disinfection. Horses or men must be used for the removal of the cadavers, and the conveyance used for this purpose must be thoroughly cleansed and disinfected. The animals removed must be so placed upon the vehicles that no part of them can touch the ground, or any blood, hair, etc., drop from them upon it on the way to the burying-place. The hides of the slaughtered animals must be so cut as to destroy their value, and the cadavers saturated in crude petroleum or carbolic-acid solution.

"A stable in which diseased animals have lived must be at once thoroughly cleansed and disinfected. The manure is to be burned, or saturated with disinfectants. Nothing in the stable is to be removed from it."

Regulations after the Pest has come to an End.

"The pest may be considered ended in any locality when all the cattle have been killed, or are dead, or when three weeks have elapsed since the last case of death, or slaughtering of diseased animals, or such as have cohabited with them, and when the thorough disinfection of the infested stables has taken place.

"The disinfection must be begun and executed according to the circumstances, so soon as all the animals have been removed. It must also take place if all the animals have been killed, though not a single case of pest has been found among them.

"The disinfection can only take place upon official notice, and under the supervision of the proper officers. The disinfection begins with again opening the stable, which must take place within twenty-four hours after the removal of the animals, and care must be taken to give the air the freest possible circulation. The manure is to be carried out and burned, or taken to places where no cattle can gain access within the next three months, and deeply buried. The fluids in the drains, or yards, are to be disinfected with sulphuric acid and chloride of lime, and then led into deep holes and covered up. The surface of the plastering upon the walls is to be scraped off; the walls must then be whitewashed. The wood-work is to be washed with hot potash-water, and, in a few days, washed with chloride-of-lime solution. The floor is to be taken out and replaced ; if of earth, dug out one foot deep and replaced with fresh earth; if of pavement, replaced with new, or the old must be completely cleansed and disinfected. Wooden floors must be taken out and burned, or thoroughly cleansed and disinfected. The cribs, utensils, etc., must be cleansed and disinfected. After all this has been done, the stable must be opened freely to the air for fourteen consecutive days. In disinfecting, only such persons can be employed as have no cattle, or have nothing to do with them. They can not leave the premises until the work has been completed, and must then change their clothes and be thoroughly disinfected. The clothes used by them must be thoroughly washed, etc.

"Even after complete cleansing and disinfection of an infested stable have taken place, and after all restrictions have come to an end in the locality, new animals can not be bought and put in them in less than three weeks from the time the place was declared pest-free, and then only with the consent of the authorities.

"Grazing-places which have been used or passed over by diseased or suspected animals can only be again used after the lapse of at least two months.

"The Government can only give permission to use the places which have been taken for the burial of the killed or dead animals.

"No cattle-markets can be held at such places within three weeks from the time they have been declared pest-free."

Most stringent regulations exist, controlling the disinfection and cleansing of freight-cars by the railroad companies *every time* they have been used for the transport of any species of domestic animals. This cleansing must take place under the supervision of a state official. The disinfection must be effected either—1. By means of scalding-hot water, after thorough cleansing; 2. By scalding-hot water and caustic potash—500 grammes to 100 litres of water; 3. Or, by other disinfectants which are acknowledged as sufficient by the Government.

All utensils, unloading-platforms, etc., must also be subjected to the same course.

THE PRUSSIAN REGULATIONS FOR THE SUPPRESSION OF ANTHRAX; THE FOOT-AND-MOUTH DISEASE OF CATTLE, SHEEP, AND SWINE; THE CONTAGIOUS PLEURO-PNEUMONIA OF CATTLE; GLANDERS OF THE HORSE, MULE, AND ASS; THE VARIOLA OF SHEEP; THE GENITAL DISEASE OF HORSES AND CATTLE ("MALADIE DU COIT"); SCABIES OF THE HORSE AND SHEEP, AND RABIES OF ALL DOMESTIC ANIMALS.

Of the Notification of their Presence, or the Suspicion of the same.

"The *owner* of domestic animals is obliged to at once notify the local police authorities of an outbreak of either of the above diseases in his stables, *and of all suspicious phenomena* which justify the expectation of the presence of such a disease.

"The same responsibility rests with those intrusted by the owner with the care of the animals; further, those persons who accompany animals in transit; and especially is this the case when strange animals are intrusted to their care and introduced into the stables, yards, or pastures of the owner.

"Veterinary surgeons, and all those persons who make a practice of treating the diseases of animals, inclusive of those employed at knacker establishments, are obliged, under penalty of the law, to notify the proper authorities, either of the outbreak of any of the named diseases, or of the appearance of any phenomena which at all justify a suspicion of their existence.

"*It is the duty of the local police* to at once notify the official veterinarian, when they have received notification, or in any other way acquired knowledge, of the outbreak of an animal pest, or of the suspicion of its existence, in order to have a technical opinion upon the same.

"The state veterinarian must ascertain, and report in writing, the nature, condition, and cause of the disease, and plainly state whether it is an infectious disease or only a suspicious case.

"In peremptory cases, the veterinary official may at once proceed, without waiting for authority from the police authorities, and order the immediate quarantining and isolation of the diseased or suspected animals, and in necessary cases appoint a guard over the same.

"When this is the case, the causes for action must be given by the veterinary official in writing to the owner, or his representatives, as well as to the local police authority.

"The selectman, or other supervising officer of the town or locality, must order the temporary guarding of the infected or suspected stable, or locality, upon requisition of the official veterinarian.

"In order to confirm a suspicion, the local police authorities may condemn and slaughter a suspected animal; the results of the autopsy must be reduced to writing (upon the official blanks) by the state veterinarian. If the presence of a contagious disease is confirmed, the police have to at once order the execution of the necessary regulations, and give notice thereof according to the prescribed forms.

"The owner may also call in the services of an approved veterinarian in all those cases where a suspected animal is condemned and killed by the authorities, in order to establish the true nature of the disease.

"In those cases where a difference of opinion as to the nature of the disease in question exists between the veterinarian of the police and that of the owner, the police may call in the services of a department veterinarian, who must make his report in writing; the opinion of the latter is decisive, and the police must proceed accordingly.

"Official veterinarians have to supervise all cattle and horse markets, or all gatherings where animals are brought for the purpose of sale or barter.

"The district veterinary authorities are authorized to extend the same regulations to cattle, horse, or animal fairs or exhibitions."

It is the duty of the veterinarian to at once notify the police, in all cases, of the presence or suspicion of infectious or contagious diseases among animals so collected, which is to be followed by ordering into action the appropriate regulations. If there is danger in delay, the veterinarian is authorized to anticipate the action of the police by isolating and guarding the diseased or suspected animals. The expenses of the supervision of cattle and horse markets or fairs by the official veterinarian must be borne by the directors of the same.

Restriction of the Travel or Use of Animals.

"The isolation, guarding, or police supervision of an animal, or animals, affected with a contagious disease, or in which such is suspected. The owner of such an animal is obliged (upon demand) to make such arrangements that it can not leave its confinement while under observation, and that it is kept free from all contact with other animals.

"Restrictions as to use, or the transport of diseased or suspected animals, or the products from the same, or of such objects as have been in relation with the diseased or suspected animals, which may give rise to the extension of the disease.

"The use of common grazing-grounds is to be forbidden animals from different stables; further, the use of common drinking-places, and all intercourse between diseased or suspected animals in any way.

"Dogs are forbidden to run about free.

"When the official veterinarian has proven the presence of a contagious disease, the stables, farms, villages, or localities in which said animals are kept may be, according to circumstances, subjected to quarantine, so that no connection may be had with them, or with objects which could serve as vehicles of the infectious elements. The quarantine can only extend to a town, or village, or district, when the nature of the pest is such as to threaten with danger the greater number of the animals (of a susceptible species) of the locality. The owner is obliged to do all in his power to support the execution of the regulations."

Inoculation.—"The inoculation of animals exposed to infection can only take place in those cases allowed by law, and under the prescribed restrictions. The inoculation can only take place under the observation of the state veterinarian."

Anthrax.—Charbon.

"When the presence of anthrax has been determined in the manner fixed by law, or when there is reason to fear an extension of the disease, the police authorities are empowered to put in action the regulations for its suppression without waiting, in each case, for the opinion of the state veterinarian."

Regulations against its Extension. — "The police authorities and the state veterinarians are obliged to make known to the owners, and those persons who have the care of, or that may come in contact with, animals diseased with anthrax, the danger which always exists of its transmission to human beings, and to warn them to have care in their relation with such animals.

"In the stables where such animals are, care must be taken that the proper disinfectants are always on hand for the use of persons who have the sick animals in charge.

"The sick animals must be at once isolated from the healthy ones, and the stables quarantined. It is the duty of owners of the animals to make such arrangements as will insure the complete carrying out of the above regulation, so that no contact can take place between healthy animals and the sick ones, their excretions, or the utensils used about them. No other persons than those engaged in the care of the sick animals must be allowed admittance to the stables. The stables in which the sick animals are isolated must be kept dark, so as to keep flies away, and daily subjected to a slight fumigation with chlorine-gas.

"When the disease acquires a pest-like extension, the local authorities are authorized to subject all the animals in the infected place, or places, of the same species as those infected, to stable quarantine. It is the duty of the owners to support this regulation. The quarantining may be limited to single divisions of the animals in question, when the official veterinarian considers such a course warranted by the circumstances. The sick animals, in such cases, are to be isolated in special stables from the healthy ones.

"All slaughtering of the diseased or suspected animals, or the sale or use of any parts of the same, the milk, flesh, or hair, is to be forbidden. All those animals are to be considered as suspicious which have been in relation with diseased ones within a period of four days. The performance of surgical operations upon animals diseased with anthrax, or in which the same is suspected, can only be made by approved veterinarians, and after the diseased or suspected animals have been carefully isolated.

"The cadavers of anthrax-diseased animals, or of such as have been killed, can only be opened by approved veterinarians, and then only with the consent of the police. Skinning of the cadavers is to be strictly forbidden. Until the cadavers have been thoroughly destroyed, they must be kept isolated and securely covered with earth, straw, or some such material, and carefully guarded, so that other animals, and especially flies and insects, can not come in contact with them.

"The regulations herein mentioned in the first part are not to be applied to such animals as are subject to the control of the state veterinary schools or academies, where they are kept for the purposes of such institutions.

"The cadavers are to be destroyed as quickly as possible, when convenient by chemicals or by burning; but, when this is not the case, by deep burying, after the hide has been so cut as to destroy its value. The flesh is to be spoiled by saturation with petroleum, tar, or some such material. The place of burial is to be determined by the local police. The cadavers can only be transported in closed wagons, or so covered that no part of the body is exposed, and so that no dropping of blood or excretions can take place. The burial-places must be dug out so deep that at least six feet of earth lies upon the cadavers. When the latter are covered with lime, the holes need be no deeper than to permit of three feet of earth covering the cadavers. The burial-places must be paved with stone, and must remain in this condition for a period of three years; where this is impossible, they must be so inclosed that no animals can gain access to them. During this time such places must not be used either for agricultural or grazing purposes. These last regulations have equal relation to wild animals which have perished or been killed from anthrax.

"Excrements, blood, and other refuse from animals diseased with or which have died of anthrax, as well as the manure, hay, and straw in their stalls, must be either burned or buried. When the disease acquires an enzoötic extension, a weekly examination of the animals in the infected locality may be ordered by the police; it must be performed by a state veterinarian. When the invasion is ended, the police have to see that proper cleansing and disinfection of the premises take place.

"The action of the above regulations ceases—

"1. In isolated cases, when the diseased animals have recovered or are dead or have all been killed, the cadavers removed, and the locality thoroughly cleansed and disinfected.

"2. In enzoötic outbreaks, when fourteen days have elapsed since the last diseased animal died or has been killed, and after cleansing and disinfection have taken place according to law."

The "Foot-and-Mouth Disease" of Cattle, Sheep, Goats, and Swine.

"When an outbreak of this disease has been confirmed under conditions which threaten its rapid extension among the above-named species of our domestic animals, the police may at once order into action the necessary protective regulations without, in every case, waiting for the opinion of the state veterinarian.

"The police authorities must notify the public, in the manner fixed by law, of the first outbreak of this disease among the animals of a district. At the same time they must warn the people against the danger of infection from the consumption of uncooked milk from diseased animals.

"The infected localities must be made known to the public by means of inscriptions, 'Foot-and-Mouth Disease,' at prominent points.

"The police must place the following restrictions upon the owner and inhabitants of the infected localities: The diseased animals—swine, sheep, and cattle—or such as are in the stables with them, must be restricted to the same. Healthy animals of the above species from non-infected stables may be used for agricultural purposes. But they can not leave the grounds of the owner without special permission from the police, which, as a rule, is not to be withheld when the animals to be removed are to be at once slaughtered. Until the invasion has been declared at an end, the manure from the infected farm can not be removed across or upon ways which are passed over by animals of the same species from other farms or places.

"Raw food can not be removed from the infected stables. Hides can only be removed in a completely dried condition. The owner can not allow strangers, or persons uninterested in the care of the sick animals, into the stable; and also must have care that those persons having the sick animals in charge do not leave the place without first washing their hands, and changing the clothing and shoes they have used about them. Dealers in animals and butchers are forbidden to enter the infected grounds.

"The grazing of the sick animals, or those in the stable with them, is to be forbidden when the situation of the fields is such that grazing them is connected with danger of the extension of the disease to other animals. The sick animals and those with them may be confined to their stables by the police, when it is impossible for the owner to comply with the restrictions necessary to the prevention of the disease extending.

"The sale of the milk in an uncooked condition for human consumption is forbidden.

"When the disease has acquired an enzoötic extension, all animal markets, except those for horses, are to be forbidden in the locality, and, when the circumstances require it, in adjoining localities. In such cases the police may forbid ruminants being driven through the streets of the infected district. The removal of these animals from them can only take place with the consent of the authorities. This permission shall not be denied when the animals are from non-infected stables, and are destined for immediate slaughter. In these cases the removal of manure can only take place from the infected stables under the control of the police. Signs bearing upon them 'Foot-and-Mouth Disease' must be placed upon the roads approaching the infected district.

"When the disease appears among animals at grass, the police must make such restrictions and post such guards that animals from these herds can not be driven off or others upon the infected pastures. When this is impossible, the diseased animals must be removed to places where they can be properly confined, and the grazing-places isolated or plowed up *with horses*. Such grazing-places must be indicated with the previously mentioned inscriptions. Strangers and cattle-dealers are to be kept distant from them.

"When the disease appears among droves or animals in the way of transport, it is the duty of the police to prevent the droves being driven farther, and the animals quarantined.

"It is the duty of the authorities to see that the infected stables or fields are properly cleansed and disinfected when the disease has been declared at an end.

"The disease may be declared at an end when no new case transpired within fourteen days from the healing, or removal of the last case in the infected localities, and when the cleansing, etc., has been carried out according to law. The termination of the disease is to be made known to the public in the appropriate organs."

Contagious Pleuro-pneumonia of Cattle.

"The investigations of the official veterinarian with reference to an outbreak of this disease must take place (as a rule) in the presence of the head man of the locality, or of an officer detailed by the local police for that purpose.

"If the existence of the disease is proven, or if strong suspicions of the same exist, it is the duty of the veterinarian to ascertain how long the suspicious phenomena have been noticed, if the diseased or suspected animal has been in relation with other cattle, if animals have been recently slaughtered from the same stable or farm, or removed, when and where the suspected animal was bought, and who the former owner was. The results of this examination are to be at once communicated to the police and the local officers, in order that they may put the necessary laws in execution. If the corresponding police regulations have not been ordered, and the police representative was not present at the examination, it is the duty of the official veterinarian to at once order a preliminary separation and isolation of the diseased and suspected animals. It is also the duty of the veterinarian to notify the owner or his representative in writing of these regulations. In necessary cases the official veterinarian can require the presence of the head man of the town."

The Regulations in Case of Suspicion.—"The cattle of a farm (or locality) which has been heretofore free from the disease are subject to the police observation when it has been confirmed; that, among the cattle, individuals are found which have been in relations with animals having this disease within the last eight weeks; when the cattle in which the disease was suspected, before the official examination, have been slaughtered, removed, or otherwise done away with. The police have to make a memorandum of the number and characteristics (marks) of the animals in the suspected locality, and to make such regulations that the owner or his representative can not remove any cattle without the permission of the police. It is the duty of the police to see that these regulations are executed.

"After the lapse of four weeks, the police must order the official veterinarian to make a second supervision of the cattle in the suspected locality.

"If the official veterinarian can not at the time positively assert that the disease exists among the animals, but if the examination has confirmed the existence of suspicious phenomena which justify the fear that an outbreak of the disease may take place, it is the duty of the police to subject the stable to quarantine. The other cattle of the place must be confined to the limits of the owner's property. No cattle can be removed from the place, nor can food materials be removed which may endanger the extension of the disease. The police may allow those animals which have not been quarantined in the stable to be used for work in the fields of the owner, or to graze when the fields or the ways to them are so situated that the cattle of other owners can not possibly be exposed to infection. These regulations come to an end when the official veterinarian declares that suspicious phenomena no longer exist."

In case the disease comes to an outbreak: "When the disease has been confirmed, it is the duty of the police to give public notice of the same in an appropriate manner. The infected localities are to be made known by inscriptions, 'Pleuro-pneumonia,' being placed at prominent places.

"All the diseased or suspected animals must be discovered as soon as possible. All cattle in the infected locality (farm or stable) are to be looked upon as suspicious, inclusive of those which are found in isolated stables. It is the duty of the police to kill at once all animals which the official veterinarian shall pronounce diseased. If a perfectly secure isolation is possible, the police may restrain the above proceedings for a period of fourteen days, if the owner urgently requests it. The suspected animals at the infected farms must be subjected to quarantine. The removal of cattle or food from such farms must be forbidden so far as there is danger of the extension of the disease, though they may be used for work if such can be done under proper restrictions. If the disease acquires a considerable extension in a district, no cattle are to be allowed to be driven from it, or introduced into it. In such case the holding of cattle-markets must be forbidden, and, in necessary cases, in neighboring places also.

"If the disease breaks out among cattle which are constantly kept upon pastures, it is the duty of the police to order the diseased animals killed; such places must be so guarded that no cattle can be driven on or from them. Such pastures must be indicated by appropriate signs. If it is impossible to isolate such pastures, then the remaining cattle must be removed to more suitable quarters. If the disease is found among droves, or in cattle on the cars or in canal-boats or other means of transport, then the police have to order the diseased ones killed, and the remainder isolated.

"In order that the slaughtering of suspected or quarantined cattle may immediately take place, the police are permitted to allow their removal by rail or other closed conveyance, to such slaughtering-places as are under the control of the state. This can only take place where no possibility exists of their coming in contact with other cattle. In such cases the police must give timely notice of the arrival of the suspected cattle. The cattle must be slaughtered subject to the supervision of an official veterinarian. This liberty is not extended to already diseased animals.

"If suspected animals are removed in opposition to the above regulations, or found in places where they have been forbidden, it is the duty of the police to kill them at once. Animals which are condemned to be killed by the authorities must be slaughtered under their inspection within the limits of the place (farm, etc.) where they are found. The lungs of the slaughtered, and bodies of those animals which have died, must be destroyed. They may be skinned upon the named grounds. The flesh of the slaughtered cattle can be removed after it has been cooled off. The hides can only be removed from such places after they have become completely dried, unless they are directly delivered at a tannery.

"The cleansing and disinfection of the infected stables must be controlled by the police, and must take place before the restrictive regulations are relaxed. The police and veterinary official must return reports with reference to the execution of the laws.

"The disease is to be declared at an end when all the cattle have died or been condemned to slaughter; when all the sick cattle have been removed, and no new case has occurred within four months from the last case of disease; when no case of disease has shown itself among the cattle of the infected locality for a period of three months after the last possible infection could have taken place. No cattle can be removed from such places, save for the purpose of immediate slaughter, until after the lapse of six months.

"The police are to notify the public that the invasion is ended, after the disinfection has been properly effected."

Glanders.

"The examination of animals (horse, mule, ass) by the official veterinarian must take place, as a rule, in the presence of the head man of the place, or a special representative of the police. If the presence of the disease is confirmed, or if there is a strong suspicion of the same, it is the duty of the veterinarian to ascertain how long the suspicious phenomena have been noticed, if horses have been lately sold from the place, or removed; if the diseased or suspected animals have been in relation with other horses; if so, where the same were bought, and from whom. The results of this examination are to be at once communicated in writing to the local police and the head man of the place, in order that the requisite regulations may be placed in operation.

"If the regulations are not yet in active operation, and the representative of the police was not present at the examination, it is the peremptory duty of the official veterinarian to at once separate and isolate the diseased or suspected horse. The veterinarian must also at once notify the owner, or his representative, of these restrictions. A memorandum must at once be taken of the characteristics and appearance of the diseased and suspected animals, and of those horses which, although not yet diseased, have been in relation with them and others exposed to infection. The papers are to be at once sent to the police, so that the regulations may be put in force."

Protective Regulations.—"The public are to be notified by the police in the usual manner. This notice may be dispensed with in places of over 50,000 inhabitants with the consent of the Minister of Agriculture."

When Glanders is proven.—"If the presence of the disease is confirmed in a horse, it is to be at once killed. It must be done in some isolated place. In the transport to such a locality care must be taken that the diseased animal does not come in contact with others of the same species."

When the Suspicion of Glanders exists.—"In the following cases the suspected animals may be killed:

"(*a.*) When it can be proved that the suspected animals have been in relation with diseased ones.

"(*b.*) When a suspicious nasal outflow, hard and swollen glands, especially the intermaxillary space, suspicious nodules in the skin, suspicious tumefaction of one or more limbs exists; especially when one or more of these phenomena are present at the same time; or when, at the same time, difficulty of respiration or staring hair is present with some of these phenomena.

"(*c.*) When, after the lapse of three months, the isolated horse can not be declared free from suspicion by the official veterinarian.

"(*d.*) When suitable room can not be afforded for the isolation of the suspected horse, or when other reasons exist to render insecure the danger of further extension of the disease.

"When, in the above cases, the owner desires the animal to be at once killed, and this regulation is in the public interest, it is the duty of the police to comply therewith.

"If the isolated horses are used contrary to the restrictions, or found in places forbidden them, they are to be at once killed.

"Horses in which suspicious phenomena have been diagnosticated must be subjected to stable quarantine until killed, or until they are declared free from suspicion by the official veterinarian. The owner must supply the necessary conveniences for such a purpose. Such animals can not be removed from the stable without the consent of the police. The grooms appointed to the care of the isolated horses must be made aware of the danger of the transmission of the disease to mankind. They must be forbidden any interference with other horses, and must not be allowed to sleep in the infected stable. The racks, utensils, and other objects in the quarantined stable can not be removed except with the permission of the police. If necessary, such objects should be appropriately branded."

Horses in which Infection is to be suspected.—"All horses which have stood in the same stable with glandered or suspected animals, or which have been in relation with them, but in which at the time no suspicious phenomena are perceptible, are to be isolated in special stables by the police. These horses must be subjected to inspection by the official veterinarian every fourteen days. This regulation is not to be applied to large towns or cities where several approved veterinarians reside, when the owner brings the horses in question to the veterinarian every eight days for examination; the officer is to report to the police, in writing, the results of each examination. So soon as a suspicion of glanders is confirmed, the horse is to be at once confined and isolated. So long as the horses thus subjected to observation are considered healthy, they may be allowed to be used *within* the limits of the place in question. Special permission from the police is necessary when the horse is to be taken outside the limits of the place; this can only be given when the use required of the horse is of such a nature that it is not necessary to put him up in any other stable or shed. Such police control is to be extended over at least three months. During this period, the horse in question must not be brought into other stables, or farms, or places, than those indicated by the police. If such permission is given, the police control must be extended to such places. If the police regulations are not strictly followed by the owner, the horse is to be immediately quarantined in its stable. It is the duty of the local police to see that the official veterinarian subjects the quarantined horses to an examination at least once a month. If the disease extends, if circumstances exist which make such an extension probable, the police may order a special supervision, by the official veterinarian, of all the horses owned in the place.

"The cadavers of horses diseased with glanders are to be either chemically destroyed, or buried after the skin has been so cut as to utterly destroy its value. The burial-places must be so deep that at least four feet of earth covers the buried bodies. The selection of the burial-place rests with the police. These regulations are not applicable to horses at veterinary schools or other government establishments, where they are required for educational or experimental purposes. The disinfection and cleansing of stables in which diseased animals have stood must take place under police supervision. A record of the same must be kept in writing.

"The disease is declared at an end when all glanders-diseased or suspected horses are dead, or when the latter have been declared free by the veterinarian of the state. When no suspicious phenomena have presented themselves during the course of the police control. When the cleansing and disinfection have been performed and attested to.

"It is the duty of the police to make this known to the public in the usual manner. This publication is not necessary in the large cities and towns, where the presence of the disease, or its suspicion, is not made public."

Variola Ovina.

"The outbreak of this disease in a flock of sheep is to be made known, without delay, by the police, in the usual manner. The infected place is to be indicated by appropriate inscriptions at prominent points. The police have at the same time to quarantine all the sheep at the infected locality. So far as circumstances will allow, the visibly diseased are to be isolated from the apparently healthy sheep. The owner of the sheep has to supply the proper conveniences for this purpose, and assist in carrying out the regulations. The passage of such quarantined sheep to the pastures is only to be permitted when the situation and nature of the pastures are such as to forbid the extension of the disease, or such that police regulations can attain this end."

The owner of the sheep has also to comply with the following regulations:

"The removal of the manure from infected stables in such ways or to such places that it would endanger the infection of sheep from other places is to be forbidden, unless this danger can be obviated by other police regulations. Hay and straw from the infected stables can not be removed. Shepherds and other persons who have been in relation with the diseased sheep can not be employed in the care of those of other owners, or other sheep which are not diseased. They can only leave the place after careful washing and change of clothing. Strangers and butchers must not be admitted to the infected stables. Common washing-places can not be used for the diseased sheep. Diseased sheep can only be washed by persons who are to be forbidden coming in relation with other sheep within the succeeding ten days. The wool from such sheep can only be removed from the place when closely packed, and then only with the permission of the police.

"Sheep are to be placed under police observation in those cases where an outbreak of the disease can not be securely determined, but when the official veterinarian declares the case to be decidedly suspicious. This observation is to be given up when, after the lapse of fourteen days, the official veterinarian declares that no suspicious phenomena have been seen in the sheep.

"When the situation of the individual outbreak is such that a complete isolation of the diseased sheep is pronounced impossible for any length of time, or when the general interest demands the speediest possible termination of the outbreak, it becomes the duty of the police to occasion the speediest possible inoculation of all the sheep in the district. The police must strictly attend to the necessary restrictions. Such inoculations can only take place under the supervision of an official veterinarian.

"When the disease breaks out in flocks in transit, they are to be at once subjected to quarantine. No inoculation of sheep by owners can take place without the consent of the police. The notification of such intention must be handed in at least eight days before the inoculation is to take place. The district police must at once notify the public that such inoculation is to take place, and, so far as the district is not under their control, they must notify the neighboring police of the fact. The above-given regulations are then to be applied to the inoculated sheep in the same manner as if the disease had broken out in a natural way.

"The slaughtering of such diseased sheep for human consumption is forbidden.

"The cadavers of sheep which have died, or been killed, on account of variola, must be chemically destroyed, or, where this is impossible, buried. The burial-places must be so deep that at least four feet of earth lies upon the bodies. Such sheep may be skinned, but the skins can not be removed except with the permission of the police, and then only when perfectly dry, or for direct delivery to a tannery.

"The infected stables or pens must be cleansed and disinfected according to law.

"The disease may be declared as ended when the official veterinarian has declared all the sheep at the infected place free from the disease.

"The regulations are, however, to be held in force for two months after the disease has been declared as ended. Sheep in full wool can only be removed from such places after four months from the time the disease was declared at an end. At the cessation of all restrictions, the same must be made known by the police in the usual way."

Rabies of the Domestic Animals.

Dogs.—"Dogs in which signs of rabies appear, or which indicate suspicious phenomena, must either be at once killed by the owner or those having them in charge, or be placed in secure confinement until the police have determined what is to be done with them.

"When a human being or an animal is bitten by a dog which is suspected as being rabid, or been in any relation with such, which renders infection probable, the suspected dog is *not to be killed, but be safely secured, when such can be done without further danger,* until the police decide upon the course to take.

"The transport of a dog in which rabies is suspected, with the purpose of confinement, must take place in a closed vehicle, or the dog must be securely muzzled and well chained with two chains between two conductors.

"It is the duty of the local police to immediately cause the examination of a dog suspected of rabies by an official veterinarian, or, when time would be lost in waiting for the attendance of the latter, by an approved veterinarian.

"If there is a well-founded suspicion that the suspected dog had been in relation with a rabid or suspected dog, the dog must be securely confined and watched for a period of six days, if the examination of the veterinarian does not at once confirm the suspicion. If the dog lives over this time, and no suspicious phenomena appear, he is to be discharged.

"If a dog suspected of rabies is at once killed, or if it dies during confinement, it is the duty of the police to order a *post-mortem* examination by an official veterinarian, if there has been any probability of men or animals having been bitten by the same, or if the said dog has been roaming over the country.

"If the presence of the disease is confirmed, it is the duty of the police to make it known to the public in the usual way. Dogs in which the disease has been diagnosed, must be at once killed. It is further the duty of the police to at once kill all dogs which have been bitten by the rabid dog, as well as such as have been in relation with it so as to render the possibility of infection imminent.

"When a rabid or suspected dog is known to be freely running over a section of the country, it is the duty of the police to order all other dogs in the district securely confined. All places in which the rabid or suspected dog has been seen are to be looked upon as dangerous, as well as a territory extending four kilometres beyond them. If the suspicion is unfounded, the confined dogs are again to be freed from the restriction; if, on the contrary, the suspicion becomes confirmed, the restrictions are to be extended over a period of at least three months. If dogs are found free in opposition to these restrictions, they may be at once killed by the police. In such places where dogs are obliged to wear muzzles, these restrictions need not be called into force. These restrictions are further not to be extended to dogs which are used for draught, when they are firmly harnessed to wagons, and are securely muzzled; shepherds may also be allowed to use their dogs. So long as the disease has acquired no considerable extension, dogs may be used for the purpose of hunting, on the condition that they be securely muzzled and led by chains or strong cords, at all times and places except those where they are hunted."

Cats.—These are to be killed.

Other Domestic Animals.—"Other animals which have been bitten or in such relation with a rabid or suspected dog as to render infection probable, must be placed under technical observation for the time fixed by law, unless the owner prefers to kill them. The duration of this observation is, for horses, three months; cattle, four months; sheep, goats, and swine, two months. So long as the animals are pronounced healthy by the official veterinarian, they may be used for work. But if they display phenomena which serve to confirm the suspicion of rabies, it is the duty of the owner to notify the police thereof. The latter have to order the examination of the animal in question by an official veterinarian; if he confirms the suspicion, the animal is to be confined to its stable. If the disease becomes confirmed, the animal is to be killed by order of the police. No attempt at treatment can be undertaken under penalty of the law."

Regulations with reference to all Animals.—"No rabid animals are to be slaughtered, skinned, or used in any manner, nor is the milk or other parts of them to be sold. The cadavers of animals which have died or been killed on account of rabies are to be either chemically destroyed, or, after the skin has been destroyed, buried. Autopsies upon such cadavers can only be made by approved veterinarians. It is the duty of the police to select the spot where such dogs shall be buried, or otherwise destroyed. The straw of the kennels, wooden utensils used about them, and wooden dog-kennels must be burned. Stall-utensils of other animals which have been rabid, and killed, must be cleaned with hot lye-water. Iron utensils must be highly heated. The stables must be cleansed, the walls and floors cleansed with hot lye-water and chloride of lime."

Disinfectants.

"*Potash and Soda.*—Potash-lye is to be prepared by cooking one part crude potash with ten of water, and by adding gradually one part of slaked lime. Instead of potash, four times the quantity of wood-ashes may be used. Soda-lye is to be prepared in the same manner. These preparations are more suitable for cleansing woodwork.

"*Freshly-slaked lime* is to be used in a dry form for covering cadavers, or as lime-water for washing over walls, mixing with manure or other refuse. Hides may be disinfected by placing them in a strained solution of one part lime to sixty or eighty water.

"*Common Salt and Saltpeter.*—Hides, flesh, intestines, bones, horns, claws, etc., may be treated with these salts, by laying them in layers or piles thoroughly mixed with them, or by placing them in a strong solution of the same.

"*Chlorine* may be used in different ways:

"As gas, in the disinfection of stables. Gas is easily and quickly prepared by pouring double the weight of muriatic acid upon chloride of lime, or equal parts of sulphuric acid upon the same. Or it can be prepared by pouring strong (commercial) muriatic acid upon a quantity of small pieces of peroxide of manganese, or by pouring strong sulphuric acid upon a powdered mixture of three parts common salt and two of peroxide of manganese. A solution of chloride of lime can be made by mixing one part of the same with ten of water.

"*Hypermanganate of potash and soda* are mixed with water, and four to five per cent solutions used for washing the hands, instruments, etc.

"*Carbolic acid* is not to be used where animals destined for slaughter or milk purposes are being kept, on account of its penetrating odor. It is only soluble in water to two per cent, but a complete solution is unnecessary for disinfection purposes. In the disinfection of wooden or iron objects, a mixture of the crude acid with four to six parts water or oil is sufficient. Coal-tar or wood-tar also act as fair disinfectants at times.

"*Heat.—Dry heat in closed rooms,* when the temperature has been raised to 70° C., makes a very good disinfectant for clothing, wool, hair, bones, etc.

"*Hot water and steam* are valuable in destroying the germs of infection.

"*Fire* is to be used to destroy contaminated wood-work, and cleansing various iron utensils.

"A free exposure for a long time to the circulating atmosphere is often valuable in so widely dispersing the infectious elements as to nullify their action."

Disinfection with Reference to the Different Contagious or Infectious Animal Diseases.

Anthrax.—"The infectious elements of this disease possess a great degree of tenacity. They are not securely destroyed by desiccation, or by the dry dissolution of the cadaver in the earth. Chemicals used in disinfection must be of the strongest concentration. Great heat, chloride of lime, and freshly-slaked lime (thick) are among the best. The bedding and manure of diseased animals must be burned. Blood or other fluid elements from the diseased animals must be treated with chloride of lime or freshly-burned lime; four or five per cent carbolic acid solutions are suitable for the disinfection of the hands, instruments, etc.

Foot-and-Mouth Disease.—"The infectious elements are quite movable and easily destroyed; therefore, the disinfection of infected stables may be limited to a thorough cleaning.

Contagious Pleuro-pneumonia.—"The infectious elements are movable, and come from the diseased lungs with the expired air, filling the atmosphere around the diseased animals, and being again taken up by the others in the stable. Where the nature of the conditions will allow it, the stables are to be treated with weak chlorine-gas; this is not necessary with animals at the public slaughter-houses. In stables where the hay and straw are situated over diseased cattle, the superficial parts must be carefully removed, and not used for feeding cattle after the diseased ones have been removed. Stables in which only animals that have gone through with the disease are confined, do not require disinfection."

Glanders.—"The infectious elements retain their vitality a long time, and are very tenacious. Stables or rooms in which glandered horses have stood, the racks and other paraphernalia which are used about the diseased horses, must be carefully cleansed and disinfected. Clothes and brushes, etc., used about the diseased horses must be burned; chains heated hot; but harnesses, etc., may be thoroughly cleaned and disinfected."

Variola Ovina.—"The infectious elements soon lose their vitality on exposure to the moving atmosphere; hence are easily disturbed. The manure and the walls of the pens, however, retain it a long time, and are to be treated accordingly."

Rabies.—"The straw, wood-work, utensils, muzzles, collars, etc., must be burned. The other disinfection is according to the usual course."

PART III.

THE MEANS OF PREVENTION.

A NATIONAL VETERINARY POLICE SYSTEM.

Aside from those animal diseases which are transmissible to man, there are contagious animal diseases which are limited to special species. We have now well domesticated with us one of the very worst of these evils—contagious pleuro-pneumonia of cattle. It is not my purpose to enter into any historical notice of this disease, either in Europe or this country. Its first most extensive ravages were felt here, in Massachusetts, between 1860 and 1868, the disease being finally crushed out at a cost of some sixty thousand dollars. In September, 1879, I received a letter from one of the commissioners of the State of New York for the suppression of this disease, in which he says that over five hundred diseased cattle had already been killed by the authorities, and some seven hundred more, which were either suspected or had surely been exposed to infection, causing an actual loss, exclusive of the official expenses, of not less than fifty or sixty thousand dollars.

This disease has now spread over many of our seaboard States, being domesticated surely as far north as Connecticut, and as far south as Northern Virginia. It has not as yet been sufficiently proved that it has crossed the Alleghany Mountains, but, unless our people wake up to the urgencies of the case, it will surely extend to the herds of the West, and then we can give up all hope of ever becoming free from it. A peculiarity of this disease, which it enjoys in common with glanders, is the insidiousness of its course during its early stages. An animal may be diseased for weeks, or even months, without showing any striking indications that a disease having such a truly devastating character is progressing within it. During all this time it is capable of infecting others. The following report, taken from the "Turf, Field, and Farm," January

16, 1880, will give an idea of what the authorities in New Jersey are endeavoring to do, and have done.

REPORT BY THE SURGEON-IN-CHIEF TO GENERAL STERLING, THE GOVERNOR'S AGENT FOR THE PREVENTION OF THE SPREAD OF PLEURO-PNEUMONIA IN THE STATE OF NEW JERSEY.

249 WASHINGTON STREET, JERSEY CITY, N. J.,
December 15, 1879.

SIR: In compliance with your instructions, I have the honor to submit my report of the details and operations under my charge as Veterinary Surgeon-in-Chief of the Bureau.

I found it necessary to organize a staff of six qualified veterinarians to assist in carrying out the provisions of the law entitled "An Act to prevent the spread of Epizoötic, Contagious Pleuro-Pneumonia among Cattle in New Jersey." (See Chapter 89 of the Laws of the State of New Jersey, approved March 13, 1879.) Much work having been done in Bergen County, and no disease having been found, and reports having come to the office that the disease was present in Hudson County, the inspectors were assigned to work there.

Every herd has been carefully examined, and when the disease has been found, the animals have either been destroyed or the stables quarantined and the stock carefully watched. The dairymen had been in the habit of pasturing their stock indiscriminately on the public commons, this being a source of spreading the disease.

It became necessary to take some steps to control it. With that object in view, the Police Commissioners of Jersey City were consulted, and they caused an order to be issued prohibiting the driving of all cattle through the streets, unless accompanied by a permit issued from this office. On July 7th it became necessary to quarantine Essex County to facilitate inspections, which, when completed, showed, as a result, that the stock was, with a few exceptions, healthy. The other counties have only been inspected in localities where the disease was reported to exist, and the herds in the immediate neighborhood have been examined to ascertain the extent of the spread of the malady. Having been made aware of the existence of the disease in Pennsylvania, and arrangements having been perfected, four veterinarians were dispatched to the western frontier of the State, one to be stationed at Bull's Island and one at Trenton, these to examine all cattle arriving between Camden and Phillipsburg, and two at Camden, to examine all stock arriving between that point and Salem, with instructions to return all stock found infected with contagious pleuro-pneumonia. On August 18, 1879, regular examinations were commenced on that border, and the results obtained have shown the necessity of the measures taken.

Four months' inspections have discovered sixteen lots of diseased cattle containing 217 head, forty of which were found infected with contagious pleuro-pneumonia, and, with the rest, sent back to Philadelphia.

These are only the positive results obtained; the farmers have been greatly benefited by receiving a much better grade of cattle than heretofore, as the dealers buy only healthy stock, knowing by experience that it would be useless to attempt to pass any other kind.

How the Work is being done.—Finding a strong feeling of antipathy existing among the people against the introduction of radical measures, and with a view of obviating that feeling, the inspectors were instructed to exercise discretion and extend courtesy toward those with whom they came in contact while in the discharge of their duties, and to report all interference on the part of the people to this office, where the case would receive due consideration.

This course, I am happy to say, has been productive of excellent results, as far as removing all feeling of opposition and inducing cattle-owners to look upon the inspectors as a source of protection.

The Method of making Inspections.—In order to facilitate the work, a detective, who is thoroughly acquainted with the city, precedes the inspectors, locating the stables, number of cattle, etc., which he reports to this office. The inspectors are then provided with lists of the same, with printed forms of quarantine notices, and instructed to proceed to the places, make a careful examination, and if any diseased animals are found, to mark them by clipping the hair from the right gluteal region, forming the letters P. P., with a cross-cut through the skin between with a sharp scalpel, while those standing contiguous to, or having been in contact with them, being thereby rendered liable to develop the malady, are simply marked with the letters and isolated to await further developments.

The stable is then quarantined by placing a printed notice on the building, and at the close of the day's labor the inspectors return to the office where, upon printed forms, a report of the number, location, and condition of each herd is made, which is placed upon file for further reference. As soon as compatible we then proceed to the infected herd, make a careful reinspection, and determine what should be done under the circumstances. The owner being first consulted by stating to him the case with its probable results, and if it is necessary to kill in order to prevent the spread of the malady, he is so informed, and the animals are taken out, destroyed, their hides slashed, and the carcasses, if in the city limits, carted away by the offal contractor; if not, they are buried.

The remaining animals, though showing no diseased condition, are looked upon with suspicion from having been in contact with the infection, and when in proper condition are sent to the butcher, where they are slaughtered under the supervision of an inspector. In some cases where the animals are in a safe locality, so that there is no danger of the disease spreading, though having passed through a slight attack of the malady, but evidently making a rapid recovery, it is considered prudent to keep them in quarantine until they can be fitted for the butcher, and the flesh utilized for human consumption.

After the manure, litter, and all material having a tendency to retain infection has been removed from the stable, it is then thoroughly disinfected, and ninety days afterward, if the owner is desirous, the quarantine is removed, and new cattle allowed on the premises.

Dealers.—One of the worst difficulties we have been called upon to overcome is the dealer, a sharp, shrewd, unscrupulous, uuprincipled person, who studies to take advantage of the unsophisticated dairyman, and even the Bureau, whenever the opportunity presents. His favorite method is to go to a stable where diseased animals are known to be kept, procure one in the early stages of the malady, take it to a healthy herd, where its presence will soon occasion an outbreak, when he will stand ready to purchase the diseased animals at his own price and put them upon the market to be used for beef.

Investigation has shown that such a course has been productive of a great deal of trouble, and we have considered it necessary to restrict them in their manner of dealing, in order to arrest the spread of the malady. With that object in view, we have introduced a system of granting *permits*, requiring all those desirous of moving cattle to call at this office, where they are required to give their name, number, or residence, number of cattle and where they wish to take them. If, upon consulting our books, the person does not appear as having cattle that have been previously inspected, an inspector is directed to the place, who makes an examination, and if the animals are found free from disease, as well as the place where they are destined to go, a printed form of permit is granted from this office allowing their removal.

By this means they may be traced at any time, and any effort on the part of the dealer to traffic in unhealthy animals is prevented.

This course proves a positive protection to the purchaser, as well as requiring the dealer to traffic only in healthy stock and secure him a good reputation, however much he may desire otherwise. All cattle leaving infected places must be accompanied by a permit which admits of their being taken only to places of slaughter, where, under the supervision of an inspector, they are destroyed, and a proper disposition made of the carcasses.

Reinspection.—When cattle have assumed a risk, but not actually presenting symptoms of the malady, and while awaiting its incubation, it has always been the custom, in this as well as in European countries, to practice occision; but, believing that proceeding to be an expensive experiment, we have adopted the rule of allowing the animals to remain in provisional quarantine; and from time to time making reinspections, by which means we are able to keep the stable under surveillance during the incubative period, when, if the disease does not appear, the quarantine is raised and the stock declared healthy. This manner of proceeding being a departure from the rule adopted in European countries, is looked upon with disfavor by foreign veterinarians, notwithstanding experience has taught us that it has been productive of a great saving to this State. Several stables, containing a number of cattle, were during the spring months quarantined in consequence of finding one or more diseased animals in them, which were removed and destroyed, and the stables subjected to an occasional reinspection until six months had elapsed, when, no further disease being manifest, the quarantine was raised and the premises declared free from all contagious disease. After carefully computing the cost of conducting these reinspections, and comparing it with the necessary expense following the destruction of the cattle, there is a handsome balance in favor of the former method.

Mistaken Theories.—Nine months' constant intercourse with "epizoötic contagious pleuro-pneumonia" has established the fact that many erroneous ideas have been allowed to creep into the minds of the people in regard to the nature, character, means of prevention, etc., of the malady, and foremost among them is *inoculation.*

A so-called preventive means of avoiding the spread of the malady is practiced with varying success. The following are the views of two eminent authorities on the subject.

Professor Liautard, Dean of the American Veterinary College, says:

"The prophylaxis of inoculation, efficient as it may be in an epizoötic outbreak, certainly has no claims for adoption in connection with the disease as it now exists, for it would only prove one of the surest methods of spreading the malady, while our aim should be to confine it to its present quarters, and then eradicate it at whatever cost the method may entail."

Referring to the subject, Clater says:

"Inoculation has been practiced with questionable success. Experiments professing to be for the object of testing the efficacy of direct inoculation for pleuro-pneumonia have been recommended and practiced with great looseness. The peculiarly subtle character of a contagious disease is not sufficiently weighed with care. It is a very general practice to recommend and adopt the remedy after an animal has succumbed to the affliction. We contend, therefore, that inoculation in such cases is no test of efficacy, as with the existence of pleuro-pneumonia upon the farm, no one can arrive at a safe conclusion whether the consequence of the malady has really resulted from a direct cause or from the artificial means employed.

"All the profitable terminations of pleuro-pneumonia have been witnessed in its unmolested march through a herd when inoculated; hence our disbelief in the sufficiency of the evidence at present before us."

The results of investigation are so conflicting, indefinite, and at variance with seeming facts, that it is not by any means established that any degree of success has ever been obtained by its use.

There is not a single instance, so far as we have been able to learn, where it has been resorted to until after the malady had actually attacked a herd, when more or less of its number might reasonably be supposed to have assumed a risk.

Now, since all authorities are agreed to the fact that its incubative period ranges all the way from ten to ninety days, we can not see how its application could affect an animal when applied at about the time it should be assuming an acute character, unless we can go a step further and claim for it a curative effect. In the face of the fact that the malady often exhausts itself with attacking but one or two animals out of a herd of many and the rest suffering immunity; also that the disease often breaks out in the same herd after inoculation has been performed, as well as the negative results following its use in England, Belgium, Australia, and other countries where the disease has existed for a long time—we think there is but little doubt, notwithstanding it has a few advocates, that it has thus far proved inert to accomplish the desired result, and that we must look elsewhere for a more substantial means of eradicating the disease.

Careful investigations recently prosecuted from this office induce us to fully coincide in the above view of the subject.

In this month's issue of the "Veterinary Journal," Mr. George Fleming, in an editorial article, takes strong ground in favor of the treatment which he bases upon the result of experiments conducted at Edinburgh, Scotland, by a Mr. Rutherford, recently from Australia. He also claims advantages following its application there, which are at variance with the true facts in the case. We have made some effort to obtain information as to how it is received there, and find it is looked upon with a good deal of disfavor.

We also know that, notwithstanding it has been practiced for a number of years, the country is still overrun by the malady. Suppose its introduction did confer immunity, we believe it would still, owing to its cost, be impracticable. We have in this State 236,000 head of cattle, all of which it would be absolutely necessary to inoculate to use this method, and when we consider the time required to reach the herd, and consumed in introducing the virus, with the cost of the necessarily diseased animals which have to be destroyed in order to obtain a supply of virus, we may safely compute it at fifty cents per head, establishing a first cost, to either the State or the individual farmer, of not less than $118,000; besides, it would be necessary for the first few years to treat the offspring of that immense number of stock, entailing an increased expense.

Other Diseases.—Many reported cases, in young stock, upon investigation, prove to be the result of the presence in the bronchial tubes of the parasite *Strongulus filariæ*, species *Micruris*. In some localities it exists to an alarming extent, causing a severe mortality.

Its symptoms being similar to pleuro-pneumonia, it is usually mistaken by the farmers for that disease. It readily yields to scientific treatment; but, owing to the immense loss it entails, should receive legislative consideration. Hog-cholera, likewise, exists in the southern part of the State, and is creating a good deal of alarm, but, not coming within the provisions of the act under which we are working, has received but little attention. It is a subject that also calls for legislative action.

New Facts.—That we meet forms of pleuro-pneumonia varying in degrees of virulence is beyond question, and to that fact may be attributed the difference of opinion in regard to the efficacy of inoculation. When, as frequently found, the malady will run through a herd, causing perhaps the loss of but one or two out of a large number of animals, and affecting the remainder to so slight a degree that the layman can scarcely appreciate it, we must admit it differs widely from that form which (under similar circumstances) causes a mortality of fifty and sometimes sixty per cent. To the former type may be traced the cause for the disputed question, Does an animal once affected ever recover? We are inclined to the negative side of the question: after having destroyed a number of cases that have passed through a mild attack of the malady, we have found upon examination lung lesions generally in an encapsulated form.

These cases we are willing to admit are perfectly safe to mingle in a herd, so long as the capsule walling up the disease-germs remains intact, but if it should break down, a condition we may very reasonably look for, and those germs be allowed to escape, shall we not have another outbreak? If it is true, as claimed, that the disease-germs are imprisoned and lie dormant in the lung for months, even years, the question very naturally presents itself, Do they in the mean time lose their infecting principle? Until this vexed question is settled beyond doubt, we advise as a means of prevention the destruction of all such cases.

Very respectfully, your obedient servant,

JAMES C. CORLIES, D. V. S.

To General W. H. STERLING, 249 Washington Street, Jersey City, N. J.

The following is a summary of the work accomplished: Number of cattle inspected, 40,309; diseased, 572, of which 315 were destroyed.

It will be seen from this report that "dealers" in cattle are a source of great trouble to those intrusted with the execution of laws against contagious animal diseases.

I wish also to express my earnest opposition to inoculation, so far as it may be advocated as a preventive means for this country. Were it absolutely necessary that every head of cattle in this country should have the disease, either in a natural or artificial form, in order to put a stop to its ravages, then this procedure would be justifiable. At present it is not. The disease has not as yet acquired any very devastating extension, although, from the want of really competent veterinarians, it is doubtful if we know exactly to what degree it has extended in all the States where it is now domesticated. We shall know in time to our cost. Were our people so educated that they could really appreciate the truly devastating character of this animal pest; were our legislators at all adequate to the demands we have a right to make upon them, there would not be an isolated case of lung-plague in this country in six months from this time. Alas! unity of action is the last thing to be expected of an American Congress. While political pettifoggers are squabbling over party-bones, the people are being daily robbed of millions of dollars by the ravages of different animal pests, and that other pest, equally dangerous, quacks.

If all the cattle having this disease could be at once killed and paid for by the Government; if all suspected animals, which includes all which have been in contact with them, could be isolated and quarantined, or else at once killed, and sold for flesh; if it were possible to subject all cattle entering our territory from Canada or from across the Atlantic to an appropriate quarantine—then we might soon be rid of this destroyer, and keep it foreign to our shores. This is impossible at present. We have not the necessary laws, and it is still more doubtful if we have at our command the necessary number of qualified veterinarians.

I wish to say a word about cattle-inspection at points of delivery. In one sense of the word it is useless. Unless an inspector knows that a given lot of cattle have come from a suspected locality, he has no more right to condemn them for pleuro-pneumonia contagiosa than for an ordinary pneumonia before an autopsy has been made. Many people seem to think that it is easy to recognize this disease in the living animal, whether one knows the history of the case or not. In truth, no two animal diseases present so many difficulties in the way of recognition of their true character as this disease and pulmonary glanders. The differential diagnosis between a developed case of lung-plague in cattle and tuberculosis is by no means difficult, although many would have it that it is so. All cattle, or other animals destined for transport, should have a "clean bill of health" signed by a State veterinarian at the place of purchase, and attested to by the proper legal official. This should be an invariable rule of animal transport. With this precaution, and careful regulation of the cattle during transport, there is but little danger of the spread of such diseases from one point to another. It is evident that, if the laws in the respective States were different in this regard, all action would be made null and void. All pneumonias are not pleuro-pneumonia; yet, how is the inspector at the place of destination or final shipment to distinguish one from the other, unless he knows the history, or has condemned one to necroscopical examination? The truth is, but few veterinarians in this country really know the pathological character of an ordinary bovine pneumonia. Cattle are so phlegmatic, they can endure so much, that but very few of them die from this disease; yet it is a fact of pathological interest, at least, that the fully developed simple pneumonia of cattle is the only form among our domestic animals which bears a strong resemblance to the cheesy pneumonia of man.

Mr. John Gamgee says that "England loses two million pounds sterling annually from this disease." *

Fleming says: "The losses from only two exotic bovine maladies (contagious pleuro-pneumonia, and the so-called 'foot-and-mouth disease') have been estimated to amount, during the thirty years that have elapsed since our ports were thrown open to foreign cattle, to 5,549,780 head, roughly estimated at £83,616,854. The late invasion of 'cattle-plague,' which was suppressed within two years of its introduction, has been calculated to have caused a money loss of from five to eight millions of pounds. But these examples and estimates, after all, give but a slender idea of the devastation, misery, embarrassment, and loss that have been due to ignorance, apathy, and neglect of the teachings of veterinary science, which must, nevertheless, claim the merit of having conclusively demonstrated that the most formidable diseases can be readily repressed, or altogether abolished, though not by attempting to cure them, and, having done this, nothing more remains than to indicate the steps necessary to make the legislation of a wise government effective in its dealings with animal plagues in general." †

It is scarcely possible for us to comprehend the monetary loss this disease has caused since its history began, not to speak of the misery it has brought upon many poor people.

There is at present but one rule for its treatment: *No temporizing.* Immediate slaughter, and redemption by the Government.

We have, fortunately, not yet been visited by the rinderpest. Should that day ever come, there will be mourning in the land—Columbia weeping for her property, and little comfort will she get from church or State, unless we mend our ways and act more intelligently.

The people of this country have no idea as to the real nature of a contagious animal disease. To this end it may be possible that they need the presence of this destroyer. The horse epizoötic of 1871 and 1872 was certainly infectious enough, but this disease is equally infectious, and so much more devastating that it is impossible for words to fitly express it. It is not slow and sneaking in its prog-

* "Report on the Cattle Diseases in the United States," Washington, 1871.

† "Animal Plagues," introduction, p. xxxiv.

ress. It breaks loose in a night; ay, in an hour; and, like a demon incarnate, it frequently sweeps the bovine family before it. Russia loses millions every year from it. Germany scarcely passes free from its ravages for any single year, though they are at present very quickly stamped out. In 1878 she lost 2,560 cattle, having a value of about half a million dollars. England lost some twenty-five million dollars' worth of cattle in the last great invasion which she suffered in 1865, 1866, and 1867.

We have in this country the "Texas disease" of cattle, the real nature or causes of which we at present know very little about. It produces no inconsiderable loss each year, however, and the States, the frontiers of which border on lands where this disease seems to be domesticated, have been obliged to make laws regulating the traffic in cattle. The Agricultural Commissioner pretends to give some statistics with reference to the losses the people suffer from swine-plague. In 1876 it was reported that the loss from this disease alone amounted to some $20,000,000. The report for 1878 gives $30,000,000 as the amount of loss to the country from all contagious animal diseases. These are estimates—nothing more. It is absolutely impossible to gain any reliable statistics in a country where there is no system of veterinary laws or an efficient veterinary police. The value of reliable statistics, with reference to the extension of contagious disease among our animals, can not be overestimated. Until we have them, it will be useless to hope for much conformable legislation. Every observing citizen must at once perceive the immense tax which these diseases impose upon the nation.

It is highly probable that, were the real facts known, their ravages have cost the people more in the last hundred years of our existence than our national debt amounts to.

Every one should know that, if not absolutely preventable, yet it is possible for a competent veterinary police to reduce these losses to a very low minimum.

Germany, with its efficient code of laws and veterinary police, is continually proving this; while Britain and ourselves as frequently give proof of the incapacity of our respective Governments in this regard.

No prevention can be hoped for until we have the necessary implements to work with. These implements are a national code of police laws, corresponding to the results obtained by modern scientific investigation, and an efficient body of educated veterinarians to execute them. With reference to the latter, men of very ordinary education can do the "pole-axe" business; the graduates of our present American veterinary colleges being equal to that, while they are utterly incapable of doing the higher state-work—i. e., making researches into the causes and nature of disease. This is no reflection upon them personally. It *is* upon conditions which do not give men desiring them suitable opportunities for acquiring an education which would fit them for this work. At present, however, we have to do with the question of a national code of veterinary police laws. This word "national" is a peculiar bugbear to many people in this country, who can not rise above party affiliations or sectional jealousy. *National* does *mean centralization*—nothing else. The question to be considered—and in politics it is a truly scientific one—is, how much centralization is necessary for the good of the whole country, and how much individuality can be allowed the respective States, without their interfering with the rights of each other. We have in this country a singular phenomenon. We have multiplied the sacred rights of the individual to such a degree that the masses have scarcely any rights left. We are continually in fear of trampling upon the rights of the individual. In doing this, we forget that the masses have still greater rights. No individual has any right to pursue a course or suffer considerations which endanger the property or interfere with the rights of the masses. Unfortunately, instead of "the masses," we act as if one individual is alone to be considered. It is this "right of the British freeman" which has been the chief obstacle to the suppression of contagious animal diseases in Britain. I do not think our American citizens are such obstinate and ignorant sticklers for their individual rights as Englishmen. In conversing with a number of intelligent farmers in the vicinity of Boston, where pleuro-pneumonia had prevailed in times past, I found that they were mostly entirely unacquainted with the true purposes of the laws for the suppression of this disease. As is well known, Massachusetts deported herself most energetically and creditably at this time, successfully exterminating the disease, and keeping it from her borders ever since. These farmers seemed, however, to have the idea that they, or their neighbors, or town, had been most unjustly treated. They had never gained the idea that, by slaughtering *all* the cattle of a few owners, those of the majority were saved, and the town spared a much greater loss. *The rights of the individual are as nothing when those of the masses are endangered; yet it is the duty of the latter to amply remunerate the former for the loss they have caused him to incur for their protection.* This is the sole and only principle which should guide legislators in drafting laws. Especially is this true with reference to those we are now considering. This principle is equally applicable to our respective States. Without such centralization—i. e., without some *one* controlling, inciting, directing power—nothing was ever yet accomplished. The question of regulation is to find the proper relation of such a power to the other elements or powers by which it is surrounded, that the greatest good for all concerned may result from their united action. This principle is one of true politics. Whether it be true republicanism or democracy I do not know, and care even less. The family can not well exist without its head. The ship can not pursue her course over the sea without her responsible captain. No business has ever succeeded without its competent and accountable head. "Too many cooks spoil the broth" is a homely but true saying. As a nation, we stand at present impotent before the ravages of the infectio-contagious animal diseases. We shall never get much beyond this impotent stage if we adhere to the State-rights doctrine with reference to the suppression and prevention of these diseases. This doctrine requires special notice at the present moment. We are approaching a period in our history when the different State Legislatures will be called upon to make some kind of laws and regulations with reference to this question. Reflecting men, those best competent to judge, are also endeavoring to urge the General Government to do likewise. The real question, which must be discussed with cool and unprejudiced brains, is, Which step is the more likely to be of most lasting benefit to the people of the whole country, as well as those of single sections? Dr. Bowditch, in his valuable essay, "Public Hygiene in America," tells us that we have at present (1876) twenty-one States without either law or regulation looking to the suppression or prevention of these diseases. In ten States there were some, and sixteen were reported as indefinite, while from one State it was impossible to gain any information. Our markets are all without the supervision of competent inspectors, notwithstanding the great danger to the poorer classes, more so than the rich, of disease of a disturbing if not fatal character, from the consumption of diseased meat. No State in this Union, so far as I know, has a State veterinarian in the true sense. In some there is a veterinarian attached to some agricultural society; in others, to a cattle commission. The few regulations which exist in some States are totally inadequate to the purpose. They almost entirely fail in properly defining the duties of the public. Quacks are in no way made responsible for the proper notification to the authorities of the presence of a suspected contagious disease in a given animal. In fact, our laws are of such a nature that, while in some cases, as in pleuro-pneumonia, they allow of quite satisfactory action, because of the very limited extension of the disease, in others, as glanders, they are next to useless, because of the great extension which the disease has already acquired among our horses. One of our greatest errors is, that we have made no use of the few competent veterinary practitioners in the country. Our laws serve only to make one man very prominent without being of the service to the State that they should be. It is in the interests of the people that the veterinary profession be made of use, and not that a single veterinary commissioner, in unison with several citizen members, have the entire work to do. It can not be done, as is sufficiently proven in Massachusetts, where we have an old and well-tried veterinarian on the cattle commission. While they did kill out pleuro-pneumonia, it has been sufficiently demonstrated that they are next to powerless in fighting glanders single-handed. We seem to think that, having organized a "cattle commission," our work is done; as if there were no other animal diseases worthy of consideration! Finally, in some States they attached a section with reference to glanders, and with that we have thus far rested content. Such a system is next to useless. It can never lead to any reliable statistics. These laws or regulations in the different States have very little in common. In many States they are simply dead letters, there being no competent authority to see them properly executed. "What is everybody's business is nobody's." In no one sense is the saying, "In union there is strength," more strictly true than in combating contagious animal diseases. It may be positively asserted that, if we adhere strictly to the principle of State-rights in this regard, all our endeavors to prevent and suppress these diseases will be weak and of but little avail.

All must admit that the manner of viewing any given subject is not the same even among a few individuals. How much less likely is this to be the case among large bodies jealous of each other! These great differences of opinion are largely dependent upon a difference in information and education by the individual members; and, secondly, upon a varying degree of appreciation of the nature of a threatened danger. A large amount of reading and reflection is necessary before men are competent to logically legislate on any given subject, and on none more so than that we are at present considering.

Hence it is that in some States we should have more or less suitable laws with a corresponding execution of the same, while in others quite the contrary would be the case. Only when a common danger exists, or when there is some central and controlling power to spur men on to their duty, and warn them of their danger, do we have energetic and uniform action. The results of this condition of things may be made more apparent by supposing that pleuro-pneumonia is present in two or more adjoining States. The authorities of one of these States, thoroughly aware of the dangers to which her bovine population is exposed, and not regardless, we may hope, of their duty to sister States, have made ample provision of money, and drafted appropriate regulations for "stamping out" the disease. They have selected special persons to execute the same. On the other hand, the authorities of an adjoining State have decided to follow the temporizing policy. They seem to fear a primary outlay, not appreciating that a small outlay, well expended, at first, may save an immense expense in the future. The regulations of this State, and the manner in which they are executed, are of that form which serve to express a fear of the ill-will of the people. Her legislators seem to have their attention more earnestly fixed upon influences likely to interfere with the next elections, rather than on their duties to the people. They appear to utterly ignore any responsibility with reference to their duties toward adjoining States. They make of their State a hot-house from which pestilential germs may be disseminated, not only to adjoining States, but even to those more distantly situated. Of what use, then, is all the outlay of time, money, and labor by the authorities of the first-named State? To prevent the disease extending over her borders, she must treat her sister State as an enemy. She must place an embargo, not only on all cattle *from* that State, but upon all *passing through* that State. She can allow no cattle to cross her frontiers from a State where the laws are less stringent, or poorly executed, without first subjecting them to inspection, and frequently to quarantine. Were this regulation carried out along a long line of traffic through different States, it requires no stress of the imagination to perceive the great disturbances which our trade in domestic animals would suffer. In the case of glanders it will be absolutely impossible to keep it properly confined within narrow limits, unless we have the same laws and regulations for every State in the Union, and equally stringent execution of the same. Otherwise, such horses can be run backward and forward across State boundaries, or the result will be that the disease will acquire an undesirable extension in those States where the laws are lax, or where they are but dead letters for the want of proper execution. The people of such a State will then suffer losses which they richly deserve. We find it necessary to have national laws to prevent the introduction of contagious human diseases from foreign countries. Is it not equally necessary that we have such a code of laws as will best protect the animal property of all the people in this country to the same degree, and not (as will be the invariable result, if we leave the States to make their own laws) have such codes as to offer but incomplete protection to the people of any State? The universal testimony of all men who have busied themselves with the suppression of contagious animal diseases is, that it is rendered doubly difficult because of the ease with which owners can get rid of diseased or suspected animals. Dealers are, in general, only too willing to take advantage of such opportunities to get cheap bargains, and they are equally regardless of the interests of the community in transporting them. A man sick with a contagious disease gladly stays at home. But if a person practicing as a veterinarian informs most owners of the presence or the suspicion of a contagious disease among their animals, the owner's first endeavor is to get them off; and experience has proved that many of them care very little about the danger of infection to which they subject the property of other men. This is absolute testimony to the necessity of regulating the duties of empirics and quacks in the practice of veterinary medicine, as well as owners. The duties of graduates must naturally also be regulated by law. With reference to the trustworthiness and public spirit of owners, a most interesting example occurred in connection with trichinosis in swine within a few weeks.

A gentleman came to me one afternoon, and in a very bombastic manner requested me to examine two pieces of pork. These hogs had been fattened by himself, and, as he expressed it, were "blooded Berkshires." It was, or is, his custom to fatten two each year, and present pieces of "home-fed pork" to his friends at Christmas. One piece was free, but the other was very badly trichinous. On showing them to the gentleman upon a hot table attached to the microscope, so that he could see the worms squirm about, he called me a "swindler," and intimated that I had introduced them surreptitiously into the specimen. Convincing him of his error, however, he somewhat recovered his temper, and remarked that he certainly could not think of presenting such pork to his friends, and that some would have to go without their present this year. "But there is no law against my sending it to market, is there?" To which I am sorry I had to answer that there was not, nor could I prevent it; but that I thought the rendering establishment the best place for it.

The answer, and the manner in which it was given, were something really worth recording. "Thank God, there's some freedom left in Massachusetts!" said this pattern of Boston aristocracy; for the gentleman is one frequently pointed out as an example of honesty and Christian virtues. "Thank God, there's some freedom left in Massachusetts" for a wealthy man to sell pork which, if a little underdone, can cause the serious illness of persons consuming it, or even death! Is there not need for *laws* to prevent the sale of improper food by technical examination? If a person of this man's worldly standing has no moral responsibility, what have we to expect from the ordinary owner of horses, cattle, etc.? Every one at all acquainted with the internal arrangements of the German Empire must know that there is far more jealousy between the different kingdoms of which it is composed than there is between the different States composing our Union. Notwithstanding this, these governments have seen the absolute necessity of an imperial code of laws for the suppression of the contagious animal diseases, experience having proved the state laws hitherto in existence insufficient for the purpose, there being here and there a dissimilarity which resulted in evil consequence to the people of one state or another. We need not copy literally the German laws, but we can study them and adapt them to our uses. It is high time that active steps were taken, in this country, in this direction.

To this end our national Congress should either select a commission of honest men, or authorize the President to select such from among the leading stock-raisers of the country, one from each of our great geographical sections. This commission should select three of the ablest *approved* veterinarians in the country, and two able and non-partisan lawyers. These five men should be paid to make a study of the veterinary police laws and institutions of such countries as are worthy of consideration, and should then draft a national code of laws and regulations in strict accord with the results of the best scientific research, and with exact regard to logic and explicitness in language. These laws should be accepted by Congress and by the respective State Legislatures. Such a plan in no way interferes with the right of States to make such special laws and regulations, in addition to them, as their local needs, positions, or other requirements may demand; and furthermore, as will presently be seen, our plan will provide each State with a competent and trustworthy body of men to execute the laws. From these three, and others, if they desire, should be selected a person to be known as Veterinary Inspector-General of the United States. This position should never be disgraced by being filled by political favorites of congressmen, secretaries, or commissioners. The present Commissioner of Agriculture would gladly have the appointment given over to his dispensation. Fortunately, Congress has not yet seen fit to give him such a liberty. A man must, at least, know something of the duties of the office to be filled, if he is to appoint an incumbent. This position must be filled on its merits, and by public competition before the members of the National Board of Health in the first place; but when the time comes, the incumbent should be elected by vote of the trustees and teachers of the national school, from among the State veterinary inspector-generals of the country. No teacher or professor of the school should ever be eligible to the office so long as they were connected with that institution. In no other way should it be possible for any man to gain the position. Science is the search after truth. A scientist who uses the ways of politicians to gain a position does not deserve the name. Science is open as the day. Politics is as dark and intricate as the passages of a coal-mine, and about as dirty. Science is not politics, as we see it displayed in America. There is such a thing as political science, but it has not yet been introduced into our legislative halls. The great men of science have been the truest servants of mankind. Scientists are patriots, not demagogues or political hucksters, ready to sell their birthright for a mess of pottage.

The Veterinary Inspector-General of the United States should be attached to the National Board of Health, as should all State inspector-generals to State boards. The whole system of veterinary sanitary police should be part and parcel of one grand national sanitary system, working in the interests of true preventive medicine.

These officers should hold their positions until sixty years old, unless incapacitated for work by sickness. They should be liberally paid; and, in case of retirement, their pay should be continued to them during life. The nation and the States need all their energies and time.

On his death, if leaving a widow or minor children, the former should have at least *two thirds* of the husband's pension during life, and the children a proportionate share until sixteen years of age. The State inspector-generals should be selected by public competition of approved veterinarians before the members of the State Board of Health. In each State there must be county, district, market, and other local veterinary officials. These men must first have passed a special examination, instituted for the purpose, with reference to sanitary police duties, at the National Veterinary Institute.

Until such an institution is organized, the competitions should take place before the members of the State Board of Health of each State. They should receive a certain amount of pay per year for official work, and in no case should they hold office after becoming sixty years old. They should not be subject to pensions, as their official positions should assist them in practice by guaranteeing to the people their superior education. Local inspectors, while belonging to the force, such as market and milk inspectors, should be paid by the respective local authorities. State inspectors, ordered to attend horse or cattle fairs or markets, should be paid for the time of service by the respective associations. The State should fix the price, which should be liberal, and allow for all traveling and incidental expenses.

We can not expect any intelligent appreciation, on the part of the public, of the value of such a sanitary system, unless we can present them with reliable statistical information on the subject. Without statistics we can not tell to what degree such diseases are domesticated in a given State, nor can we judge of our success in combating them from year to year. To this end, returns should be made quarterly by the district and local veterinary officials to those of the county, and semi-annually by the latter to the State Inspector-General, who should make an annual report to the inspector-general at Washington, who in his turn should prepare a condensed annual report of the condition and work done in the whole country—the same to be a part of the report of the National Board of Health. It must not be forgotten that this work of inspection is never to be limited to contagious diseases of animals alone, but that most especial attention must be given to the study and observation of those diseases and conditions which are either known, or are supposed, to exert harmful or dangerous influences upon the health of mankind. The true veterinarian is fully as much a guardian of the public health as the medical hygienist. The curing of sick animals is by far the most insignificant part of his work. *Prevention* is the true strength of veterinary science. In this regard the veterinarian is of far more importance to humanity than the medical practitioner. The tables are exactly turned about in the two branches of medical science. The doctor is strongest in practice, the veterinarian in the prevention of diseases.

By the plan which we have proposed for a national veterinary police code and organization, it is self-evident that the extension of any disease over the country, or from one State to another, can be very strongly combated. In case a contagious animal disease—we will assume the rinderpest—breaks out at any place, say Columbus, Ohio, the law requires the owner, attendant quack, empiric, or regular practitioner, to at once notify the next veterinary official of the State of the suspicion or actual appearance of the disease. If the former is very strong, or becomes at once confirmed, he at once notifies the inspector-general of his State, who at once notifies every official veterinarian in the State, and the inspector-general at Washington. The latter notifies each State general inspector, who in his turn notifies the State veterinary officials. What is the result? An absolute quarantine of every head of cattle in this whole country. Not a single one can be moved without the permit of an official veterinarian. All transported cattle are watched from place of shipment to destination. Extension, under such circumstances, is reduced to the lowest possible limit. The same is true of every other contagious animal disease. Smuggling or removal across State boundaries of suspected or diseased animals becomes useless, for notification is at once transmitted from the one State to the other. There is no opposition between the authorities of different States. The laws are the same. The officials belong to one organization. They are appointed for a term of years. Truly, every one must see that in this case we have unity in purpose and strength to execute the laws. State rights are respected, individual rights honored, yet both State and individual receive the fullest amount of protection for their animal property which it is in the power of science to bestow. I have said that the national veterinary inspector should be attached to the National Board of Health, and that the whole veterinary sanitary organization should be a part of a grand national system of preventive medicine. We have a National Board of Health. Others have expressed their ideas of its work, therefore it may be allowed me to close this section of my book with some of my own, crude as they may appear.

The National Board of Health was called into being simply on account of the yellow fever. Its work, up to the present time, has been chiefly limited to the study of that disease, and in seeking for means looking toward its prevention. This much-needed work should be amply supported, and obstinately persevered in, but we may be sure that many years will elapse before any marked success will crown our efforts. Success will come, however, if the American people can keep their balance long enough not to cry out for a false economy, which is the last cry one should hear in this important branch of our Government. The work of a National Board of Health has, however, scarcely begun when it is limited to yellow fever. Such an institution must be the focal stimulus which shall gradually cause the organization of one grand national system of preventive medicine. It must seek to incite reforms where they are needed, and among these none is more important than one standard medical examination for the country, and one similar course of study at every medical school in the land. No good work can ever be done except as the result of organized effort. Centralized, that is, concentrated effort, is always rewarded by better results than isolated, sporadic endeavor. Many of our States are still without effective boards of health, as is also the case in many large cities or towns. In only one State, Massachusetts, have we anything like State medical officers. In this State we have the "medical examiners" taking the place of that useless inheritance from England, the "coroner." In effective work it is absolutely necessary that the whole country become subjected to one code of sanitary laws, suitable to the general needs, while in every State, county, city, or town, such special laws must be made, and are in general, as the local needs demand. These special laws and regulations should always bear a proper relation to the general. It is the drafting of the latter which will devolve upon the national board. Once having such laws and regulations, the next thing is their execution. To this end competent sanitary officials are necessary. These appointments should never be made until candidates have passed a special examination, to be fixed for the purpose by the National Board of Health for the whole country—the examination to consist in questionings upon the pathology, etiology, etc., of the diseases included among those generally spoken of under the headings of preventive medicine. The examinations should be made by the members of the respective State boards of health. The organization of the sanitary system in each State should be similar to that which I have portrayed with regard to a veterinary organization. These positions should be points of ambition for our best young men. They should receive pay for official work. In cases where the necessities of the public demanded their whole time they should be liberally paid, and open to a pension in the same manner as above considered. We should therefore have a National Board of Health in connection with State boards, which should be in connection with local boards and health officers. These officials must be thoroughly educated in the principles and practice of modern research, and in pathological anatomy and necroscopy. The professional members of the State boards of health should be appointed by the Governor from among the most competent of the sanitary officers. They should all be paid, and hold office until sixty years of age, or during activity. Those members who are required to devote their whole time to the service of the State should be pensioned on retirement. The State can never afford to be a "bummer." Men who can afford to work for honor alone are seldom fitted to serve the State well. This principle of working for the State for honor alone, so common in certain positions in this country, can not be too strongly condemned. It is death to young men, and equally detrimental to the public good. A State which is too poor to pay competent men for the work it requires of them is too poor to exist. It had better secede out of this Union, or be merged into another which is capable of paying for work well done.

Boards of health are too much limited to gathering statistics. Again, these statistics are often too much limited to those of the so-called infectious diseases. The latter class of statistics has a very subordinate value. It matters but little whether one thousand or ten thousand men perish from a given infectious disease, so long as the cause is present, yet unknown, and prevention thus far impossible. It is far more necessary that observations and experiments in these two directions be made than that exact statistics be gathered annually. Statistics as to causal influences, however, can never be too highly appreciated. These accumulated statistics have one good purpose: without them, in this country, it would be impossible to get means enough from the Legislatures to carry on the necessary studies and experiments by which we may in the end hope to find means of prevention. Boards of health should always have the necessary means to carry on an experiment station, and to amply reward specialists for experimental researches in any desired direction.

There is, however, another form of statistics, the careful collection of which would send a thrill of horror over the human family, and it is from this form that we may, in the distant future, expect very valuable results. To obtain them we need far better practitioners, much less prejudiced thinkers, than we at present have in the medical profession.

I allude to statistics with regard to the really preventable diseases of life; the diseases due to ignorance, not only on the part of the diseased, but of practitioners as well. An ignorance of duty with reference to the latter, for the medical adviser who *treats* only is simply fit for confinement among idiots. I allude further to the diseases due to the ignorance of the people in the employment of quacks, and further to the still more to be condemned American craze, the use of those disgraces of our civilization, *legalized patent life-destroyers, discoveries of the devil or his agents—patent medicines.*

Another disease which requires statistical attention is tubercular consumption. It kills more people in ten years than any invasive disease of the present day is likely to do. Our climate has been made to play a much too important part among the causes of this disease. Climate, employment, etc., all play the sufficient or producing causes, but very seldom the primary cause. The primary cause is to be sought in the senseless inbreeding of weak lungs from generation to generation among human beings, until at present the very irritation of normal breathing is often sufficient to send a child into an early grave from tubercular consumption. The medical profession acknowledge the influences of our climate. Perhaps they can see the other also. But truth is ever unpleasant; and to tell parents that their children dare not marry at all, or dare not intermarry—to tell young lovers they dare not marry, because they would condemn their children to an early grave—would seriously interfere with one's yearly income. *Who of the medical profession stands up as a man of truth and proclaims to the world that consumptives dare not marry, or that children of families with such tendencies must not intermarry?* We must *out-breed* this tendency to weak lungs by sensible and exact marriage, or we shall find still more reason to condemn our climate than we now have. Why do these men study medicine? It is certainly not to think, not to speak, the truth. To make a living, regardless of the good of humanity. Medical practice has fallen to a business in this country, instead of being conducted as a science. Can these men think? Can they observe what every breeder of fine cattle has long since known? I scarcely believe it. Blind! blind! Education is a myth! Ignorance only exists! To think, the evidence of true education seems to be the thing we must seek after. We may find it among the lost arts. *Until then, humanity will go on damning its children, for a longer or shorter time, to a living hell of misery and pain. There is but* one *cure for consumption* (quacks to the contrary): *Consumptives, descendants of consumptive families, dare not intermarry.*

Syphilis is a disease of similar character. It can scarcely be rooted out from an organism when once its terrible germs have gained access. Does the medical profession do its duty in this regard? Does it tell young but unfortunate patients that they dare not marry? "Marry, doctor?" "Oh, yes." "Perfectly cured?" "Oh, yes." But the child produced not only brands the medical adviser as a liar, a stupid and irresponsible ignoramus, but publishes the father's "cured" condition (?) to the world. Statistics would indeed teach a valuable lesson with regard to these inherited diseases and disease tendencies. After these numerical statistics have been gathered, still another form of no secondary importance demands our attention. It is not enough to know the number of deaths which occur in a country from a number of given diseases. We do absolutely nothing, except to establish an annual percentage with such figures. To complete the work, it is necessary that all natural influences should be most carefully observed by competent men. We must have accurate reports with reference to the condition of the ground-water in all sections of the country, its temperature, and seek to accurately define the relations of the same to typhus and typhoid diseases. We must know the influences exerted upon the eruption and extension of diseases by the water-courses and prevailing winds. We must know what diseases prevail mostly or most severely in the valleys and upon high and exposed table-lands, as well as wooded districts or low and marshy lands. We must know accurately the influences exerted by changes of temperature, seasons, wet or dry, and the connection between the diseases of the different species of the animal kingdom. When all this is done, our National Board of Health should publish, once in every ten years, pathological geographical maps, with reference to the extension of all forms of disease in the United States; not one is to be excepted, whether due to transmitted influences, to infection, or to external influences. This, with the annual reports, in unison with investigations at the hands of competent experts, and the work of the veterinary department, constitutes, in my mind, the work of a national organization for the purposes of preventive medicine.

A NATIONAL VETERINARY INSTITUTE.

In the preceding parts of this work we have endeavored to make our readers individually appreciate that mankind is constantly threatened with several serious and in many cases fatal diseases, from contact with diseased animals in life, or from the consumption of flesh, milk, or other materials derived from them. We have also shown that the prevention of these evils, as well as the ravages of the strictly contagious animal diseases, can not be attained, or hoped for, without a well-organized system of veterinary police, and a carefully drafted code of laws and regulations. It should be evident to every one that this much-desired prevention, and the collection of those valuable statistics, in a trustworthy manner, by which the people can alone determine as to the extension which the contagious and infectious animal diseases acquire each year, do not come within the province of the medical practitioner. We have shown that, in the majority of the States, no laws exist for the suppression and prevention of contagious animal diseases, and in no State are they what they should be, or at all conformable to the latest results of scientific research. This work can only be well performed by the veterinarian who has been thoroughly schooled in the principles and methods of scientific medicine at a well-regulated institution. It is the same in medicine. The thirst for knowledge for itself is the sole incentive to original research. Monetary rewards are not gained in the medical laboratory which is devoted to the study of physiology and pathology. The practitioner who is always boasting of his cures, who prides himself in a knowledge of the by-gones, if not too lazy; who always treats the earnest endeavors and researches of some brother practitioner with scorn; who echoes the popular voice, by speaking of him as a theorist, "a very learned man, but fails in not having had *my* practical experience," is to be invariably put down as a humbug and first-class ignoramus. The man of experience alone is always an ignorant man in the light of science. How often do the boasted men "of great practical experience" fail! They sink into a well-deserved oblivion before the genius of the first-class practitioner, who unites in himself the two elements, theory and practice, the one inseparable union which shall endure forever. *Scientia est potentia* ("Science is power"). Without science, i. e., without theory, where would the world be now? Science holds the keys to the money-vaults of the world. She opens to our view the hidden treasures of the earth. She adapts to our uses the raw materials which she teaches us to win from nature. She has given us all the means of comfort and luxury which we have; but, greater than all these, she is the fair goddess whose rules and teachings, faithfully applied, lead to health. Science alone can discover the means of prevention—crude experience, empiricism, never! The workers in the many fields of science have been among the noblest benefactors of the human race, and among these none have excelled those of medicine for their untiring devotion and self-sacrifice. These men constantly neglect the very laws which they are begging humanity to follow; no devotion is too great to dampen their zeal; every means, even to unnecessary experiment upon themselves, which have too often led to sacrifice of life, have been donated to the service of humanity. With right France immortalizes the name of her Bichat, Germany her Virchow, England her Hunter, Holland her Boerhaave, Austria her Rokitansky. With right and justice, and a grand appreciation of the value of such men to the world, as well as their native countries, do the Continental governments support them in the days of their activity, and relieve their minds from all anxiety for the future of themselves and their immediate dependants, by properly pensioning them when the period of decay comes on.

All hail, then, the day when veterinary science shall find a fitting place wherein to develop among the people of this country!

To the purposes of prevention and suppression of the ravages and extension of the diseases which have been considered, it has been frequently observed that veterinarians are necessary. Having portrayed their work, it becomes us to consider how we can best produce them. The material is ready, the field planted. We have, I truly believe, better material, young men, to work upon than any other country in the world. All they are waiting for is *the means* by which they can acquire a suitable education. It is the duty of the people to supply these means. But, to this end, there must be, somewhere in the country, a properly endowed, organized, and regulated institution for the study of veterinary medicine. There are several ways by which veterinary schools have been established, but only two of these are worth a moment's earnest consideration; still there are two others which it becomes our duty to consider, in order that we may be made well aware of their utter fallacy. The first two plans, which we will not at present consider, are—1. State schools, controlled and regulated by each State, to which we will oppose a national school, answering all the purposes of the nation; but, instead of being controlled by the Government, regulated by a board of trustees and its teachers, the former to be elected from a national association, which should be organized for the purpose.

There are two plans which are to be condemned and combated as evils, the nature of which the people of this country have not as yet any conception of, but of which they must gradually learn. The first of these is an irregular number of chartered, uncontrolled, irresponsible institutions in each State; and the second is known as the *subscription plan*, which may be rightly included in the first, but for special reasons deserves individual treatment.

The first of these—that is, one or more chartered, uncontrolled, and in many instances irresponsible schools in each State—needs no exercise of the imaginative power in order that we may study it in all its bearings. It is more than amply illustrated by the condition of medicine in this country at the present time. In 1876 we had fifty-nine uncontrolled, chartered medical schools in this country. In some States the executive powers were not content with chartering one, but willingly increased the number conformably to the pleasure of applicants: as, in New York State, there are seven; in Ohio, six; and in the District of Columbia, one. But, not even content with thus disgracing the science of medicine to a most mercenary business, we find in some cities three or more schools, as is shown by the following cutting from a daily paper:

"The city of Chicago contains *six medical schools*—allopathic and homœopathic—and, according to the 'Times,' they turn out graduates with greater rapidity, and of poorer quality, than any other medical colleges yet known. No preliminary education is absolutely required as a condition of admission. An attendance upon two courses of lectures, each of twenty weeks, suffices in some of them to secure a diploma, under which the holder is authorized to begin practicing upon his fellow-citizens. The 'Times' further alleges that in some instances diplomas have been obtained for money, or through the personal influence of friends who were on good social terms with the professors."

It is a very singular phenomenon, in a country the people of which place so much stress upon the value of public schools, and where the State controls them, and requires every child to have an education, and where the quality and quantity of the education given at schools of certain rank is guaranteed by the State, to see all responsibility avoided by the State, with reference to the academical or collegiate education of our youth; this lack of responsibility even extends itself to the medical schools, whether connected with colleges or individual institutions. While no very harmful results, other than superficialness and snobbishness, have been brought forward with reference to the universities and colleges from this neglect on the part of the State, it is quite the contrary with reference to the schools of medicine. As to the universities and colleges, it may be truly asserted that, were they State institutions, strongly funded, and free from the curse which is making America the laughing-stock of nations—politics; and were teachers appointed on their merits, not on account of their connections, science would have been much further developed than it is now.

Some singular results may be observed to follow this neglect of its duties by the State with reference to the medical schools. If a young man is a graduate of a certain high-grade public school, and applies to a merchant for a position, with his certificate of graduation, the latter, if at all posted, is able at once to form an approximate idea of the degree of education the youth has acquired, and of his fitness for the position he has to offer him. On the contrary, if a young graduate of a medical school settles in one's neighborhood, and hangs up his sign as an "M. D.," how much do we know? Absolutely nothing, save that we may generally assume he has a diploma. But until we see it, until we find out, not only from what city he came, but frequently from which school in said city, and not until we have ourselves investigated into the character and responsibility of said school, do we know whether the "M. D." of the young man is worth more than the tin it is painted upon. The State takes no responsibility in the matter. She is absolutely neglectful of her duties. Many of the fifty-nine medical schools in this country deserve no other destiny than to be immediately closed by law as common nuisances—i. e., producers of unqualified vampires, destined to prey upon an innocent and trusting community. This neglect of the higher education on the part of the State, and leaving it entirely to the charity and public spirit of the community, is a great mistake, and one which tends largely to the detriment of the development of science in this country. It is one of the greatest evils of a popular form of government that no great improvement or reform can ever take place until the people have first become in a measure educated up to it. This retards all movements, unless they are so essentially practical that the results by which the public are to be benefited "stare them in the face." The rewards of science, however, are only developed slowly, and by the labor of countless workers. In monarchical or parental forms of government the above is not the case. As soon as the government sees that a certain thing is necessary to the welfare of the nation, *it does it*, irrespective of public opinion, which is invariably slow to see the reasons for changes, especially when the benefits follow slowly. With reference to their medical institutions, there is scarcely a Continental country from which we could not learn an immense deal. The governments are, in this thing at least, true to the interests of the people, when they control the schools and regulate strictly the quality and quantity of education of each graduate. With us, as is well known, the contrary is the case—"the more the merrier," seems to be the motto of our States with reference to the establishment of medical schools; and until public opinion itself demands a change, we may be sure none will take place for years to come, unless our own poor endeavors, unaided as they have yet been, succeed in leading the way to a reform which shall extend to the medical schools, by the establishment of a veterinary institute upon purely scientific principles.

It may be axiomatically asserted that it is as much the duty of the State to protect its people against incompetently educated men and impostors in medicine as it is to protect them against frauds in other departments of life. This can only be attained by the State's regulating and controlling the entire system of education, and the terms of graduation of the medical school or schools within its territory. While most parents display a creditable degree of anxiety with reference to the education which a son is to acquire when fitting for a mercantile position in life, it is only too true that many parents look upon a medical education as a sort of luxury, and, utterly regardless of the welfare of their fellow-men, desire their son *put through* the medical school in the shortest time and at the least expense possible. While there is a certain degree of uniformity in the printed catalogues issued by the fifty-nine medical schools in this country, yet it is very doubtful if the conditions upon which diplomas are conferred are held up to by all the schools. In fact, experience goes to prove the latter to be the case. In most of them the conditions necessary to obtaining the diploma read *three years* of study, two full courses (one year) at some medical school, one of which must be at the institution in question. In reality, we have here a demand for but three sessions' study in a medical school. As these three sessions are supposed to extend over a year and a half, one is somewhat at a loss to know what the regulation three years' study means. The regulations frequently say "three years' study with some regular practitioner," which, if insisted upon, would make the full term of study four and a half years; and, as students may graduate at twenty-one years of age, many students would be but sixteen and a half years old when beginning the study of medicine—too young by far for most youths to have acquired that education and drilling in the natural sciences by which alone the study of the professional branches can be followed with any profit. The "three years with any regular practitioner," whether he be of good or irregular standing, may have been a necessity in the early days of our history, but is to be looked upon now as a disgrace to any civilized nation. It is injurious to the young man, injurious to the people, degrading to the profession, and puts incumbrances in the way of the scientific advancement of the profession, which will only be overcome with immense difficulty, and at the cost of much ill-feeling and great self-denial. It can only succeed in building up a class of self-conceited, scarcely semi-educated empirics, who, having acquired a certain amount of practical experience in the company of Dr. Old Fogy, the much-overestimated "regular practitioner," look upon the school as an uncomfortable hindrance, which keeps them from jumping into a lucrative practice, and which is only to be used in order to gain the legitimizing "M. D." with as little study and expense as possible.

There is not a strictly scientific medical school in the United States. There are fifty-five too many. The needs of the country demand about four large and well-regulated medical institutions; but as this is and will be impossible, it is necessary that we do our utmost to reform the existing institutions. To this end, the State must assume control of them, as it does of the public schools. The corps of teachers should be selected by public competition, and it must never be forgotten that not every man who can write well or who has distinguished himself in original research is fitted by nature to teach. The ability to logically and practically detail the results of the world's knowledge is the requisite to be sought in a teacher; if these can be united with great original ability, all the better; but at a school there must be *teachers* as well as investigators. There should be in each State a board of health, the technical members of which should also constitute the medical board of examination. The members of such boards, as well as the teachers of the medical school and other State officers in connection with science, should be well paid. It is an American disgrace and misfortune that men of great original ability can seldom afford to work for the State. Too many such positions are filled by *dilettanti*—rich men's sons who dabble in science, and take such positions for the honor of the thing. Or else they are men who, having grown old *and experienced* (?), are thought especially suited for such honorable positions; whereas the period of combativeness and activity has passed away with them. A man is only of use to the world so long as he is combative. The same is true of our colleges. Men of ability, but poor, must seek a living elsewhere, and are obliged to turn their backs upon the laboratories they would delight in, and upon institutions they would honor, in order to prepare for their old age, while snobbishness and mediocrity too frequently fill the places they should be honored with. Hence, we seldom find men of vast scientific ability filling the chairs of American colleges. At the medical schools the conditions are in general still worse. We find many of the teachers struggling between their duties to a dangerously sick or dying patient in one part of the city, and an impatient and neglected class in the medical school at another part. The scenes of "hurrying to and fro" are often ridiculous in the extreme. It is self-evident that the students must suffer. Too many medical schools seem only to have been established to give a certain class of ambitious men a false reputation, and a certain degree of imposability before the people. Professor Æsculapius Wormwood is always *going* before the people as a very learned man, while in truth he is generally a most consummate humbug, one of his most frequent specialties being the removal of parasites, which, like himself, prey upon the vitalities of his patients.

The publications in which most of these medical schools make known their respective advantages are certainly as uncreditable to scientific institutions as is the ridiculous race for students in which nearly all the schools indulge. They are embellished with numerous striking woodcuts of the main buildings, laboratories, etc., and in more ways than one resemble the publications issued by hotel proprietors at summer resorts. The promises and opportunities are unexceptionable; but, once having you fairly in their grasp, with the fees secured, it matters very little in the one case about the intellectual and in the other about the corporal food one gets.

As I have previously said, the States have not been content with chartering one medical school within their respective limits. State charters for medical schools seem to be far more easy of attainment than liquor-licenses; in fact, it is very questionable if our inquiries as to the character of applicants for the latter are not more stringent than those which are made with reference to those who would originate a school for medical education. The law requires no absolute testimony of character or ability on the part of persons desiring to establish schools for medical education. Our legislators never ask, Have we not enough such schools? They seem to assume that the more we have the better, and look upon them from the same stand-point as they do institutions for general charity.

Chapter XXXII, section 1, of the Massachusetts General Statutes, reads: "Seven or more persons within this State, having associated themselves by agreement in writing for education, charitable, or religious purposes, under any name by them assumed, and complying with the provisions of this chapter [which say nothing as to their individual fitness], shall, with their successors, be and remain a body politic and corporate." The conditions are the same in nearly all our States—at least, I know of no exception to the rule. A friend writes me from Philadelphia: "As you are writing upon the establishment of veterinary schools, it may not be inappropriate for me to inform you that there are *two so-called* 'colleges' in this city, which are unfortunately chartered by the State. The men composing these 'colleges' are all *quacks;* they do not attempt to teach anything—were that possible for them—yet they *sell* diplomas or degrees to men who wish to practice. It is said they do pretend to require a sort of an examination before they issue these valuable papers." . . . In the city of New York there are three chartered, non-regulated veterinary schools.

Let us endeavor to look for a moment at the results of this purely American system of medical institutions:

1. From the want of uniformity and the lack of responsibility on the part of many institutions, the "M. D." of the young graduate is rendered next to worthless until we have made inquiries into his antecedents.

2. Most of them being poorly endowed and in many cases beggarly institutions, one may observe a most disgraceful rivalry for students, which is borne witness to by the business character of their catalogues.

The entire reason for these disgraceful conditions is to be sought in the lack of appreciation for true science which exists not only in the profession, but with the people as well. The curse of America is her overestimated "practicality." The most unmitigated of humbugs is often spoken of as "a man of great practical ability." *Superficial* betokens the Americanism of to-day. Sterling integrity, which is said to have been a characteristic of our forefathers, seems soon to be destined to a place among the lost arts. Fraud prevails! It is nourished, and, if successful, the stigma is soon buried beneath the glitter of the externals. The American people seem to love fraud. In no other country, unless it be England, can disgraceful quacks and humbugs flourish in every department of life as they do here. "A free fight and no favor," seems to be the motto governing our legislators, who apparently have entirely forgotten that the people they are supposed to represent—which they seldom do—are being consumed and plundered by these impostors. Humanity, as a whole, is still a babe in "swaddling-clothes." It still needs protection from itself. Only a few individuals have as yet been able to stand alone; and still fewer to furnish serviceable props for others. The second cause of these evils, with reference to the medical schools, must be charged to the State. We have too many. Education in them has become a business instead of a science. In no State should there be more than one medical school.

It is a great misfortune that we can not reduce the number to four or five large, well-founded, scientifically-founded sectional institutions, under one system of regulations for the whole country. The chartering of special schools for the promulgation of any special doctrine, as homœopathy, or for the education of special classes—women—is to be most vigorously condemned. In the first place, the fundamentals of medical science are the same, and if, on graduation, a practitioner chooses to start off upon a theoretical side-track, it matters not to the State. As for special schools for women, that is another absurdity. If the women desire to enter into the struggle for existence, good: give them a free chance; but, when they do this, they must know that they descend from the reverenced throne which American women in general sit upon, and that they have forfeited all rights to any special consideration *as women.* They must be ready to take the bitter with the sweet, the rough with the polished, the profane and vulgar with the chaste: unless they are willing to do this, *back* to their homesteads! The Trustees of Harvard College deserve nothing but condemnation in refusing the women admittance to their medical school. They say, "Endow another and a special school"; but they entirely fail to say a word about its qualifications and restrictions. They certainly know—not to their benefit, I think—that the State will charter anything; but they should also know that she as yet exercises no control over the chartered organizations. Harvard snobbishness is probably endangered by petticoatism; else why this fear? Who is to protect the people against incompetently educated graduates? That matters not, so long as Harvard keeps to her exclusiveness. Let the women be educated; but, if the legislators and women of Massachusetts have their senses with them, let them break down these doors of exclusiveness and enter Harvard. The men (?) there will be even more benefited than the women. It is possible that a true manhood might get an opportunity to develop, when women have trimmed the skirts of Harvard exclusiveness.

The first great step toward medical reform in this country is to do away with the superfluous schools, by having but one in each State; by having them under the control of the State, represented by its board of health as the examining body; by introducing the competitive system in the selection of teachers, and in opening the schools to free teaching by young aspirants, from which the competitors for the special branches are to be finally taken—in fact, in making these scientific institutions, instead of empiric hot-houses, grinding out yearly the largest possible number of half-educated, half-drilled fledglings. There should be a delegation appointed by the board of health of each State, with the consent of the respective Governors, to determine upon a universal course of study, to be extended over four years, and a national or universal system and standard of examination, so that, other things being equal, the "M.D." of each school should have a corresponding qualitative and quantitative value. Should this much-to-be-desired end prove impossible of attainment, then there is but one course left. It will then become the bounden duty of each State to *protect* the graduates of its own school as well as its people from the services of men graduating from schools in a neighboring State, or States, where the education is not recognized as equal to that in the first-named State. Unless they do this, all regulation of the home-school is but nonsense. A law will therefore have to be made, by which graduates from inferior schools in other States must make the State examination in a given State, before they can be allowed to practice as "M. D.'s," although the quack and empiric fields are still open to them. No graduate should be allowed to practice in any State until he has received a license for the purpose from the State Board of Health. A careful record of all licenses should be kept for reference.

The practice of medicine, or the advertising of practice, or of medicines, under false pretenses, should be most stringently regulated by the State. Several attempts have been made in this direction in different States, but in only a few have they been at all successful. Massachusetts holds a most unenviable position in this regard. Legislators labor under a great mistake with reference to the desires of the medical profession on this point. They assume, unjustly, that in some way the profession desire to interfere with the rights of the individual to have such medical attendance as he chooses to select. While this is not the case; while the profession, as represented by its best men, has no desire to institute a medical monopoly, it is very questionable if the rights of so-called matured persons can be allowed to interfere or trifle with the health of minors or irresponsible persons that the accidents of birth have placed in their charge. While I may have a certain right, under *civil* law, to poison myself by the use of tobacco or opium, I have no right to teach my child the use of such drugs; in fact, the law would prevent it, were outsiders to become acquainted with such a purpose on my part. It is the same with the employment of the empiric or quack. But there is still another side of this question which seems to have entirely escaped the attention of legislators. The graduate of the school acquires his right to the title "Doctor," or "M. D.," by hard labor and expense. He has, therefore, the right to a certain degree of protection, but only with reference to the title. This is all he asks. The people are, in general, thoughtless and trusting; they scarcely ever stop to question the right of the displayer or the advertiser to the title "Doctor," or "M. D." The first is much more frequently usurped. It is unquestionably the duty of the State to guarantee to the graduated student the exclusive use of these titles; and, also, to make them evidences of real worth to the people, that they may then select whom they please, by forbidding the use of them to all other men but graduates who practice medicine. This in no way interferes with the freedom of choice of the individual, nor does it restrain the quack or empiric from practicing the healing art; but it does reach the necessary end of giving the people the means of distinguishing the accredited man from the swindler, which is their right, and it will strike a heavy blow against fraud in medicine. Forbid, under penalty of the law, non-graduated men the use of the title "Doctor," or "M. D.," in any way whatsoever, either by sign, card, or advertisement, and we at once take away the charm by which they are alone enabled to swindle the people.

In using the words empiric and quack, we should always make a distinction. Not every empiric is of necessity a quack, nor is every quack an empiric. It is the deportment of the person which makes him a quack. There are empirics that have never graduated from a school, or even studied at one, but whose conduct can well be measured by the strictest code of medical ethics; such men are not and never will be quacks. Quacks are swindlers, misrepresenters of facts—promisers of things, such as cures, which they know to be impossible. While some empirics are not quacks, there are hundreds of men claiming to be graduates of licensed schools who are quacks of the blackest dye. It is impossible for the law to reach these scoundrels. We find them advertising cure-alls in every form. This mania for specifics and curative compounds is, I am sorry to say, gradually extending to members of the "regular" profession. Practitioners' offices are becoming littered up with sample bottles of "Dr. ——'s Viburnam" and other compounds, which, although not patented, are nothing else than quack medicines, being advertised in the same manner, having on one label the diseases it is supposed to be good for and on the other the dose. In fact, this evil is becoming so extended, that practicing M. D.'s, either too lazy or too ignorant to correctly compile a prescription, now frequently write "Dr. ——'s Compound," "one bottle—take as directed." What lessons are we to draw from the foregoing pages with reference to the establishment of veterinary schools in this country?

1. It would be an unpardonable sin to curse the people of this country with another set of private, unregulated, irresponsible medical institutions.

2. Under such a system of schools the title "Veterinary Surgeon," or any other to be selected, would be, as it is now, *worthless*, being assumed alike by graduated men, empirics, and veritable quacks.

3. It neither protects the people, by giving them a reliable means by which they can distinguish the approved man from the impostor, nor does it protect the honest and hard work of the school graduate.

4. It can never, until eternity, answer the manifold needs of the country, or produce, what is more needed than in human medicine, really scientifically qualified veterinary practitioners, who, while capable of attending to the practical demands of the public, are no less capable of meeting the scientific requirements of the State, in taking an active part in the study of and prevention of those animal diseases which carry misery and desolation to mankind, as well as threaten their health and life in some cases.

Equally to be condemned with the above *are private veterinary schools supported by subscription.* They would not deserve any additional consideration were it not that this plan has recently received the indorsement of no less an authority than the Universities of Pennsylvania and Harvard.

In considering the development of veterinary medicine, and the foundation of the Continental schools, we have endeavored to impress upon the reader the fact that these institutions were established by the respective governments, and have always been controlled by them, thereby guaranteeing, so far as possible, the quality of their graduates to the people. The result has been, that all these institutions have been steadily improved, until at the present day, and for some thirty years back, many of them have acquired the right to be called scientific institutions, though veterinary medicine has not, in my opinion, yet arrived at that stage in which it can be called a science. This remark requires an explanation from me. In the great veterinary schools of Europe the scientific method of study and research has been more or less perfectly introduced; but it has been adopted, almost wholesale, from human medicine. Veterinary medicine has never yet produced a great medical thinker. We have not yet got beyond good observers.

When we shall have produced a medical dictator, a Virchow or a Bichat, who will revolutionize all medical thought, or at least reform it, it will be time enough for us to speak of an individual veterinary science; and not till then will there be any such thing. Until then we shall be nothing more than a parasite drawing our best nourishment from human medicine—although, at present, we are making brave efforts to stand on our own feet.

Another fact, which is well worthy the attention of the citizens of the most "practical" land in the world, is—*not one of these Continental schools pays in the American sense;* i. e., they yield no direct dividends. We have seen that the Berlin school exceeded its income, in 1878–'79, by some $16,600. But, while yielding no direct returns in money, their indirect returns have benefited their respective countries and the world at large to such a degree that we can not estimate it in dollars and cents. To the teachers at these Continental schools do the veterinarians of Britain and America owe the greater part of the material of which their text-books are composed. To whom do we owe the greater part of our knowledge with reference to the contagious and infectious animal pests? To whom but Continental veterinarians! The names of Hering, Hertwig, Haubner, Roell, Brückmüller, Chauveau, Reynal, Bouley, Collin, Leisering, Wehenkel, Schuetz, Feser, and many others, are fast becoming as well known to English-speaking people, thanks to the efforts of Mr. Fleming, as they are to those of the Continent.

It is of the utmost importance to us, as American citizens, *to inquire why it is that this valuable information has been gained by Continental veterinarians, to the exclusion of those of Britain.* The answer is simple, and one which it is the duty of every American to study earnestly.

These schools are so established, and the teachers so carefully selected, and their present and future welfare so well cared for (for they are moderately paid during active life, and liberally pensioned when the period of decay comes on), that they can give their entire energies to the proper instruction of students and to scientific research.

These grand results can never be hoped for in countries where there are only to be found private, uncontrolled, and irresponsible schools—in proof of which we have already noticed the medical schools of this country, and have yet to consider the veterinary school at London, the representative one of Britain, on the subscription principle.

In sketching briefly the history of some of the principal veterinary schools of Europe, it must have been noticed that we omitted to speak of those of Britain. We neglected them for two reasons: first, because the London school, which we select as the best representative, has never yet deserved to be classed with those of the Continent; and, secondly, because it has been especially quoted as a favorable example of the "subscription plan" for the support of such schools.

In Britain we find directly opposite conditions to those of the Continent. Here we find the Government strangely blind to the interests and welfare of the people. America, the child, nobly follows the ignoble example of the mother. Britain has allowed her noted and valuable flocks and herds to be repeatedly decimated by pests without taking a single step to educate properly qualified veterinarians. Here we find no state responsibility; no state regulating the standard of education at the schools; no critical selection of teachers; no contribution to their support, by means of which the discovery and improvement of methods for checking and preventing the ravages of animal pests may be hoped for.

Being myself so bitter an opponent of both private and even state schools for the education of veterinarians, it may appear fairer for me to let a less partial judge speak for me on these matters.

Mr. George Fleming says: * "It was not, however, until 1792 that England had a veterinary school [established by Saint-Bell, a Frenchman], but this was of a private and speculative character; deriving no benefit from the state [and conferring none upon it], but allowed to push its own way from the fluctuating support or patronage of private subscribers and the fees of students." This school succeeds, at present, in the American sense—it pays. The director and some of the leading teachers—they call themselves professors, without ever having done anything worthy of the name—enjoy fat salaries, in return for which they energetically oppose every suggestion for improvements which could only be to the advantage of the Government and the people.

It is probably unknown to most of the readers of this book that certain representative gentlemen of Pennsylvania, or, more correctly expressed, Philadelphia, as well as the authorities of Harvard University in Massachusetts, have lately displayed quite an active zeal in the cause of veterinary medicine. It would have been better for them, better for their States, infinitely better for the whole country, had they taken greater care to acquaint themselves with the history of veterinary medicine and its results in other countries than England, before giving to the public "An Appeal to the Citizens of

* "Animal Plagues," p. 176.

Pennsylvania for the Foundation of a Veterinary Department in the University of Pennsylvania" (Philadelphia, 1879).* The "Appeal" is issued by the "Pennsylvania Society for the Prevention of Cruelty to Animals." It begins thus:

"*To the Citizens of Pennsylvania.*

"By resolution of the Board of Managers of the Pennsylvania Society for the Prevention of Cruelty to Animals, I have been requested to call your attention to the pressing need there is, at the present time, for some well-organized system of teaching veterinary medicine and surgery to those who are willing and anxious to avail themselves of such instruction. There is no veterinary college in active operation in this State [and there is absolutely no call for one; in fact, the teachings of the history of veterinary medicine emphatically forbid it, as I shall presently show.—B.] In New York State and elsewhere [where?] much attention is being given [the State of New York *per se* gives none] to this subject, and the veterinary practice of medicine is taught in some colleges [which produce a class of semi-educated wolves, called empirics]. During January, 1878, the Trustees of the University of Pennsylvania passed resolutions looking toward the establishment of a veterinary department as soon as money could be obtained to defray the expense. The Pennsylvania Society for the Prevention of Cruelty to Animals has made a study [a very limited one] of the methods of effecting some organization to bring about so desirable an end, and has held communication with a committee appointed by the trustees of the university having charge of this branch of science.

"The Hon. John Welsh, our minister at the court of St. James, writes from London under date of February 26, 1879, to Dr. William Pepper, of this city: 'At this moment, the importance of well-instructed men in this [veterinary] branch of medical science is particularly prominent, for the opinions of the Privy Council in regard to the American live-cattle trade are entirely controlled by them. The diseases of animals are becoming of great interest to the public, and for some years past the efforts of the English Government have been directed toward 'stamping out' rinderpest, pleuro-pneumonia, and other contagious diseases among cattle, sheep, and swine. [With but very limited success, as can easily be seen by studying the history of these efforts, and reading the correspondence and editorials in the "Veterinary Journal" of London. There is little better

* The criticisms which are here made are equally applicable to the attempt of Harvard University to establish the same kind of a humbug school at Boston.

organized effort in this direction in England than in this country. Glanders runs free over the land, and quacks treat it on all sides as they do here, openly defying whatever law may exist against it.—B.] At this time there seems to be great probability that the live-cattle trade with the United States will be suspended, because one cargo of oxen which landed here about a month ago had thirteen cases of pleuro-pneumonia, although some eighty thousand were brought here before, and some three thousand since, in good health.'" The "Appeal" goes on, saying, "The offer made by the University of Pennsylvania should not be permitted to fail for want of means to carry out its wise and humane project."

Then follows the plan proposed whereby to raise the necessary funds, which is fraught with still greater danger to the future of American veterinary science than even State veterinary schools. In fact, the gentlemen issuing this "Appeal" know so little about the subject upon which they have written, that I must seriously warn every public-spirited American against being influenced by them. They have become filled with a grand idea, and then, with most incomplete preparation, have, as the Germans would say, "let loose" upon it:

"In order that the burden of this project may fall as lightly as possible on the charitable-minded citizens of this Commonwealth, a plan has been agreed upon [a poorer could not have been selected] whereby each contributor may receive an ample equivalent for the money he will invest in this laudable undertaking. [Where the burden upon the charitable-minded citizens is then to come in, I, for one, fail to see. Self-interest, not patriotism, not love of animals, not interest in the development of science, and an honest pride in the *reputation of one's country* in this regard, is made the basis of this 'Appeal.'] It is proposed to establish a rule such as is in force in connection with the Royal Veterinary College of London [a school which has done nothing for students or for the advancement of veterinary science in England, but, like 'a dog in the manger,' has opposed every attempt at progress, as I shall sufficiently demonstrate from the most trustworthy English authority].

"Each subscriber of one hundred dollars is to be known as a life-subscriber, and is, in return for his subscription, to be entitled to certain advantages. Thus: he is entitled to accommodation in the infirmary so far as space will permit, and in preference to non-subscribers [who, being of the poorer classes, are to be excluded, and, as their animals also offer much better opportunities for the clinical study of the student, the latter is to suffer, as he does in

London, for the benefit of the 'charitably-minded' owner of fine horses, who finds it as cheap, or cheaper, to send a horse 'a little off' to the school for a week or so, than to keep it at home], for such animals, his own property [an occasional horse belonging to a friend will not be objected to, the professors are so accommodating; and if they are not, they will not know it], as may need medical or surgical treatment, at a price to be fixed, closely approximating the actual cost of feed and care. He may also demand free examination of ten horses or mules each year, as to soundness, with a view to purchase. He can also secure free advice in case of animals brought to the infirmary, but which he proposes to keep in his own stables or kennels. Rules and regulations looking toward the protection of the university and subscribers will be made, to prevent abuse of these privileges, and firms will be permitted to register as subscribers on the condition of one member only being named to act as the representative of the firm, in its correspondence with the authorities of the veterinary department."

The worthy President of the P. C. A. Society must have had some adviser more interested in becoming a "professor" than in the future of his profession, or the welfare of his brother practitioners, when he penned the above lines. It is with extreme regret that I feel myself, as a devoted servant to my countrymen, obliged to most earnestly oppose the above "appeal and plan" in its most essential parts. It contains many words of wisdom and truth, and is deserving the earnest study of every patriotic American; but the above plan, if carried out, would lead to the establishment of a school run entirely in the interests of a select number of subscribers, opposed to those investigations by which science is alone advanced, conservative in the worst form, opposing always the interests of its own graduates by keeping up a constant opposition in practice which the private practitioner is unable to compete with.

The "Appeal" is made nominally "to the citizens of Pennsylvania," but it will virtually result, if at all successful, in an "appeal" to those persons who alone are by the "plan" to derive the benefits, viz., the well-to-do and wealthy horse-owners and large firms of Philadelphia alone.

What interests have the citizens of Pennsylvania or Massachusetts in an institution, the direct benefits of which are only accessible to the residents of Philadelphia or Boston, or their immediate vicinity? I could fill a small book with the testimonies of British veterinarians of unquestioned reputation with regard to the futility and injuriousness of the above plan, and the injury which the quoted

London school has been to the British veterinary profession, but will limit myself to some remarks from the most eminent veterinarian of England. My esteemed friend and colleague, Mr. George Fleming, expresses himself in the "Veterinary Journal," London, in an editorial in the November number for 1879, vol. ix, p. 318, as follows:

"Our readers will have observed that for some months an agitation has been going on among the members of the veterinary profession, chiefly metropolitan practitioners, *with reference to the unfair competition maintained toward them by the Royal Veterinary College (London) known as the 'subscription system.'* As is well known, and as so many veterinary surgeons find to their cost, that school advertises that for two guineas a year it will examine twenty horses for soundness, give advice with regard to an unlimited number, receive into the school-hospital and treat sick horses, as well as sell medicine at cost price, shoe horses for a smaller sum than the ordinary farrier can, etc., while for five guineas per annum an indefinite number of horses will be examined, and all other privileges guaranteed. In fact, it offers to do what no practitioner could afford to do, and undersells its own students to such an extent that it is not only impossible for them to compete with the cheap establishment, but the bread is actually taken from their mouths by this so-called *Alma Mater* of theirs. It has been said by some political historian that the French Revolutions eat up their own children. The London Veterinary School does this, and more; for it first charges them heavy fees for teaching, then starves and swallows them. The system can certainly boast of a long history. The school was commenced as a subscription establishment by an obscure agricultural society, nearly ninety years ago; but then it only had ignorant and illiterate farriers to compete with, and two guineas in those days were very much more than they are now.

"*Had the school never been begun on this system, there can be no doubt that later it must have been established by the country for the benefit of the country. In this case veterinary medicine would have all along stood in a very different position to what it has done and does now, and millions of pounds would probably have been saved. The 'subscription system'* [proposed at Philadelphia] *has undoubtedly proved a most serious drawback to veterinary science in England, as history proves. The school has done little if anything to promote that science; it has never produced a scientific teacher, and never will on its present footing; its teachers have been little more than practitioners, whose principal functions were to 'doctor' sub-*

scribers' horses, or to attend to subscribers' interests; the students who entered the school have suffered all along from their and subscribers' interests clashing, and of clinical instruction there has been none worthy of the name, as the subscribers' horses could not be made available, and no others were admitted within the gates: neither in the form of text-books, nor in other ways, has the school benefited the profession, AND ITS EXISTENCE AS A SCIENTIFIC INSTITUTION IS IGNORED BY OTHER COUNTRIES.

"The teachers, to exist, have been compelled, it would appear, to practice their profession beyond the walls of the school, and thus neglect the students, who seem to be only a secondary consideration in the speculation, and are chiefly valued as contributors of fees.

"*A desire to get hold of money has been the bane of the school, as it has been its chief aim; hence the degrading 'subscription system,' and the determination to continue and extend it, no matter who suffers, whether it deprives the veterinary surgeon or the blacksmith of their means of livelihood.* [The universities of Harvard and Pennsylvania would plant this British parasite on our shores, and, if the thing 'paid,' numerous other associations of less responsibility and respectability would be sure 'to follow suit and trump,' so easy is it in this country for everything and everybody to get a 'charter.'] Surely the noblemen and gentlemen who lend their names and patronage to these schools are not aware of the fact *that it is not a scientific institution, nor yet a college, but merely and mainly a great co-operative horse-doctoring and horseshoeing concern, devised to benefit wealthy subscribers, having nothing to do with the introduction of humane or improved methods of treating diseases or accidents, and doing its business on shamefully cheap principles!* [Certainly the trustees of the universities mentioned must have been most lamentably deceived or wofully ignorant when they consented to the adoption of the subscription plan.]

"We may be told that the 'subscription system' is necessary to the existence of the establishment, and that without it it must perish of inanition. If such a statement is correct—and we do not deny its correctness—then it reveals a very discreditable state of affairs. No other veterinary school in these islands requires to resort to such ignoble stratagem to live; no medical school does or dares to undersell practicing physicians or surgeons; in fact, *the London Veterinary College is the only medical or veterinary school in Europe which, like a huge parasite, lives and grows at their expense, past and present.*

"Not only does the subscription system most seriously injure the practice of the metropolitan practitioner, it also affects the provincial veterinary surgeon, as subscribers are all over the country, and avail themselves of the degradingly cheap services offered by the school.

"It is impossible for any one who cares for the reputation and advancement of veterinary medicine in this country, and the deserved prosperity of its practitioners, not to sympathize with the movement which has been begun, even at this late period.

"*The cheap subscription system has been the curse of our science, and its malignant influence can be traced through long years and in many directions.* It is unprofessional, in every sense of the term, is derogatory and damaging to veterinary medicine, most injurious to metropolitan and suburban practitioners—its own alumni—in every way disadvantageous to the students, and a discredit to the governors of the school and the country. Had the profession not been for so many years blind to its own best interest, surely the action [for reform] now commenced would have been begun long ago."

When the above was written I did not know that a striking example of the injurious effects of this *subscription plan* would be so soon offered to public consideration. The following letter needs no further comments on my part:

HARVARD VETERINARY SCHOOL.—AN OPEN LETTER.

To the President and Overseers of Harvard College.

GENTLEMEN: A question which has been and still is troubling the minds of the thinking members of the veterinary profession is, "*What purpose had Harvard in establishing a Veterinary Department in connection with the Medical School?*" Was it to educate young men to become creditable members of a profession which should rank as high as human medicine in the public mind, or was it to run an animal hospital on a strictly business basis?

The first sermon that I have any remembrance of listening to was by that most eminent preacher, Dr. Bartol. I probably remember it on account of the striking nature of the text, which was, "'Twon't pay." Now, sermonizing is not exactly my forte; nevertheless, I am going to try and show you that you have started upon a course that "won't pay" in the establishment of your veterinary school.

"'Twon't pay" for you as the head of the leading educational institution of our State to establish any new branch of education upon anything but the best possible foundation. You would not be American if you endeavored to open this department on anything but a *paying basis.* Unless a thing *pays* its expenses, it is an utterly unpractical venture in this land of eminent practicality.

But medical schools and business enterprises can not be looked upon from the same stand-point. A business enterprise is a private affair, undertaken to make money; if it "won't pay," it goes under. A medical school is an educational affair; whether it "pays" in money or not is a matter of no importance whatever. It is a public servant, just the same as the public schools. The only dividend the public can expect to receive is that the graduates of the school are thoroughly educated in both the scientific and practical parts of their profession. Naturally, it remains for you, as the founders of this movement, to endeavor to find some means by which you can make such an institution pay its way.

To do this you have adopted the London plan of "subscriptions," by which, for a minimum sum of money per year, you promise to render services to each subscriber which no private practitioner could afford to guarantee to do for three times the amount. In adopting this subscription plan you have yet to learn that you can not, as overseers of a great public institution, afford to do what a private speculative affair like the London School has done, though not without the greatest opposition from its own graduates.

Gentlemen, you have yet to know that it "won't pay" for you to draw down upon your most worthy and necessary undertaking the opposition and ill will, not only of the few educated members of the veterinary profession of the present day, but of all time, including every man that graduates from your school.

The time will surely come when other members of the profession will openly oppose the plan upon which you are conducting this venture. Gentlemen, your advisers were bad. They knew no more about the establishment of a veterinary school than an iron-foundry, perhaps not half as much.

They had but one purpose in view, *and that was self*, not Harvard College or the State. I look upon this "subscription plan," as carried out by you, as disgraceful to Harvard College, and as bound to exert a most baneful influence, by its example, on the future of American veterinary medicine.

I have said your advisers were not the men they should be, and I now tell you that it "won't pay" to let them conduct the school in the manner they are now doing.

What are you trying to give us, gentlemen—a *medical school* for the best possible education of veterinarians, or an institution for the development of English "flunkeyism" on American soil? One would think the latter! The people can rightly hold you responsible for the public acts of your subordinates.

In the Boston "Sunday Globe," of some two weeks since, appeared an article upon your Veterinary Department, which I make bold to assert was a disgrace to Harvard College, and outdoes the advertisements of any of the noted medical humbugs and fraudulent hospitals of quacks in Boston or any other city.

This advertisement reads thus:

SICK HORSES' PARADISE.

THE HARVARD UNIVERSITY VETERINARY HOSPITAL.

Accommodations for Patients in the New Building on Village Street.

Pronounced Success of the Latest Harvard Enterprise.

"'Our horders is wery strict 'ere, sir, not to hadmit any one vithout permission. 'Fraid you'll 'ave to wait for the doctor, sir.'

"Thus spoke one of the grooms at the Harvard University Veterinary Hospital to a 'Globe' reporter yesterday, when he rang at the office-door.

"'Both of the doctors be avay just now, sir, but we hexpects them back directly'—and at that moment Dr. Charles P. Lyman, F. R. C. V. S., the professor in veterinary medicine and chief surgeon of the hospital, drove up and alighted from his English dog-cart, while his English driver conducted his English horse into the stable. Once inside, and the air of this excellent branch of fair Harvard is oppressively English. It has been established a little over a year, and actual work in the department, at least the hospital part, has been in progress only since August 10th. Such an institution is a novelty in Boston."

"Such an institution is a novelty"; indeed it is, gentlemen—a "novelty" which, as an American citizen, I am very sorry to see engrafted upon Massachusetts soil.

Again, in the Boston "Herald" is an advertising column headed "Horses, Carriages, etc." This column has become noted all over the United States for advertisements of the very worst set of "horse sharps" that infest any city in the country. Somewhere we have heard that "a man is known by the company he keeps." You will learn yet, gentlemen, that "'twon't pay" to have an advertisement of your school appear, as it does, in such a column and in company with such advertisements.

What does it show you, gentlemen? It should demonstrate to you the utter unfitness of the man for the place whom you have honored with the position of head of this department.

Are you conducting this hospital for the benefit of the school, or for that of the veterinarians attached to it? Undoubtedly you say, "For the school!" Then why allow them to use the name of Harvard University in order to gain private practice? Is such conduct in accordance with medical ethics?

In this "Herald" advertisement, as well as those appearing in other papers, you may read, "Calls for outside visits will be attended to promptly by day or night." I may be Quixotic, but it is my opinion that no one connected as teacher with such a school can, *as a professional*, make such a use of his position.

Again: *Is it an honorable thing for you to cut prices, for services at your hospital,* 100 *per cent less than the regular practitioner charges; less than those your own graduates will have to charge in order to make a living, or to keep on collegiate terms with other professionals?*

In this regard I would call your attention to the following:

"RATES OF CHARGES AT VILLAGE STREET HOSPITAL."		RATES OF CHARGES MADE BY THE REGULAR PROFESSION.	
Board, treatment, and medicine, for sick horses per day......	$2 00	Single visits, medicine extra....	$3 00
Board, care, and medicine for surgical cases—horse, per day,	1 00	Repeated visits to any case—cow, horse, or dog, each.....	2 00
Board, treatment, and medicine for dogs per day............	0 50	All operations extra; no horse cast less than...............	5 00
Board and treatment for cattle per day....................	1 00	These charges have reference to city proper.	
Examinations and advice at hospital......................	1 00		

What is meant by "examination and advice at hospital"? Do you mean examination for soundness, for which the profession charges $5 for each horse examined? In your contract with subscribers for $10 per year you agree to examine ten horses and do other professional work—in other words, you agree to do, for this paltry sum, work for which any professional would receive $50 for examinations for soundness alone.

Gentlemen, this looks very much as if you were trying to run the veterinary profession of Boston and vicinity into the ground.

What would you think of a father who, after having taught a son all about his business, and that son had started in business for himself, should cut the prices of goods in this manner? You would say it was abominable. Should the son pay for his instruction and devote three years of his life to learning the trade when he might be earning money at something else, you would say that the actions of the father were more than abominable; yet this is exactly what you are doing.

When we see the University of Harvard, of which we rightfully expected so much, taking a stand far below that of any of the private schools of New York, or anywhere else, we can not find words to express what we consider is but righteous indignation.

By public discussion of many writers the field has been prepared for you, but you have only gathered the chaff and left the wheat for others to gather.

The University of Pennsylvania is setting a good example by proceeding slowly in this matter. She will beat you in the race of providing a really good school unless you "tack ship" and "come round" on a more "weatherly course." *

Every word which President Eliot spoke about the work of a medical school in his late address at the dedication of the new building is applicable to the Veterinary Department; but not one is being applied. He spoke of the necessity of gathering funds to pursue the work. With regard to this veterinary school, the matter has never been written up in the papers as it should have been done; no public interest has ever been awakened. Had the question been taken up and publicly advocated, we know of what we speak in saying that a permanent fund of at least $100,000 could have been raised, and not with any great amount of labor.

The Village Street Hospital is a serious mistake, though it can yet be turned to advantage for the school. The accommodations at Bussy Farm are, or can easily be made, much better suited to a hospital clinic than the city place. Charenton, Alfort, is much farther from Paris than Bussy Farm from Boston proper, yet the hospital there is always full enough, and at Bussy there would be no difficulty in getting from seventy-five to one hundred patients in the hospital the greater part of the year. There are a class of patients that can pay expenses, which no practitioner really wants, and which are essentially fitted for school instruction. These you could easily have, and without in any way antagonizing the veterinary profession. In fact, they would cheerfully assist you.

At Village Street you have not the necessary conveniences for a free clinic; you should have a shed to protect the horses and men

* With reference to the University of Pennsylvania, it would seem that our words have not fallen upon barren ground. Under the date of January 8, 1884, the dean of the Veterinary Department wrote me: "*I, like you, am absolutely opposed to any subscription plan, and expect to run a large hospital and clinic without it.*" From which we may assume that it has been dropped for this school.

from the weather, and a paved and unpaved run upon which to lead horses in order to examine them for lameness. A pathological laboratory is as necessary as an anatomical laboratory. This you have not at either place. Nor have you a single man capable of teaching pathological anatomy, the great weakness of veterinary medicine, and practically adapting it to the needs of veterinary students. To do this requires a practical knowledge of the diseases of animals, and a most exact knowledge of human and zoöpathology, so far as the latter is written up. With regard to the Village Street Hospital, the money is not wasted, for the building can be let for stable-purposes, and yield a better income than the money it cost would. This income could be available to pay some of the expenses at Bussy. The students must necessarily waste much time in going between the three localities where they are to receive instruction.

The veterinary profession of the country earnestly desire the success of your venture, but not as at present conducted.

Summing up, then, let me say: "'Twon't pay" to take a dishonorable course in conducting your venture.

"'Twon't pay" to allow your teachers to use the fair name of Harvard College to advertise themselves in order to gain private practice.

"'Twon't pay" to place the school before the public as a transplanted weed taken from English ground, with all the evils of British flunkeyism.

'Twill pay in every way to drop all these things, and act in accordance with the most exact principles of medical ethics.

'Twill pay to respect the feelings and position of every member of the American veterinary profession.

Trusting these words will be received as they are written, in the true interest of Harvard Veterinary School, and the future of the veterinary profession, I remain your obedient servant.

STATE VETERINARY SCHOOLS.

In the previous section, it has been my endeavor to show the folly of private schools for the study of medicine, and that the evils connected with them were largely due to neglect of its duties on the part of the State.

We come now to speak of well-endowed—either by public spirit or otherwise—institutions in each State, but in all respects controlled by the State.

The question we have to consider is one of expediency, not of State-rights. No one denies the right of each State to a veterinary school if properly endowed and controlled. What I do, however, emphatically assert is, that such a system is not in the interests of the citizens of any one State, section, or whole country. There are some thirty-eight States in our Union at present, with every prospect of a constant numerical increase for many years to come. Being now thirty-eight, if this plan were to be carried out, there would be that number of schools. Even though these schools were regulated by the respective States, one may positively assert that there would be even less uniformity in reference to the term of study and examination requisite than at present nominally exists in the numerous private medical schools. It is useless to suppose there would be much if any uniformity. The legislators in the different States would never look upon these questions with such unanimity as to lead to any great similarity between the schools. In fact, as the case at present stands, there are scarcely any legislators, among the great number of men at present occupying such positions in the different States, that are sufficiently educated with reference to the history of veterinary medicine to legislate sensibly upon the subject. Another argument, and one of the strongest, is, that unanimity in veterinary schools is even more necessary than in human. Unless it exists—unless the education and term of study are the same in each State—how will it ever be possible to attain that oneness of purpose in all States which we have shown to be absolutely necessary for the control and prevention of animal pests? This absolutely necessary end will never be attained by State schools. State schools can turn out good practitioners, but, for the above reasons, they would never turn out men properly educated for State purposes. State schools would mean State laws; yet every one who knows anything admits that State laws for the purpose we are considering would be almost worse than useless. The manner of instruction would vary; the students would be led to look upon the pathology of the contagious disease from too many stand-points. We should soon have the country divided up into about as many opposing cliques as there were schools, each jealous of the supremacy of the other, and, although State schools, we should find the contemptible rivalry for students which now disgraces the medical schools. There being no hope that the standard of education would be the same in each State, certain States would have to make laws to protect the graduates from their own schools against the competition of graduates of inferior schools in neighboring States. Further, there are not competent men in the whole world, who can be had at any price, to furnish teachers enough for two new and thoroughly organized veterinary schools. In fact, even for one national school, we shall find it hard to procure the requisite number of scientifically educated and competent teachers. I have scarcely seen a veterinarian in this country whom I would call to fill a chair in a veterinary school. There are some who are well enough practically, but when we come to seek the scientific foundation, united with a healthy *skepticism* (by that I mean a critical mind, and with ability for original research, united to the greatest necessity of all, *ability to teach*), we shall find it hard to discover enough English-speaking men the world over suitable to our purposes.

It has suddenly dawned upon some people in power in this country that veterinarians are necessary. In one State, at least, they are already preparing a mill for grinding them out even faster than they do doctors in the medical mills. This unenviable State is Iowa. There they propose a State school which shall turn out graduates after eighteen months' study. "These graduates must be *eighteen years of age, and have completed the entire course of study.*" To illustrate how much these Solons know, and to prove my assertion that but few, if any, legislators in this country are at present sufficiently instructed upon this subject to legislate properly, we are informed that the "sessions begin the first of March (each year) and continue till the latter part of November, with a vacation of two weeks in July." If one is to judge from the above, the students are either not to study any anatomy, or the laws of Nature are different in Iowa from other places in the same latitude, for everywhere else the time especially devoted to the study of anatomy is between November and March; but here we see the school does not continue in operation between November and March, or perhaps these are hot months in Iowa, and putrefaction, etc., prevent the students studying anatomy, so that it is studied in the months between March and November, excepting two weeks in July, when the students are probably dismissed on account of the extremely cold weather. The published "curriculum" of this school, which appeared in a pamphlet called the "College Quarterly," is one of the most amusing yet saddening proofs of human imbecility it has ever been my lot to read. This school was to be opened March, 1880, yet in September, 1879, the writer of this "*curriculum*" uses the present tense, and tells us what the *future* students are already doing; among other things, "hundreds of animals *are presented* at the hospital for examinations" held at the school "*one* half day each week."

It will be remembered that the Berlin school has the largest clinic of any school in the world, yet we never saw "hundreds of animals" at any one day in the school hospital or free clinics; although the number upon the grounds on a given day might, inclusive of dogs, be about two hundred and fifty. Yet a small Western town (Ames, Iowa) is to furnish "hundreds" of patients for clinical exercises which take place "*one half day each week*." Among other wonderful accessories of this school is a pair of "scales, capable of weighing *one twenty-thousandth of a gramme*"—a thing beyond the present range of human ability. The faculty of this Iowa veterinary abortion consists of seven persons, only two of whom seem to know anything of medicine, and one only of veterinary medicine. This latter prodigy is the graduate of a Canadian school, and I make bold to say that the president of it would not dare affirm that he gives an education suitable to prepare men for teachers. This man, whom the editor of the "National Live-Stock Journal" describes as "a young man with comparatively little experience as a veterinary surgeon," is supposed to head this institution, so far as the veterinary profession finds any representation. He is to teach the *whole of veterinary medicine*, which includes the following technical branches: General pathology, general surgery, special pathology and therapeutics of all the diseases of domestic animals; pathological anatomy, special surgery, operative surgery and practice; the pathology of the contagious animal diseases and their prevention (veterinary hygiene and police), forensic medicine (veterinary), obstetrics, horseshoeing, veterinary history, and meat and market inspection—and conduct the clinics, and, according to the curriculum, also attend to a "large practice, which the students will have the privilege of assisting in." I have heard of such a thing as a "servant of all work"; the great Boerhaave was the man *par excellence* in this regard so far as medicine is concerned, but we think even his spirit must be tortured with envy at the supposed ability of this young man "of comparatively little practical experience." The work this prodigy is expected to do can not be well done by less than *eight specialists*, and they supported by eight more specialists in the different natural sciences which are necessary to the comprehension of the purely professional branches. If this *school* is not even a "humbug" before its opening, then I fail to know the meaning of the word. I must say that the adjoining States have no other course than to order a severe quarantine against the graduates of this school. The old-school empirics, the empirics of years, of which we have so many, will be found far more worthy of confidence than the eighteen-year-old graduates of this veterinary sprouting-house. It seems to me that no other evidence is needed to show the fallacy of State schools, for here we *have one* in *optima forma*, chartered, funded, and controlled by the State. Suppose the thirty-seven other States should all follow suit, each after its own fashion! Doubtless some would be found thinking one year's study would be sufficient, others thinking two, while in some isolated cases extremely wise legislators might insist upon three; but I am not yet ready to believe that our people have got very far beyond the idea that "anything is good enough for a horse-doctor." At least, the experiences of daily life continually confirm me in that opinion.

A NATIONAL VETERINARY SCHOOL.

For advocating this idea, the president of the Iowa abortion declares me to be "visionary," whereas I think about all there is in his contemplated school is the result of a vision of something else than the teachings of veterinary history. Another remarkable critique declares me to be "lacking in a knowledge of public affairs"; to which, if he means American politics, I plead guilty, and trust I may continue so.

Some four years ago, I was myself a firm friend of State schools; finally, the evils of such a system became so conspicuous that I thought sectional schools would be better; but the earnest study of all the peculiar relations of veterinary science to the public wants finally convinced me that they could only be most profitably adjusted by one school. My whole purpose in educating myself especially for this work has been to serve my country to the best degree possible. What Continental governments do for the people, by educating young men especially for the positions of teachers, and sending them to study in foreign countries, I have done at my own expense, not only of money, but almost of my life. Therefore I feel I have a right to speak as one having authority. Naturally, I expect opposition, but my opponents should have *arguments* instead of mere words or accusations wherewith to show I am wrong. There is no need of being in a hurry in this matter. "Haste will make waste," as surely as the people of the different States go heedlessly forward, and endeavor to inaugurate veterinary schools upon erroneous principles, such as those adopted at Harvard and Philadelphia, but which will produce an even more damaging failure in Iowa.

To every man who would *faithfully serve his race* and his profession, there are two paths open. The one is the beaten one, full of weeds, crooked ways, and cross-fences, in the form of adhesion to old ideas and old ways. We may select this and seek to make it better, to clean up the rubbish and let in daylight, so that truth and right may have an opportunity to develop. This path may be likened to a man who would rebuild and remodel an old house, which he finds entirely unsuited to his desires and to the times. This is generally found to be a very costly method. In reference to the establishment of veterinary schools in this country, fortunately for us, no such necessity exists. The old, to be culled over, is all to be found in the older countries. Why, then, should we begin where they began, as these Iowa, Harvard, and Pennsylvania authorities are about to do? Why not first take time to "look before we leap," and only begin when we have found out not only where they now are, and accepting the best of that, but, cleared from all their rubbish, endeavor to start with those advancements toward which the best Continental schools are tending as fast as their antiquated incumbrances will allow? This is the other plan, and the only one which the people of this country should pursue. That I am an idealist is willingly admitted, but that I am "visionary" is about as wide from the mark as possible. Every man who desires to lead, must not only of himself do the best he is capable of, but he will never attain that point unless he has an *ideal better* which he is constantly aiming at. Who ever heard of a person, endeavoring to spring over a ditch, jumping for the immediate edge of the opposite shore? Truth is always ideal; we seek it continually. Having made one form our own, we turn our attention immediately in search of another. She is ever before us. Her history is more unwritten than written. Perfection is always before us. She is the guiding star, without which the human race would soon sink into barbarism again. The common ruts, if continually followed, lead on to a self-conceited nonentity, pomposity, and ignorance. They are always blocked up with false ideas and musty superstitions. Truth and perfection are the twin sisters to clear this maze away. Truth and perfection are both extravagant, and by too many always declared visionary, impracticable. Their apostles have been cursed, hanged, and burned at the stake. They are the men who have made us what we are; their lives and works constitute the history of the world. Buddha, Confucius, Moses, Jesus, Paul, Loyola, Luther,

Spinoza, Galileo, Newton, Descartes, Knox; the fathers of American independence, Washington, Paine, Jefferson, Otis, Adams, and others; Vesalius, Bichat, and Virchow in medicine; Darwin, Tyndall, Huxley, in science; and the fathers of America's second independence, Garrison, Parker, Sumner, Whittier, and others, have all been condemned in their own day and generation as visionary, impractical, extravagant; and yet, one after the other, succeeding generations have raised monuments to their memory and pronounced them most practical men.

The first bugbear which threatens our purpose is to be sought in some secret meaning which is supposed to lie behind the word "national." It is assumed by some that I desire to put my hands in the public Treasury, and retire, to be the envy of the Kearneyites, a "bloated bondholder." Others suppose that by the word "national" I mean a school *endowed* and controlled by the Government at Washington; and they immediately see a whole mountain of political evils overclouding their vision. Beyond these views, no one seems yet to have proceeded, notwithstanding five years' public advocacy and repeated restating of these ideas.

The only sense in which I have ever used the word *national* is in reference to a plan for a school which shall best serve the requirements of the central Government, the State governments, and the people individually, as if each one of these bodies were but a single individual whose entire interests were to be served. Any other definition of my meaning is but a perversion.

One school for the nation is what I am advocating, until the necessities of the country shall require another.

Nothing more need be said of the evils of private or State schools. It is to meet all these evils that I advocate one school. The work of this school should be as follows:

1. To educate veterinarians who shall be equal, both to the demands of the State and the public.

2. To supply a suitable number of qualified specialists who, in the event of an outbreak of contagious animal diseases, or a suspicious connection between those of animals and man, may proceed, at the order of the National Board of Health, or at the request of any State board, to the invaded district, and make there the necessary researches and observations. These persons should always occupy the position of assistants, or tutors, at the school.

3. It should be an institution at which all manner of feeding, inoculation, or other necessary experiments could be made, by

which alone there is any hope for finally arriving at the causes of disease, or the means for their prevention.

4. It should be an institution where carefully detailed experiments could be made with different kinds and mixtures, as food for animals, in their relation to their use as beef, pork, mutton, milk, etc., as food for human beings.

5. It should be an institution which the Government could always use for any necessary purposes, or to which farmers or other persons could send suspected food, dead animals, or portions of the same, or other things in relation to their health, for experiment, research, or proper investigation.

6. It should be an institution which would supply men properly educated to become veterinary teachers in the respective State agricultural schools.

(*a.*) With relation to the veterinary instruction suitable to students at agricultural schools, it is my opinion that it should be limited to anatomy and physiology of the domestic animals, hygiene and dietetics, horseshoeing, a good education in relation to the contagious animal diseases and their prevention, and forensic medicine, which means examination as to soundness, etc. All instruction in special pathology, or therapeutics, as well as surgery, is to be carefully avoided, for it only leads to the increase of the already too extended number of empirics, or, what is still worse, quacks.

7. It should supply the necessary number of veterinarians for State work of every kind.

While these are the principal demands which we have a right to make upon such an institution, there are many advantages connected with it which, although negatively stated heretofore, should now be repeated in a positive manner.

While, in advocating *one school for the nation*, I do not deny the right of States to individual schools, yet I truly believe that if such a school is founded in correspondence to the plan herein stated, both State schools and private schools, chartered by States, must soon suffer a speedy death, if ever allowed even a moment's existence.

In *one school* we have but *one* standard of *education*, and that the highest practicable. It may be argued that "opposition is the soul of progress." To which I answer that the opposition should be seated in the minds of the teachers, assistants, and tutors of the school, as well as its numerous graduates, all of which would tend to keep the school alive and active.

By having a uniform course of study, and only one grade of

graduation, the people have no difficulty in at once ascertaining as to who is an accredited man.

Unless we have one form and grade of education for the whole country, it will be absolutely impossible to ever have any effective veterinary police, or to have any uniformity in the laws, or to meet the requirements set forth when considering this part of our subject. It is really a scientific question to decide, how all these ends can be met by one institution. Yet it is possible. The first question is, How can we have an institution, national in its purposes, yet free from the evils of American politics? Naturally, it must receive its charter from the central Government. Unless the institution can serve the needs of the Government, it is absolutely useless. In discussing "a national veterinary police code," I have shown the relation of the government to the schools, and said that the Veterinary Inspector-General of the United States should be a member of the board of trustees, and one of the board of examiners. This gives the Government a technical representative. If, however, such an officer is appointed by political nepotism, then the less he has to do with the school the better. He must be selected in the way I have said, or all our work is useless.

I propose, then, that an association be formed and chartered, with the right to hold property, personal and real, to the amount of two million dollars; and that said association be called the *National Association for the Promotion of Veterinary Science in the United States.* The work of this association is at first to be limited to opening subscriptions for funds. In the earlier pages of this book we have endeavored to make our readers cognizant of the very near relation which exists between many animal diseases and human health. Every man and woman of means in this country, whose education will permit of their grasping the idea of preventive medicine, should contribute accordingly to the foundation of this institution. It is an object which should especially appeal to the self-interest of every breeder and owner of domestic animals in the country. The humanitarian, the enthusiastic friends of our domestic animals, those interested in the reform of animal transport, are all knocking at the wrong door, and endeavoring to push an almost immovable load up-hill without the aid of intelligent and highly educated veterinarians.

The late Commodore Vanderbilt saw fit to endow a university. We think a large veterinary institute an object which the country has much more need of than more universities at present. It seems strange that an object which should appeal at once to the generous spirit of every wealthy American should have been openly advocated for a period of more than five years without finding a single public supporter. The object is certainly noble; the plan proposed is not visionary, for it has found able support from several medical men of eminence. Then why this apathy? Is it because the veterinary profession has not upheld it? There is no such thing as *the* veterinary profession in this country. There are a few isolated men of variable degrees of school education, but these all seem more afraid to tackle this subject, *pro* or *con*, than they would be of the "rinderpest," which they would not fear much, in all probability, as it would increase their yearly balances. Probably it is because there is no money in it. "Millions in it" is the only thing which could awaken a profession dead to all professional ambition, and without the first spark of a genuine scientific spirit.

To form such an association, it is only necessary for a limited number of representative breeders and patriotic citizens to call a preliminary meeting at any of our large cities, there to draw up a preamble, and a few regulations calling a large public meeting at a later date. Hundreds of responsible men are interested in this undertaking, but all seem afraid to take the lead. Once having formed a permanent association, a board of trustees should be selected, so as to represent the great geographical sections of the country, and for a period of ten years each. They should themselves select their own officers. The treasurer, who in the future should be an officer of the school, should be the only paid man; the others, when all is going (if it ever will be), should receive only traveling expenses. There is one position in connection with such an association which will be replete with work, and that is the position of secretary.

The locating of such an institution is a matter of immense importance. All things considered, it seems as if the city of Cincinnati were especially indicated for this purpose. It is sufficiently central in every direction. It is large enough to furnish all the elements for a clinic. It seems to be more or less excluded from the contemptible jealousies which are occasionally cropping out between our other large cities. While I am, in general, in favor of uniting such an institution with a university, our conditions seem rather to warrant us in keeping it an entirely separate institution. Such a connection might save a little in expense, by the teachers in several of the natural sciences being taken from the university; but, on the other hand, the natural sciences, with the exception of botany, need to be peculiarly adapted to the use of veterinarians;

and as this work is still scarcely begun in any country, it is sufficiently indicated that we should endeavor to found an institution where they may be especially cultivated; and, in selecting teachers, we must endeavor to obtain men of real genius. It must never be forgotten that we are not advocating a school for the production of horse-doctors, but, on the contrary, an institution for the development of those natural sciences which serve as the foundation for the study of medicine, the development of veterinary science in all its branches, and the education of scientifically qualified veterinary practitioners.

The school *must* have the scientific spirit permeating all its work. It is because our medical schools are almost all entirely wanting in this particular that we have never produced a great medical scientist. We have developed the hand-work by borrowing the elements upon which it is founded from Germany and France. What we want is American science as well as American practice. Science can never be developed except with state support. Sporadic upheaval may be witnessed from private endeavor, as may be seen in England. It is absolutely necessary that the theoretic and practical in a medical school be permeated, saturated with this scientific spirit. No one who has not lived in such a spirit can realize how it gradually stimulates even the drones among the students. It is like the deacon and his wonderful trotters—the spirit of emulation gradually extended to the deacon also. The students soon begin to think and seek the causes of things; researches, experiments, take more of their thoughts, and, instead of learning practice by rote, they begin to feel the desire to improve it, even as students. "The reason why" becomes an innate part of their being. Unless this spirit is shared by *every* teacher of such a school, in so much is it a failure. Only men having this spirit, and the practical ability to let it be seen in their works, are suited to be teachers.

Such an institution as we have in mind requires considerable land, ten acres not being by any means too much. It will require stables for hospital use—isolated stables to quarantine animals infected with, suspected of, or kept for experimental purposes, with contagious diseases. It will require a special dog-hospital, also a special stable for the use of animals to be kept for feeding and other experiments. It will also require buildings for the residences of the teachers, servants, and pupils, as well as for the different educational purposes.

In order that such an institution may fully fill all the demands we have a right to make upon it, great circumspection must be exercised with respect to every move we make. While there is no way by which we can prevent State schools, and, if we may judge from the past, private schools also, so long as our legislators are as ignorant and heedless as they now are with reference to the proper relations of our medical institutions, by which I mean schools, practitioners, etc., we must make every effort to discourage their establishment. We may be certain that the young veterinary aspirants will go to that school which gives them the best education at the least expense. There is but one way in which a national school can hope to kill out private and State institutions of a similar character. *That way is to make it free* to the students. By *free* I mean conditionally. I would have the annual fees, including everything, fixed at one hundred dollars, payable semi-annually. Each and every student should be obliged to pay them. But the conditions upon which each student may receive his education free, should be that all students who pass a successful examination at the first trial for the diploma of the institute should receive back all the fees paid in, inclusive of the examination fee during the course of study required by the school; any students failing in their first examination, or retiring from it, except for sickness, or not completing the course, to forfeit all fees paid in. I am a bitter enemy to the prize system, which selects one, two, or three students, who may accidentally pass a better examination than their fellows; but the above plan, being open to all, is certainly in the interest of parents and students, and should offer an extra stimulus to study. The prize system is degrading, for an examination is seldom a just criterion of the competing student's ability; the parrot students generally win this prize, while the men of character and individuality win those of the world. A school examination is a hard thing for men of real character. It is generally *too much book*, and not enough inclined to draw the real knowledge from the student. To carry out this plan, and pay the expenses of the school in the manner which we shall in part detail, requires a large interest-bearing fund, but the *income to the country* at large will more than justify the investment.

The course of study must extend over four full years, of ten months each, with an interval at the Christmas holidays. This may seem excessive, in comparison to the two-session course of many American medical schools, but a *proper education*, an education equal to the demands of the time, and in the spirit of modern science, can not be obtained in less. While, at the period of my studies at Berlin, the full session was limited to three years, mine was the last class to graduate at the end of three years; I found it necessary to remain nearly a year longer to fill up the vacuums, which were perceptible to myself, in my education to fit myself for the work I had undertaken, and to feel warranted in claiming that I really had an education with a scientific foundation; and had not my health and means both been pretty well exhausted, I should have certainly added a year more to my school-days. Still, they are not ended; the real student is always at school, whether in his own laboratory, or busy about practice, or enjoying a vacation. The educated mind is never without material for study. A scarcity of immediate objects of interest is often necessary in order that time may be gained for skeptical reflection. The word "skeptic" is used in the sense of critical, not in an anti-religious sense, as unreflecting people seem always to think necessary. The same is true of the word "radical," which means "root," or one who endeavors to go to the root of a matter; but the highly educated representatives of the American press seem to think it should only be applied to spiritualists, free-lovers, or other similar eccentricities of weak-minded men and women. Pardon these few digressive words.

An inexcusable mistake of all veterinary schools, and many medical as well, is, that the school-year for freshmen is arranged to begin in the fall. Every teacher that has had experience, and who makes a study of his work—that is, how he can best present his subjects to the students (and no other men should ever be teachers), if capable of making any practical observations upon the difficulties which students have to overcome—must realize that to jump them into the studies of a general first winter course, as they now are, without any preparation, is but a waste of time and source of anxiety to the student, and aggravation to the teachers. The time for students to enter upon the study of medicine should be fixed for about the middle of March, and the four-years session should end at the same time. The studies of this first term, from March 15th to August 1st, should be *osteology*, chemistry, physics, and botany. The manner in which osteology is at present taught in most schools is little more than a farce; the student learns the bones, it is true, their protuberances, muscular insertions, and cavities, but beyond this he seldom gets. Bones are indeed a dry subject. This is all wrong. There is no branch of medical study which can be made more interesting and instructive than this, and, unless it is taught in a truly scientific manner, the name might as well be stricken from the curriculum of a school. It should first begin with the development of bone-tissue in general, demonstrated by the teacher upon the board;

this will all be repeated in histology, if the school is a respectable one. The manner in which each bone develops, how the bone grows, how the tuberosities and cavities are formed, the comparative anatomy of each bone, its varying uses, and, what has not yet been invented, wooden or hard-rubber skeletons, with elastic muscles, to illustrate *osteology*, as well as myology. I am opposed to the teaching of elementary chemistry in medical schools; this, elementary physics and botany, should all be placed in the matriculatory examination; but, so long as that is at present impossible, we must do the best we can, and give the students a very thorough education in chemistry and physics. With reference to the former, each theoretic lecture should be repeated the next day by the students in the laboratory, so far as it had direct relation to the practical uses of the students. Theory must be made practical, or else it is not science. It is but words—empty words! A teacher who has not the genius which enables him to apply the abstract sciences, such as chemistry or physics, to the practical needs of the students, is unfit to teach. In most medical schools this fact seems to be entirely lost sight of. Chemistry is taught as chemistry *per se*. Many a man is suited to teach chemistry for chemical students, but there are few who have the genius to apply it to the practical needs of medical students. To this end, the teacher of chemistry should have first studied medicine, and have graduated as an M. D., or veterinarian, and then have studied and made a specialty of chemistry and physics.

With reference to botany. A good knowledge of its elements, the classifications, and the determination of the species of plants, *must* be insisted on in the matriculatory examination, else much valuable time would be lost at the school. The botany taught at medical schools is entirely out of place. Students no longer need to go out in the woods to gather herbs. In pharmacognosy and materia medica the endeavor should be to make the student thoroughly acquainted with the principal medicines in dried, crude, and prepared forms; but the teaching in botany should be limited to vegetable anatomy and physiology, with microscopic practice, and a careful comparison of the structure and functions of the vegetable with those of the animal world. The students of to-day (and, I am sorry to say, many teachers) do not realize how this course opens the way to the study of the anatomy and physiology of the animal world. It not only opens the way, but gives one such an introduction as to make the study of the latter branches doubly interesting.

I will not critically consider the whole course of study, but will rather give a course of study to be extended over four years, as I at present look upon the question:

First Session (*Spring and Summer*), March 15th to August 1st.—Introduction to the study of veterinary medicine, by the director; osteology; chemistry, inorganic, theoretical, and practical; physics; botany (theoretic, as described); zoölogy; horseshoeing (practical).

Second Session (*Fall and Winter*), October 1st to March 15th.—Zoötomy * (lectures and practice); chemistry, organic, and practice; materia medica and pharmacognosy; history of veterinary medicine; horseshoeing, theoretic, history.

Third Session (*Spring and Summer*).—Physiology (part first); histology, with practice; comparative anatomy and embryology; materia medica; toxicology; exercise in chemical laboratory.

Fourth Session (*Fall and Winter*).—Anatomy, lectures and practice; physiology (part second); nerve physiology; dietetics; hygiene; breeding (theoretic, with especial regard to evolution); reviews by assistants of chemistry, materia medica; comparative anatomy and physiology.

At the end of this session the students are to be examined in the above branches. Students failing to pass, to be put back one year.

Fifth Year (*Spring and Summer*).—General pathology (with sketch of the history of medicine); general therapeutics; general surgical pathology; special surgical pathology; special pathology and therapeutics of the diseases of the domestic animals; practice in pharmacy; practice in writing prescriptions.

Sixth Session (*Fall and Winter*).—Clinic, percussion and auscultation; pathological anatomy, demonstrative and microscopic; operative surgery (theory and practice); special surgical pathology; special pathology and therapeutics; exterior (lectures on form and soundness); practice in pharmacy.

Seventh Session (*Spring and Summer*).—Clinic; pathological anatomy, as above; obstetrics (theory and practice); veterinary sanitary science and police (contagious animal diseases and their prevention); forensic medicine; operative surgery (practice).

Eighth Session (*Fall and Winter*).—Clinic; physiology (part first); general pathology; sanitary science and police; forensic medicine; meat and market inspection.

The work of this last session should be to fasten as much as possible the principles of medicine in the minds of the students, and

* All lectures upon special branches should be introduced with a short sketch of the principal events in their development.

give them time for reviewing. The members of the graduating class should also be allowed to oversee the students in the anatomical laboratory—a certain number at a time—in order that they may have a final opportunity to refresh their minds in this important branch before appearing for examination.

This plan of study is doubtless open to improvement, but I venture to say that it is better than any at present followed. Its aim is to unite theory and practice to the fullest possible degree.

At the end of the eighth session the students will appear for their final examination. Written examinations—with the exception of a portion of the clinical—are a farce. The aim of an examination is to ascertain the real ability of the candidates. Originality of expression should be cultivated, and the teachers should endeavor to place the "*parrots*," or book-repeaters, where they belong. Grade examinations, "good," "better," "best," are another farce. The school should have but one standard—either a student passes a *satisfactory* examination, or it is pronounced *unsatisfactory*. The fate of the "first men in their classes" in the arena of the world is too often otherwise than that which is expected. All students passing an unsatisfactory examination should be put back one year, and forfeit all rights to the refunding of their fees for any part of the term. The director should signify the special lectures they must attend.

A list of each year's graduates should be published in the school organ, as well as in the leading agricultural and sporting papers. The secretary of the Board of Health of the State from which each graduate comes, as well as the presiding officer of his native place, are to be notified of the candidate's graduation, which must be published in a public print of the place. All State boards of health should also receive an official list of each year's graduates.

The writer would also seriously recommend the idea of endeavoring to introduce into the country a more intelligent and trustworthy class of grooms and coachmen, and to this end would suggest that the attendants in the stable be young men from fifteen to nineteen years old, who can read and write; that their pay be merely nominal, but enough to feed and clothe them, and that they have, from the superintendent of the clinic, lectures on treatment, on stable hygiene, and feeding, carefully illustrating the dangers of inconsiderate and inopportune feeding; from the lecturer on horseshoeing, special general lectures on the care of the foot in health; and from the lecturer on physiology, some general lectures on physiology. Such a course would, it seems to me, be nationally beneficial, and pay not only the hearers, in years to come, but the community at large. These lectures should be open to the public at a nominal price, and gentlemen could have the privilege of sending their grooms or coachmen, and farmers of attending during the winter months. Thus, and only by carrying out a plan such as this, can we expect to build up our science in America.

While I am so earnestly opposed to State schools, on account of the seeming impossibility of ever arriving at a uniform system of education for one and all of them, and a uniform grade of examination, yet I do not assert that *one school*, or institution, is sufficient to cover the entire needs of the country. It *can* supply the required number of veterinarians, and it can do an immense amount of scientific research, but, to fulfill all the requirements which may be made in this direction, another form of institution is necessary.

These are: research, experiment, stations, one in each State, at the service of and under the control of the State Board of Health, represented by the Chief Veterinary Inspector of the State. The value of such an institution to the people of each State can not well be appreciated in a country where no such thing exists. They should be small, neat stables, with a quarantine stable for infectious diseases; they also should have a microscopical and chemical laboratory, and each should have about two acres of land with them. In each State there should be *meat inspectors*, especially pork inspectors; part of the duty of the State veterinarian should be to give a course of lectures each year upon these subjects, with the necessary demonstrations. In case this official could not be spared for such a purpose, the State should engage a competent man for the purpose from among the veterinarians in the State.

With such an institution at its command, the Board of Health can constantly make feeding experiments with suspected milk, or with reference to *tuberculosis* of cows, or any other subject of importance to the people of the State. Without such an institution at its command, the hands of such a board are more or less tied.

The National School should be at the command of the National Board of Health, or National Inspector-General, for similar purposes.

The Teachers.

Sooner or later "civil service reform" has got to be introduced into our higher institutions of learning, as well as the Government. With reference to the institution we are considering, it can not and will not ever be successful if its teachers are selected and rewarded as such persons now are in this country. With reference to the selection of the first corps of teachers, were the school in readiness, I must confess I am myself somewhat at a loss what course to pursue. Still, I think that the competitive method in vogue in France, which *must* be adopted in all future cases, could also be made available here by giving public notice in this country, France, Germany, and England, of the chairs to be filled, said notice to be given at least nine months before the competition is to take place. In addition, the duties, accommodations, and remuneration should all be distinctly declared. Foreigners should be allowed a certain fixed sum for traveling expenses. Another plan would be to select a committee of three and send them on a *search;* but this is really impracticable, in my opinion.

As opposed as Americans have ever been to the *pensioning system, it must* be adopted in the scientific and higher schools of this country before we can hope to make any progress in science. Moderate pay during active life, and a fair pension for themselves or their immediate family for a fixed period, and under fixed conditions, is the only plan upon which we can ever hope to control the real geniuses among scientists for educational purposes. There are but very few men of original genius who would not gladly sacrifice all hope of great earthly reward, and who would most joyfully devote their whole services to the State, were they only secured a comfortable living during the active period of their lives, and a just pension to themselves when old or worn out, to be secured to their widows during life, and proportionately to minor children until sixteen years of age. Americans may "kick against (these) pricks" all they please; come to it they will and must, be it anti-American or not. There are a great many things that a bigoted and ignorant Americanism at present pronounces "anti-American" which a more intelligent and liberal future will adopt. It is not a support for laziness which we are demanding. It is the just rewards for genius. Every man of any education and liberality knows that most men of true scientific genius are scarcely fit to take care of themselves so far as monetary matters go. They have no time for such trifles. The costs in the end to the State, or to the association, which in this case will have to assume them, will not exceed those which would accrue from higher salaries during active life. Residences for the teachers, servants, and pupils should be found on the grounds. For the two former they should be free; for *the latter* at a reasonable rent. Every teacher should be retired and pensioned when sixty years of age, no matter how active he may still be, and his place filled by young power. Every vacancy *must* be filled by public competition of the candidates before the teachers as a body, and some representative members of the board of trustees. It must never be forgotten that genius for research united to great knowledge is not sufficient to constitute a man a teacher suitable to the young (or old). Genius for teaching, *enthusiasm* in teaching, and ability to apply one's knowledge practically, is an absolute necessity. Without this ability the most gifted genius is useless to a school as a teacher, however valuable he may be to the country at large as an original investigator. We must endeavor, to the best of our ability, to obtain men uniting these three qualifications to a high degree.

The Students.

On account of the great extent of this country, and the variation existing in the different States with regard to the standard of different schools bearing similar names, a matriculatory examination will be an absolute necessity. This should extend to a thorough examination in all English branches, which a graduate of a high-school should have perfected himself in, as well as a knowledge of Latin grammar, and ordinary translations. As to Continental languages, there is no doubt that a knowledge of German, especially, and French, is more indispensable to the veterinarian than to the medical practitioner. While much of the best foreign literature is soon translated for the benefit of the latter, the veterinarian has to wait years, and loses much of it altogether. It is impossible for the American veterinarian who does not read these two languages to estimate the great difference which exists between the German and French reviews and those of England. As to the American, they are scarcely worthy of the name. Again, a good rudimentary knowledge of zoölogy, chemistry, physics, and botany is absolutely necessary to the young student entering upon the study of medicine; without this he is constantly feeling his way in the dark. Each applicant must be at least eighteen and not over twenty-five years of age. Not every youth is fitted either to become a veterinary or medical practitioner.

As I am now drawing my "Buchlein" to a close, I may be allowed the liberty of ending it with a few remarks upon the general principles of education, which I hope will not be without interest, and perhaps benefit, to the reader.

The ground covered by the word education is covered by but one other, and that is life. From the day of birth until we pass away beyond earthly scenes we are in a constant process of education. The history of the rise, progress, and development of education is the history of man. Commerce and intercourse have been the two great factors. Education includes marriage, parentage, and all life's responsibilities within its limits. Solemn subject, which never ends but with life! Subject—the beginning of which is so subtile that no man dare indicate the moment when the first reflective brain-action begins, other than that it begins with the worldly life of the individual. It is the attribute of all the higher forms of animal life, differing only in degree and quality. The so-called instincts are not alone the attributes of the lower animals; man has them also. They may be defined as action, which follows so quickly on thought that thought and action, cause and effect, are not, even by the individual, to be distinguished from one another. This remark has no reference to those intellectual peculiarities which distinguish mankind from the lower animals. No action takes place in the animal organism without the irritation of specific nervous centers. Hunger is among the attributes which we enjoy in common with the lower animals. The attempt to stay it is not instinctive in the lower animals any more than with man. The manner of staying it is different. In both species it is dependent upon a certain form of irritation of the trophic nerve-endings in the stomach (perhaps intestines also), which is transmitted to certain centers in the brain, and irritates them, causing *reflection* (in lower animals as well as in man), and, as a natural result, the seeking for food.

There rules in the community an idea that the different grades of intelligence—the so-called "gifts" (illustrated by the expression "that one person is more gifted than another," one animal possessing a greater development of its instincts than another)—are something special; some mysterious, spiritual force or forces, which such organisms have received from the Creator. They seem to entirely overlook the true conditions which lead to these differences. These differences are founded upon variations in the anatomical structure of the centers of intelligence in different individuals. It is not known whether chemical differences in the elements forming these centers are present or not; the anatomical variations, while axiomatically true, have never as yet been demonstrated. This work belongs to the science of the future. Changes in the anatomical structure of the nervous centers of intelligence are immediately followed by variations in the functions of these parts, and finally demonstrate themselves by changes in the phenomena produced, varying in degree according to the anatomical changes of the elements.

The unit of animal, as well as vegetable life, is the cell. Beyond that we do not need to go. "Omnis cellula e cellula," says the great master of medicine, Virchow. While we look upon the cell as the unit of life, we have to pay our attention to the *units* of which it is composed. A cell is a mass of protoplasm, with or without an inclosing membrane, with or without a nucleus or nucleolus. Changes in this protoplasm cause variations in the functions of the cell. The work of the cell, the part it takes in the animal or vegetable economy, is dependent upon the composition—molecular relations and chemical nature—of its protoplasm. This is the constitution of the cell. If the constitution is normal, the functions of the cell are normal. If the relations and nature of any of the elements vary to any great degree, so that the influences of the variations, on the part of one or a group of cells, can not be equalized by the action of the others, then the functions of the cell become abnormal to a corresponding degree. Abnormality can only take place in three directions—viz., a plus, a minus, and an entire cessation of functional activity. The sum of the cellular functions constitutes *life*. The variable phenomena of life, in different individuals of one and the same family, are invariably dependent upon variations in the anatomical relations, or in the protoplasm of which the cells are composed, or in those organs in which such differences are observable. This doctrine may be traced in the early medical writings. We find it intimated by the grand Greek, Hippocrates, the father of medicine. His four humors—blood, black gall, white gall, and mucus—gave rise to the constitution of the individual. The temperaments were dependent upon the relations of the humors to one another. The cell being considered as a unit, an indefinite number of these units, collected together for one purpose, form an organ, a greater unit; and the union of a certain number of these larger units, each with its special functions, each with its work to do for itself, for its own existence, as well as work to do for the benefit of each of the organs united with it, constitutes the functions of that complex unit—if I may be allowed the term—the organism. Considered as a unit, the organism does not differ from the cell. Its constitution is dependent upon the anatomical relations and chemical composition of its elements. Its functions are dependent upon their normal relation to each other for their perfect completion. Its temperament upon the same. Man's organism has work to do to keep itself in condition, as well as its part to keep the machine (unit) in existence, which we call humanity.

The diversity of intellectual "gifts" is neither special curse nor special blessing. It is based upon variations in the structural relations, molecular proportion, or chemical conditions of the different nervous centers situated in the brain. Cheerfully admitting that this is *a priori* reasoning, yet I do not lose hope that the investigators of some future day will be able to discover and describe some of these changes. Why one child is born brilliant and another weak in intellect, from the same parents, and, so far as we know, under the same conditions, is not dependent upon punishment from God, but upon variations in the molecular construction, or chemical components (?) of the protoplasm of the cells, or upon anatomical variations of a coarser kind. The causes of these variations are generally present at the moment of the fructification of the ovum of the mother or in the sperm of the father, or are due to influences which are exerted upon the fœtus while being carried by the mother. The elements of these nervous centers in such conditions do not suffer such marked changes that we have been able to discover them, although it is true that exact investigation in this direction is but in its infancy. In extreme cases, variations in cranial formation may be present, but they are not necessary; nor do they occur when loss of intellect or disturbances take place during life from over-exertion, shock, or other causes; yet, in such cases, we *must* assume that changes have taken place in the active elements of those centers in the brain, a disturbance of which is indicated by the abnormal phenomena which have attracted *our* attention.

Every child is a unit—an organism composed of a certain number of small units, the organs, which themselves are composed of untold numbers of still smaller units, the cells. The normal relations and actions of all these parts regulate the *constitution* of the child. The functions of the brain do not differ from this rule; they are dependent upon its anatomical structure in part or as a whole. *It is impossible to make a child anything different intellectually than this anatomical structure of the brain will allow.* This is, however, somewhat dependent upon the relations of the brain to the other parts of the body. Incomplete action of one or the other of the important organs may, and does frequently, lead to changes of importance in the brain, but in their nature so subtile as to escape our present means of observation. While the brain functions of the child are in reality thus limited, the limits are of such a nature that in the normal child they are never attained. They will answer all the demands which can be made upon them, but the result is always dependent upon their structure and appositional relations. Why one child *will be* a veterinarian or a breeder of animals, another a merchant, another a seaman, or a minister, or a student of some one of the natural sciences, against the earnest will and wishes of its parents, is neither dependent on "pure cussedness" nor upon any special influence of the devil or any of his agents, nor upon obstinacy or ill-will, as many parents suppose, but upon fixed and unchangeable anatomical conditions in its brain. The same is true of many unfortunates who from early childhood develop a tendency to destroy and torture animal life, and who sometimes bring up as murderers. The causes of such conditions are in a measure at present beyond our knowledge. They have been undoubtedly strengthened by heedless marriage. Marriage is indeed a solemn thing; the world scarcely realizes how solemn. Marriage, as in general conducted, is a senseless thing. It is dependent upon fancy; upon certain supposed affinities, which do not exist save in the unreflecting minds of excited lovers. Love itself is based upon certain centers in the brain. *Love and sensuality have no relation or connection with one another.* The thing called *love*, which at best is but mere *fancy*, may exist, but the genuine article is entirely free from it. The situation of the two centers is widely separated. Some day mankind will instigate as careful investigations into the pedigree of each other with relation to inherited diseases as they do now in endeavoring to trace a connection to some broken-down sprig of Continental snobocracy. Some day we shall exercise as much care in selecting our partners as we do now in selecting animals for breeding. The purpose of marriage is to continue the race. For no other purpose are we made male and female. The same is true of every member of the animal kingdom. Tubercular consumption is not only increasing in extension, but the average age at which such people die is decreasing in the human family. We charge it all to the changeableness of our climate. The climate, the irritations of life, are simply sufficient causes to set the disease in motion. The *true cause* is to be sought in the weak lung-tissues which we transmit to our children. This weakness has been constantly and ignorantly increased at the expense and misery of the children produced. We talk about our boasted civilization. The breeders of cattle know this fact, and exclude from *breeding* animals which, were they human beings, would marry if they took a fancy. Were they to do this, they would do what humanity does for itself—condemn its children to lives of misery and an early grave. How does the medical profession deport itself toward this question? Is it true to the scientific spirit of preventive medicine? No—a thousand times no! Its members marry as heedlessly and headlessly as the people. Few members of it dare enter a family and warn young couples, intending to marry, of their duties and the dangers to which they are unquestionably going to subject their children. Were children not the result of marriage, it would then make no difference. The Church "Out-Herods Herod." Her ministers neither set a becoming example, nor do they warn, as prophets of the true God, the people of their duties in this regard.

The purpose of marriage (natural) is to produce children. "So God created man in his own image, in the image of God created he him; male and female created he them."

"And God blessed them, and God said unto them, Be fruitful, and multiply, and replenish the earth." *

The science of parentage is an undeveloped branch of universal science. It is still awaiting the appearance of its first prophet. Its primers are as yet unwritten. Man scarcely knows the meaning of the first letter of its alphabet. It is *the science par excellence.* All others sink into insignificance in comparison with it. *They all* form but stepping-stones to its development. Thousands and thousands of years old, *yet cultivated 'man does not know enough to marry.* The real duties of parentage are still too much for humanity to bear and faithfully carry out.

Physical fitness is the indispensable necessity. The "affinities" (an inexact term), a matter of secondary importance. Respect for each other's intellectual capabilities, and interest in the life-work of each other, is a far better foundation for a true marriage than the fancy mistakenly called love, which now, too frequently, leads to it. In every child, soon after birth, the elements of these character-centers in the brain begin to assume a certain fixity of form, which, under normal conditions, gradually increase with the years. This fixity in the elements of the centers referred to gives occasion to the idiosyncratic ability of the individual. This point is the pole, the center around which the entire personality of the individual is to revolve during life. *Its development,* the ultimo of the science of parentage. The study of it, by means of its developing phenomena, the so-called "tastes" of the child, the imperative duty of every parent and every teacher of youth. It is the *objective point* upon which each parent should fix his or her attention from the day of birth to that of the maturity of each child. It is the *magnetic needle* which Nature places in each child to indicate to parents the course they should pursue in the education of the child. The development of this one point is not, however, the single duty of parents in directing the education of a child; but, like a skillful general, who supports his crack corps in a desperate attack with all his other

* Gen. i, 27, 28.

forces, so must parents support this special brain, intellectual affinity of a child, for a certain occupation in life, by the most complete and studied education in other branches, so that in every way its strongest point is well supported by collateral education. Such a child is well fitted to fight the battle for existence when the years to begin it come on. Many and many a gifted child has been made a good-for-nothing man, "a rolling stone," from the ignorance or stubbornness of parents who had not sense enough to know their duty, but believed in the doctrine, which has cursed more men than it has ever blessed, that the child must bend to the will of the parents. A one-sided education is a poor thing. It too frequently leaves the unfortunate man deeply buried in the "slough of despond." This most earnest study of the developing characteristics of a child is the imperative duty of parents. The child is not the property of the parents, to be used either as a toy, an ornament, or a means to personal gratification. *It is not an object belonging to parents to be bent to their wills. On the contrary, it is a trust received from Nature to be sacredly guarded. It is an individual whose developing will is to be respected as its peculiar and inherent right, but which is also to be studied, directed, and the lesson of self-control gradually taught it, so that it may be fitted for the work of life.* Morals are not "gifts from God"; they are the results of experience. The comprehension of *right* can only develop with the intellect, and the broader the latter is developed, the more sharply defined its action, the more exact will be the child's idea of right. Right and wrong are at first in no way moral sentiments to the child. They are at first founded in a degree of fear or love of parents; and the child's opposing actions, looked upon by parents too frequently as the results of ill-will, are but the gradually developing will, individuality of the child, coming into collision with the wills, it should be with the matured judgment, of the parents. The gradual development of this will in a proper direction is the highest duty of parents. It is *not* to be controlled by them, but directed. The child is to learn that the will of its parents—which is its first idea of moral law—is to be followed with trust, not fear. He is to learn that it saves him from many evil consequences, until, by the development of his own intellect, he becomes gradually able to distinguish between a right and a wrong peculiar to himself, and the relation of his own organism to his surroundings, as well as the relation of each part to the other parts of which it is made up. The right and wrong of an intelligent and developing understanding gradually takes the place of a conflict between—to the child—non-comprehended forces and the matured understanding of the parents. *The aim of education is to prepare the child so that it may take care of itself in the struggle for existence.* This axiom answers a question which many are asking, though but few seem able to answer. *How many children may a couple generate? The answer is, No more than their means will allow them to fully educate for this struggle for existence.* Many persons, who unfortunately marry without the least idea of their new duties, are not fitted to have any children. Their own parents, having been unsuited to this noblest of duties, have transmitted their own incapacity to their children. "Verily, the sins of the fathers are visited upon the children" in more ways than we at present are aware of.

Education! What is it? What form does it take? In my opinion, education has three forms. First, the preparatory education of the school and college days. Second, the so-called "cultivation" which is the result of one's general reading. Both of these forms are but gleanings from the work of others. *Third, education proper, or that which the individual works out of himself by reflection upon what he has read, observed, and heard.* It will be at once seen, and daily experience proves it, that a cultivated man is not necessarily an educated one; nor is every educated man a cultivated one, although this exception is more rarely the case than the former.

We often read in the daily papers that the public schools of the present day are too much inclined to develop philosophers, and not enough toward practical ends. It would be a blessing indeed did they seek to produce good, clear, radical (not in the sense of ignorant newspaper writers) thinkers. A philosopher is one who thinks deeply upon any subject. He is quite frequently found, in a crude form, shoveling coal or pegging shoes. The polished form sits oftener in the professor's chair. The diamond is frequently spoiled in the polishing. So it is with many crude but sharp thinkers. When polished, the clearness is lost behind a multitude of words. Reading and writing by no means constitute an education. People seem to think they do, however. They are but the means. Ability to think logically is the attribute of an educated man. A foolish person may be taught to read and write, but no one would dare say he is educated. They lack the one pearl of price—the ability to think; but the capability to read and write greatly increases the reflective abilities of an otherwise crude thinker. It is the essential quality failing in our present humanity. The occasional individual thinks, the masses never. One would suppose, judging from personal observation, that the ability to think must have been one of the lost arts. Our aim should be to create good, logical thinkers—men capable of observing closely, and drawing radical conclusions. On that depends not only their individual success, but the advancement of our country as a whole. Let us, then, all do *our part* in pushing forward such a work. Among other things to this purpose, none is more needed than a *national institute* for the scientific education of veterinarians and the other purposes mentioned in this book.

GENERAL INDEX.

Lightning Source UK Ltd.
Milton Keynes UK
UKHW010744280219
338010UK00004B/422/P

9 780428 957704